BASIC PRINCIPLES OF PERIPHERAL NERVE DISORDERS

Edited by **Seyed Mansoor Rayegani**

Basic Principles of Peripheral Nerve Disorders
Edited by Seyed Mansoor Rayegani

Published by InTech
Janeza Trdine 9, 51000 Rijeka, Croatia

Publishing Process Manager Romana Vukelic

Technical Editor Teodora Smiljanic

Cover Designer InTech Design Team

Additional hard copies can be obtained from orders@intechopen.com

Basic Principles of Peripheral Nerve Disorders, Edited by Seyed Mansoor Rayegani
p. cm.
ISBN 978-953-51-0407-0

For EU product safety concerns:
IN TECH d.o.o., Prolaz Marije Krucifikse Kozulić 3, 51000 Rijeka, Croatia,
info@intechopen.com or visit our website at intechopen.com.

Meet the editor

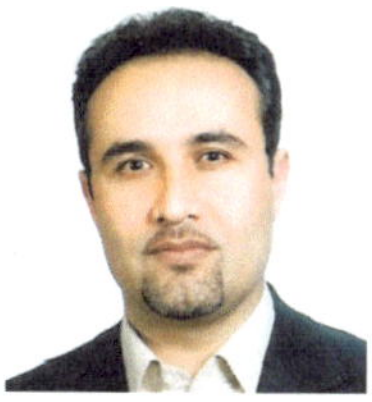

Professor S. Mansoor Rayegani, MD, 47 years old, is an academic physiatrist who has completed his residency training in PM&R from Shiraz medical university, Iran 1992. He started his academic activities as assistant professor of PM&R in Shohada medical center, Shahid Beheshti university of medical sciences just after passing Iranian board of PM&R examination in which he gained 1st rank. He is one of the founder pioneers for establishing residency training program in the field of PM&R in Tehran, capital of Iran. Professor Rayegani fields of interest include; electrodiagnostic medicine, entrapment syndromes, pain, spinal cord injury and medical education. He supervised more than 20 postgraduate residency theses and published about 19 indexed articles in PubMed and ISI and also more than 30 articles in local medical journals. Professor Rayegani is president of Iranian society of PM&R, director of Iranian board of PM&R and chief of the PM&R research center at Shahid Beheshti university of medical science.

Contents

Preface

Peripheral nerve disorders are comprising one of the major clinical topics in neuromusculoskeletal disorders. Sharp nerve injuries, chronic entrapment syndromes, and peripheral neuropathic processes can be classified in this common medical topic.

Different aspects of these disorders including anatomy, physiology, pathophysiology, injury mechanisms, and different diagnostic and management methods need to be addressed when discussing this topic. The goal of preparing this book was to gather such pertinent chapters to cover these aspects.

Because different approaches are provided by different disciplines for managing peripheral nerve disorders, an overview of pertinent topics is needed.

Basic topics such as pathophysiology, regeneration, degeneration, neuropathic pain, surgical intervention, electrodiagnosis and rehabilitation medicine were covered in this book.

Multidisciplinary approach to the management of peripheral nerve disorders made participation of different specialties as a critical and mandatory task. I think this aspect has accomplished.

The book includes contribution from an international well known group that are known for their teaching ability and commitments to these topics. I am grateful for their participation.

S. Mansoor Rayegani, M.D
Professor of Physical Medicine and Rehabilitation,
Shahid Beheshti Medical University, Tehran,
Iran

1

Pathophysiology of Peripheral Nerve Injury

Tomas Madura
Blond McIndoe Laboratories, Plastic Surgery Research, University of Manchester, Manchester Academic Health Centre, Manchester, UK

1. Introduction

Peripheral nervous system (PNS) is a complex construction, which serves dual purpose. Firstly, it disseminates information from the central nervous systems and ensures that this information is interpreted to the target end - organs. Secondly, it collects information from the periphery, translates it to nerve signals, processes it and feeds it back to the central nervous system. The PNS consists of a complex arborisation of peripheral nerves. In order to set a stage for the information that will be presented further on, I will shortly review the relevant anatomy first. The peripheral nerves are long extension of neuronal cells, which cells bodies are located in the spinal chord and dorsal root ganglia (spinal nerves) or in the brain (cranial nerves). The peripheral nerve consists of nerve fibres and supportive connective tissue. The connective tissue is organised longitudinally surrounding the nerve fibres and serves a double function. Firstly, it provides mechanical support for the nerve fibres to withstand stretching and compression during the body movements. Secondly, it contains blood vessels - vasa nervorum, which ensure trophic support for the fibres (Gray 1995). The connective tissue is organised in three "layers". The outermost layer - epineurium - is a thick layer of connective tissue which ensheaths the nerve and isolates it from the external environment (Fig.1). The vasa nervorum are continued within this layer and these vessels communicate abundantly with the network of arterioles and venules found in the connective tissues in the depth of the nerve. The amount of epineurium differs depending on the individual, thickness of the nerve and location. There is an evidence that epineurium is thicker around joints (Sunderland 1978). Deep to epineurium, the axonal fibres are organised in one (unifascicular) or more (multifascicular) fascicles. The fascicles are enclosed within the second layer of connective tissue - perineurium (Fig.1). The perineurium is a thick and mechanically strong layer, which is composed of epithelium-like cells and collagen fibres. The cells are typically organised in several layers separated by collagen with ample vascular structures running longitudinally (Thomas and Jones 1967). This stratification gives perineurium a great endurance and ability to withstand a pressure in excess of 200 mmHg (Selander and Sjöstrand 1978). Deep to perineurium the endoneurium is found (Fig. 1). It consists of loose collagenous matrix enveloping the nerve fibres and providing further protection from mechanical forces. The endoneurium also contains several important cell types. The most abundant one are Schwann cells, followed by fibroblasts, endothelial-like cells, macrophages and mastocytes (Causey and Barton 1959). It is important to note that endoneurium contains ample extracellural matrix and fluid, which is contained at a slightly higher pressure that that surrounding perineurium (Myers et al. 1978). The reason for that is unknown, although we can speculate that it protects endoneurial space from possible contamination by toxic substances external to the epineural space.

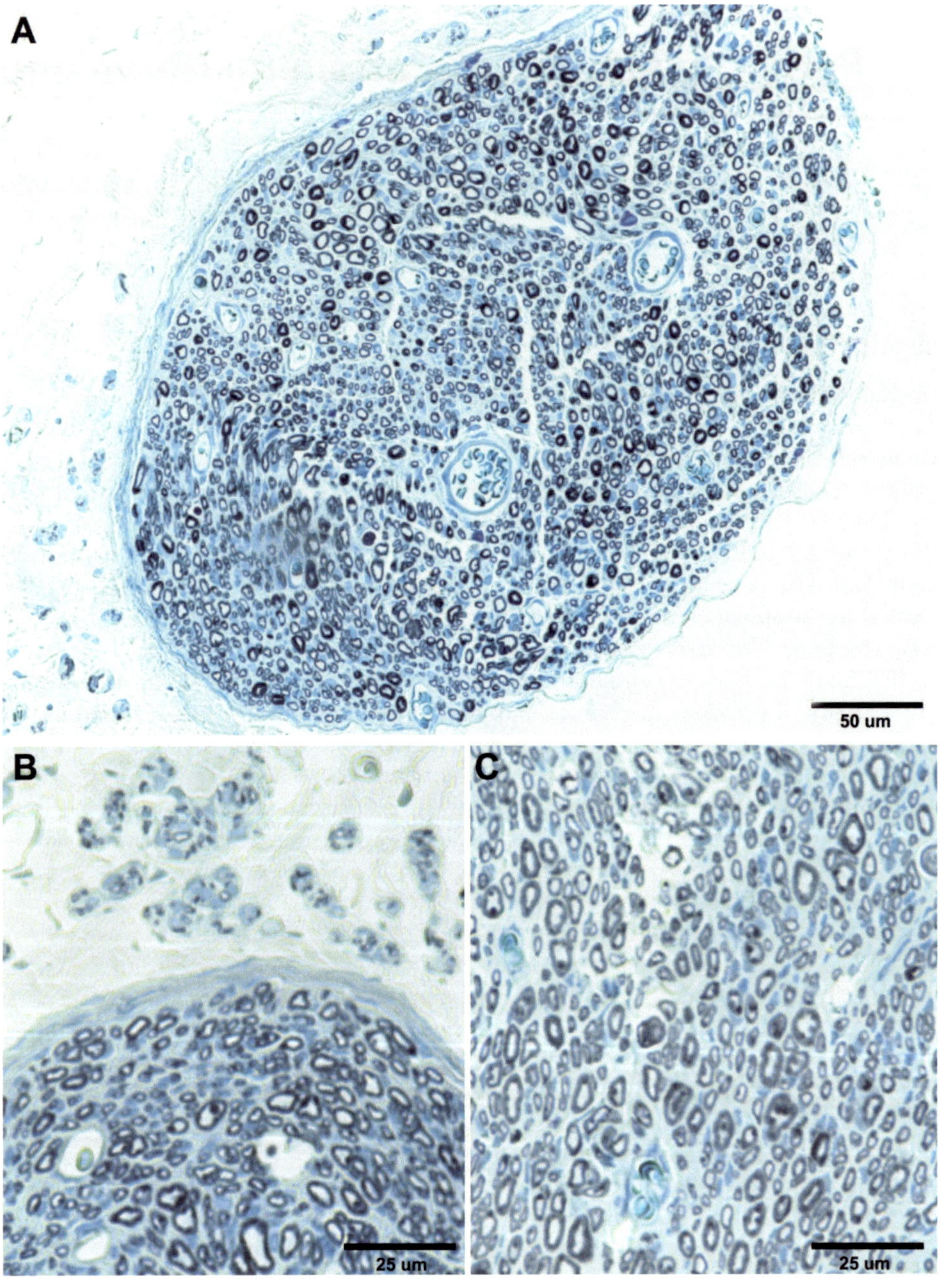

Fig. 1. Ultrastructure of the peripheral nerve.

(a) Toluidine blue stained transverse section through peripheral nerve of rat.
(b) Detail on thick epineurium enveloping the nerve
(c) Detail on area with peri- and endoneurium.

When talking about the injury to the nervous system, it is essential to consider all parts of this system and also end organs, which are dependent on it. Thus, this review will focus separately on neural cells, sensory organs and muscle.

1.1 Response of the neural cells

The damage to the neural cells is the most obvious consequence of the injury to the peripheral nerve. As mentioned above, the nerve is essentially a multi-strand cord-like structure, which keeps the nerve fibres organised and protected from the external forces. With the cell bodies being located in the spinal cord and dorsal root ganglia, all the injuries to the nerves are happening at the level of cellular processes - axons. Perhaps the only exception to this statement is roots avulsion from spinal cord, for example during brachial plexus injury. The nerve injury divides neurons into a part, which is proximal and a part, which is distal to the injury site. These two parts differ significantly from each other, as far as the reaction to the injury is concerned.

1.1.1 Distal to the injury site (Wallerian degeneration)

More than 160 years have passed since the first report describing the reaction of distal nerve stump to axotomy. The original work was performed by Augustus Waller and was presented to the Royal Society of London in 1850. Waller was studying injuries to glossopharyngeal and hypoglossal nerves in frogs. It is obligatory to quote an excerpt from his original report here (Waller 1850):

"During the four first days, after section of the hypoglossal nerve, no change is observed in its structure. On the fifth day the tubes appear more varicose than usual, and the medulla (term used to describe axons) more irregular. About the tenth day medulla forms disorganized, fusiform masses at intervals, and where the white substance of SCHWANN cannot be detected. These alterations, which are most evident in the single tubules, may be found also in the branches. After twelve or fifteen days many of the single tubules have ceased to be visible, their granular medulla having been removed by absorption. The branches contain masses of amorphous medulla."

This process of disintegration of distal axonal stump after injury is termed Wallerian degeneration. It is a recognized consequence of a mechanical (but not only) insult to the nerve. Wallerian degeneration starts almost immediately after axotomy and lasts 3 – 6 weeks (Geuna et al. 2009). The first sign is disintegration of axons, which starts during first 24 to 48 hours (Stoll et al. 1989). The beginning of this process is characterised by granulation within axoplasma caused by proteolysis of microtubules and neurofilaments (Lubińska 1982, Schlaepfer 1977). This is caused by a rapid activation of axoplasmatic proteolyses, which occurs as a response to intracellular calcium influx (George, Glass, and Griffin 1995, Schlaepfer and Bunge 1973). An early activation of ubiquitin-proteasome system has been also shown to play an important role here (Ehlers 2004). Among all the cytoskeletal structures, the microtubules are thought to disintegrate first (Watts, Hoopfer, and Luo 2003, Zhai et al. 2003). The loss of microtubular structures then leads to impediment of axonal transport and further accelerates the degeneration process. The disintegration of neurofilaments follows shortly and is usually completed within 7 – 10 days. During this time, the partially disrupted neurofilaments can be detected in the axoplasma only to completely disappear shortly afterwards. One more important point, which needs to be made, is the direction of the Wallerian degeneration. It seems that the process is bidirectional. It starts in the zone just below the injury and progresses distally while at the same time starts at the distal axonal termini (Waxman 1995). Despite the very brisk initiation of degenerative changes, the distal nerve stump preserves its excitability for a considerable period of time. When the transacted axons are stimulated distal to the injury zone, it is often possible to record nerve potentials for up to 10 days. Therefore, it is very important for this period of refractory excitability to finish, before accurate estimate of the nerve injury extent can be made by electrophysiological methods.

The processes, which we have discussed so far, were limited to the axon and its inherent ability to degenerate after injury. To have the full picture of the Wallerian degeneration, we also need to talk about other cells, which participate and play an integral role in it. In particular, the role of Schwann cells and macrophages is critical for the Wallerian degeneration to take place. The Schwann cells are very sensitive to the loss of contact with axon. In case of dennervation, the Schwann cells change from "supportive" to "reactive" phenotype. They stop producing myelin (LeBlanc and Poduslo 1990). The continuing proliferation of Schwann cells leads to formation of Bands of Bungers, which purpose is thought to be guidance of the regrowing axons (further discussed in the regeneration subchapter) (Liu, Yang, and Yang 1995). It seems that this phenotypic switch is, at least partly, a response to neuregulin secretion from the transacted axons (Esper and Loeb 2004). Activated Schwann cells were found to secret a wide range of immunologically active substances. In particular, Interleukin (IL) -1B, IL - 6, IL - 10 and Leukaemia Inhibitory Factor (LIF) were detected abundantly at the injury site in the first few days after injury (Bolin et al. 1995, Jander et al. 1996, Jander and Stoll 1998, Kurek et al. 1996). These substances are responsible for attracting immune cells into the distal nerve stump and orchestrating their function. It was shown, that in the first two days after nerve injury macrophages and T cells start to infiltrate injury zone, which culminates in infiltration of the entire distal stump by day 4 (Brück 1997, Perry, Brown, and Gordon 1987). They are responsible for phagocytosis of the axonal debris and myelin sheaths residua released from the disintegrating axons and thus finishing the breakdown and elimination of axons.

1.1.2 Proximal to the injury site (proximal end degeneration)

The immediate consequence of axotomy is partial retraction of the proximal stump (Cajal 1928) leaving empty endoneurial tubes lined by Schwann cells. The distance to which the proximal stump retracts is usually one or two nodes of Ranvier, but that depends on severity and character of injury. Within the same timeframe the injured axons also seal their injured axolemma to prevent axoplasma leakage. Shortly after retraction and as early as hours after axotomy, the proximal stump starts to produce regenerative sprouts (McQuarrie 1985, Meller 1987, Friede and Bischhausen 1980). While these sprouts are forming the cut tip of the axon swells up, containing endoplasmatic reticulum, mitochondria and microtubules. This swelling contains products accumulating in the tip of the stump because of disrupted anterograde axonal transport. One important event happening in the area of the swelling is reorganisation of microtubular cytoskeleton. In the normal axon the microtubules are organised longitudinally and all point distally along the axon. After axotomy the arrangement of microtubules changes and they point against each other (Erez et al. 2007).

This swelling is very probably giving the basis for development of axonal end-bulbs, which occurs within 24 – 48 hours after the injury. The relation between axonal endbulb and axonal growth cone remains not fully understood (Goldberg, Frank, and Krayanek 1983). A recent report suggests that depending on the local environment, the injured axons either form regenerative growth cones or incompetent endbulbs (Kamber, Erez, and Spira 2009). The successful formation of the growth cone is the ultimate goal of the proximal nerve stump, as this will be the starting point of the nerve regeneration (see below).

1.1.3 Cell body response

The neurons, which axons were injured and ended up in Wallerian degeneration have lost a substantial part of their cellular mass. Although we expect them to re-grow their lost parts and re-establish the functional connection with their end organ, the situation is not always so favourable. It seems, that the outcome is influenced by location of the lesion in relation to cell body, type of neuron, physical age and local availability of trophic factors. The most extreme outcome of nerve axotomy is cellular death of the injured neuron. The proportion of neuronal cell death in dorsal root ganglia after sciatic nerve lesion in rodents has been reported to be 10 – 30 % (Ygge 1989, Groves et al. 1997). The number is much lower in motoneurons, where no significant neuronal death has been observed (Vanden Noven et al. 1993). However, the situation is dramatically different if the nerve (or ventral root) has been avulsed from the spinal chord. In this case the motoneuronal death can be as high as 80% (Martin, Kaiser, and A C Price 1999, Koliatsos et al. 1994).

There are several morphological changes in the surviving neurons after axotomy. The most obvious one is chromatolysis, which is dissolution of the Nissle substance (Cotman 1978, Kreutzberg 1995). The Nissle substance is a synonym for rough endoplasmatic reticulum containing mRNA, which has blue and dotty appearance on haematoxylin eosin stain. It is normally located in the centre of the neuron. The chromatolysis starts within hours of injury and peaks from 1 – 3 weeks. It usually resolves with reinnervation and the process is more prolonged and intensified if the distal reinnervation does not occur. The chromatolysis seamlessly continues either to regeneration or to neuronal death (Martin, Kaiser, and Price 1999). It is not entirely understood what makes the neuron to initiate chromatolysis. It seems that local synthesis of regulatory proteins on the axonal level and their linking to the dynein retrograde motor are at the start of the process (Hanz and Fainzilber 2006). Another early event after axotomy is swelling of the neuronal body and increase of nucleolar size. Later, the nucleus is displaced under the cell membrane and if the reinnervation does not occur, the neuron undergoes atrophy. One more important morphological change after neuronal injury is a reduction of dendritic arborisation. This dendritic retraction leads to a decrease of the number of synaptic connections of the injured neuron and to a functional isolation of it (Purves 1975, Brännström, Havton, and Kellerth 1992a) There is an evidence the motoneurones rebuild their dendritic complex following the reinnervation of target muscle (Brännström, Havton, and Kellerth 1992b). In contrast, in permanent axotomy this does not happen (Brännström, Havton, and Kellerth 1992a).

Apart from the morphological changes discussed so far, there is also a great shift on the functional cellular level. After axotomy, the surviving neurons switch from signal transmitter "program" to regenerative "program", or as Fu and Gordon put it from "signalling mode" to "growing mode" (Fu and T Gordon 1997). The survival of the cell and the mode switch are the first critical steps taken by the neuron towards regeneration. The switch brings changes to protein expression levels in the way that signalling-associated proteins become downregulated and growth-associated proteins and structural components of the cell become upregulated. Gene expression studies have demonstrated changes in expression patterns of hundreds of genes - the function of many is still yet to be explored (Kubo et al. 2002, Bosse et al. 2006). There seems to be a similarity between these newly found expression patterns and protein expression in developing neurons during embryological development. A group of growth-associated proteins, such as GAP-43 (Skene et al. 1986), are upregulated during the axonal growth phase up to 100 times and then their expression drops down upon reinnervation (Karns et al. 1987, Skene et al. 1986). Also, the expression of cytoskeletal component genes follows the developmental pattern. The production of neurofilaments gets tuned down (Oblinger and Lasek 1988, Hoffman et al. 1987) whereas the production of tubulins steeply increases (Miller et al. 1989, Hoffman and Cleveland 1988). Following is the recapitulation of changes in gene expression in the most important gene categories (Navarro 2009). Upregulated genes include:

- Transription factors (c-fos, c-jun, ATF3, NF*k*B, CREB, STAT)
- Neurotrophic factors (NGF, BDNF, GDNF, FGF)
- Neurotrophic receptors (Trk, Ret, P75)
- Cytokines (TNF*a*, MCP1)
- Growth associated proteins (GAP43)

And the downregulated genes are:

- Neurofilaments
- Neurotransmitters
- Postsynaptic receptors

This is by no means an exhaustive list, but should serve only as a demonstration of the philosophy behind gene expression alteration following nerve injury.

1.2 Response of the end organs and connective tissues

The multitude of functions that nerves fulfil is only possible because of a fine-tuned crosstalk between the nerve and its end organs. It is important to note here, that the nerve acts merely as an interface between the central nervous system and peripheral organs. Thus, for the nerve to function as intended it must be connected to the end organs. The end organs must not only function properly, but also have to effectively communicate with the nerve. After the nerve injury this co-dependent communication circuit gets disrupted. If we look at the nerve regeneration as a process of re-establishing this communication, we also need to consider the end organs and their reaction to the nerve injury. This will be in discussed in this subchapter.

1.2.1 Response of muscle

Reaction of the muscle to the dennervation takes place on several levels. The dennervated muscle changes its structure and its electrophysiological and biochemical properties. It has not been fully explained why these changes occur. It is probably a mixture of inactivity and loss of trophic stimuli from the neurons (Midrio 2006). The principal structural change is atrophy of individual muscle fibres with loss of muscle weight. The weight may decrease to as low as 30% of the muscle original weight (Fu and T Gordon 1995). Under light microscope the muscle fibres form nuclear knots, which are chains of nuclei with very little surrounding sarcoplasm. On ultrastructural level we can detect disruption of myofibrils and disorganisation of sarcomeres. Electrophysiological tests will show decline in Compound Muscle Action Potential (CMAP), which normally recovers with reinnervation. During regeneration the muscle motor units can significantly enlarge. This happens due to collateral sprouting, where one neuron will eventually innervate a higher number of motor plates then it did originally (Fu and T Gordon 1995). On biochemical level, the dennervated muscles show decreased uptake of glucose, impaired binding of insulin, decrease of intramuscular glycogen and also alteration of glycolytic enzymes (Burant et al. 1984, Donaldson, Evans, and Harrison 1986, DuBois and Max 1983).

1.2.2 Response of sensory organs

The response of the sensory organs is much less studied and understood than that of the muscle. A successful reinnervation of cutaneous sensory organs depends of a small subset of Schwann cells found at the terminal ending of neural fibres. The dennervation of the sensory organs results in the survival of these Schwann cells along with the capsular structures of sensory organs (Dubový and Aldskogius 1996), which are thought to guide the axonal regrowth towards their appropriate targets.

2. Axonal regeneration after peripheral nerve injury

As discussed above, the first wave of axonal sprouting occurs as soon as hours after axotomy (Fawcett and Keynes 1990, Mira 1984). The transected axons produce a great amount of terminal and collateral sprouts, which are progressing down the endoneurial tube while being in close contact with the Schwann cells (Nathaniel and Pease 1963, Haftek and Thomas 1968). This first wave of axonal sprouting is followed by a second wave about two days later (Cajal 1928, Mira 1984, Cotman 1978). It has been observed that axons may branch once they reach the distal stump, where one axon may give rise to several branches (Jenq, Jenq, and Coggeshall 1987, Bray and Aguayo 1974). The early regenerating axons are growing in the environment, which contains Schwann cells with their basal lamina, fibroblasts, collagen, immunocompetent cells and axonal debris from degenerating axons. The Schwann cells and their basal lamina play a crucial and indispensable role in the nerve regeneration. It was shown that if the Schwann cells are not present in the distal stump, the regeneration occurs very slowly. This is only thanks to a support of the Schwann cells migrating from the proximal stump and accompanying the regenerating axons (Gulati 1988, Hall 1986a). If the migration of the Schwann cells into the distal nerve stump is prohibited (such as by a cytotoxic agent), the axons fail to regenerate completely (Hall 1986b). As mentioned above, the Schwann cells react swiftly to the loss of axonal contact by proliferation and assisting in breaking down the myelin sheaths. While multiplying, they also migrate and align themselves into longitudinal columns called bands of Bungner (Waxman 1995, Duce and Keen 1980, Lundborg et al. 1982). The bands of Bungner are physical guides for regenerating axons. The axons first grow through the injury zone and then into the bands of Bungner. In order for the regeneration outcome to achieve the pre-injury state, the axons should ideally grow back into their corresponding columns. However, the studies on early behaviour of regenerating axons showed that this is not happening. Axons send several regenerative sprouts, which can grow in multitude of directions and encounter of up to 100 bands of Bungner (Witzel, Rohde, and Brushart 2005). Some of the axons then grow into them, whereas others may grow freely into the connective tissue of the nerve, or take an extraneural course. In this setting, the choice of final regeneration pathway becomes only a matter of chance. This process is termed axonal misdirection and can significantly hamper the regeneration process. If we consider a situation where a motor fiber grows into the pathway belonging originally to a sensory neuron, this will lead into the failure of functional restoration (Molander and Aldskogius 1992, Bodine-Fowler et al. 1997). It seemed, that there was a preferential affinity of motoneurons to reinnervate motor pathways (Brushart 1993), although a more recent report did not detect any differences in motor against sensory regrowth (Robinson and Madison 2004). One way to reduce the misdirection, which is fully in our hands, is a meticulous surgical technique. It is imperative to use an operating microscope to minimise the impact of a gross misalignment of nerve stumps.

Apart from providing a mechanical guidance for the regenerating axons, the Schwann cells are also responsible for humoral stimulation of the neuronal outgrowth. The expression of NGF is stimulated in Schwann cells shortly after nerve injury (Heumann 1987). This happens very probably as a response to Interleukin-1 secretion by macrophages (Lindholm et al. 1987). Also, the expression of Neurotrophin 3, 4, 5, 6 as well as Brain - Derived Neurotrophic factor sharply increase (Funakoshi et al. 1993). The advancement of axons is further facilitated by growth - promoting molecules, such as laminin and fibronectin (Baron-Van Evercooren et al. 1982, Rauvala et al. 1989). Several studies also demonstrated positive involvement of adhesion molecules, such as neural cell adhesion molecule (NCAM), neural - glia cell adhesion molecule (NgCAM), integrins and cadherins (Walsh and Doherty 1996, Seilheimer and Schachner 1988, Bixby, Lilien, and Reichardt 1988, Hoffman et al. 1986).

In case of myelinated axons, myelination starts as early as eight days after the injury. The remyelination is thought to recapitulate events from the embryonic development. The trigger for the start of myelination is axonal radial growth and reaching a certain diameter. In development it is around 2 μm (Armati 2007). The Schwann cells then rotate around the axon in their endoneurial tube and form a myelin layer around a length of axon, which will correspond to an intermodal segment. It is important to note, that there is a constant relation of 1:1 between a number of cells and internodal segments - i.e. one internodal segment is always myelinated by only one Schwann cell. The internodal segments tend to be shorter in regenerated nerves, in comparison to the developing nerves (Vizoso and Young 1948, Ghabriel and Allt 1977, Minwegen and Friede 1985). This is probably an explanation for decreased conduction velocity in regenerated nerves (Cragg and Thomas 1964). The information whether the myelination will occur or not is stored in the axons. The Schwann cells have an ability to detect that and selectively myelinate appropriate axons (Aguayo et al. 1976, Weinberg and Spencer 1975).

3. Classification of nerve injuries

3.1 Seddon's classification

Under normal circumstances, the nerves remain connected with their innervation targets during the whole life of an individual. The most common disturbance to this status quo is a nerve damage by mechanical forces, which results in a loss of ability of the nerve to transfer stimuli. These forces can act through compression, traction, laceration and direct injection into the nerve. Moreover, the nerve can get damaged by thermal noxae, electric current, radiation and metabolic disorders. As a result of the injury the CNS completely, or partially, looses the ability to communicate with the neural end organs. The extent to which this happens is greatly variable and depends on the degree of damage to the nerve. The first classification of the severity of nerve injury was published by Seddon (Seddon 1943) and was based on his extensive experience with war victims. He classified the nerve injuries to three degrees, neuropraxia, axonotmesis and neurotmesis and defined the terms as follows:

1. *Neurotmesis* describes the state of a nerve in which all essential structures have been sundered. There is not necessarily an obvious anatomical gap in the nerve; indeed, the epineural sheath may appear to be in continuity, although the rest of the nerve at the site of damage has been completely replaced by fibrous tissue. But the effect is the same as if anatomical continuity had been lost. Neurotmesis is therefore of wider applicability than division.
2. *Axonotmesis*—here the essential lesion is damage to the nerve fibers of such severity that complete peripheral degeneration follows; and yet the epineurium and more intimate supporting structures of the nerve have been so little disturbed that the internal architecture is fairly well preserved. Recovery is spontaneous, and of good quality, because the regenerating fibers are guided into their proper paths by their intact sheaths.
3. *Neuropraxia* is used to describe those cases in which paralysis occurs in the absence of peripheral degeneration. It is more accurate than *transient block* in that the paralysis is often of considerable duration, though recovery always occurs in a shorter time than would be required after complete Wallerian degeneration; it is invariably complete.

3.1.1 Neuropraxia

Neuropraxia is a situation where the nerve (or more commonly a segment of it) losses its ability to propagate action potential while the structural continuity of the axons is fully preserved. The condition is associated with segmental demyelination of the nerve fibers. Because the degree of myelination differs depending on the type of nerve fibers, so does the extent of functional loss and return. The motor fibers are the most susceptible and their function is lost first and regained last, whereas pain and sympathetic fibers are the opposite (Sunderland 1978). Typical example of this type of nerve injury is sleeping with the pressure on the nerve, also called the "Saturday night palsy". This type of injury usually recovers within 12 weeks without any intervention.

3.1.2 Axonotmesis

Axonotmesis is an injury resulting in the loss of axonal continuity without any damage to the connective tissue structures within the nerve. Full Wallerian degeneration and axonal regrowth occur here and a Tinnel's sign accompanies the regeneration. The recovery of function is usually very good, although not as good as in neuropraxia. Surgical intervention is normally not necessary.

3.1.3 Neurotmesis

Damage to the neural connective tissue structures, including endoneurium, perineurium and / or epineurium is termed neurotmesis. Again, Wallerian degeneration and axonal regrowth occur and Tinnel's sign is possible to elicit over the injured nerve. The regeneration process here is hampered by axonal misdirection, loss of nerve/blood barrier and intraneural scarring. Injuries interrupting peri- and epineurium require surgical intervention. The outcome is generally worse than in axonotmesis. This, however, also depends on the relative location from the innervation target and in general it is difficult to predict.

3.2 Sunderland's classification

Early work of Sunderland brought about a much deeper understanding of the nerve ultrastructure (Sunderland, 1947, Sunderland and Bradley 1949). This offered an explanation for a wide variety of clinical findings and outcomes in the neurotmesis category. Natural following of this line of thought was extension of the Seddon's classification, which was formalised by Sutherland (Sunderland 1978). In the new classification the types I and II correspond to neuropraxia and axonotmesis respectively. Type III is an injury involving axons and endoneurium while perineurial and epineurial structures are intact. Sunderland's type IV injury is associated with division of axon, endoneurial and perineurial structures. This is a more significant injury, which often leads to intraneural scarring and requires surgical intervention to ensure the best possible outcome. Finally, type V of Sunderland's classification is a total division of the nerve trunk where all the neuronal and connective tissue structures are interrupted. It is important to note that in real clinical situation nerve injury is often a combination of more than one type of injury. This mixed pattern injury has been classed as a type VI, which was added to the original classification at a later date (Mackinnon 1988).

3.3 Correlations among the grade of injury, clinical and electrophysiological findings and potential for functional recovery

The correlations are found in the following Table 1:

Seddon	Neuropraxia	Axonotmesis	Neurotmesis	Neurotmesis	Neurotmesis
Sunderland	Type I	Type II	Type III	Type IV	Type V
Pathological findings	Anatomical continuity preserved Selective demyelination of the injury zone	Axonal continuity disrupted (together with myelin sheath)	Axonal and endoneurium continuity disrupted	Axonal, endoneurium and perineurium continuity disrupted	Complete division of the nerve
Wallerian degeneration	No	Yes	Yes	Yes	Yes
Motor paralysis	Complete	Complete	Complete	Complete	Complete
Sensory paralysis	Often partially spared	Complete	Complete	Complete	Complete
Autonomic paralysis	Much of the function spared	Complete	Complete	Complete	Complete
Muscle atrophy	Very little	Progressive with time	Progressive with time	Progressive with time	Progressive with time

Seddon	Neuropraxia	Axonotmesis	Neurotmesis	Neurotmesis	Neurotmesis
Sunderland	Type I	Type II	Type III	Type IV	Type V
Tinnel's sign	Absent	Present	Present	Present	Present
Electrophysiological findings	Normal conduction proximal and distal to injury site No conduction through injury site No fibrilation waves	No conduction distal to injury site Fibrilation waves present	No conduction distal to injury site Fibrilation waves present	No conduction distal to injury site Fibrilation waves present	No conduction distal to injury site Fibrilation waves present
Spontaneous recovery	Complete	Complete	Variable	None	None
Surgery needed?	No	No	Varies	Yes	Yes
Rate of recovery	Days (up to 3 months)	Slow – 1 mm per day	Slow – 1 mm per day	Only after surgical repair - 1 mm per day	Only after surgical repair - 1 mm per day

Table 1. Classifications of nerve injuries and their correlation with clinical, pathological and electrophysiological findings.

4. References

Aguayo, A J, J Epps, L Charron, and G M Bray. 1976. "Multipotentiality of Schwann cells in cross-anastomosed and grafted myelinated and unmyelinated nerves: quantitative microscopy and radioautography." *Brain Research* 104 (1) (March 5): 1-20.

Armati, Patricia. 2007. The biology of Schwann cells : development, differentiation and immunomodulation. Cambridge, UK: Cambridge University Press.

Baron-Van Evercooren, A, H K Kleinman, S Ohno, P Marangos, J P Schwartz, and M E Dubois-Dalcq. 1982. "Nerve growth factor, laminin, and fibronectin promote neurite growth in human fetal sensory ganglia cultures." *Journal of Neuroscience Research* 8 (2-3): 179-193.

Bixby, J L, J Lilien, and L F Reichardt. 1988. "Identification of the major proteins that promote neuronal process outgrowth on Schwann cells in vitro." *The Journal of Cell Biology* 107 (1) (July): 353-361.

Bodine-Fowler, S C, R S Meyer, A Moskovitz, R Abrams, and M J Botte. 1997. "Inaccurate projection of rat soleus motoneurons: a comparison of nerve repair techniques." *Muscle & Nerve* 20 (1) (January): 29-37.

Bolin, L M, A N Verity, J E Silver, E M Shooter, and J S Abrams. 1995. "Interleukin-6 production by Schwann cells and induction in sciatic nerve injury." *Journal of Neurochemistry* 64 (2) (February): 850-858.

Bosse, Frank, Kerstin Hasenpusch-Theil, Patrick Küry, and Hans Werner Müller. 2006. "Gene expression profiling reveals that peripheral nerve regeneration is a consequence of both novel injury-dependent and reactivated developmental processes." *Journal of Neurochemistry* 96 (5) (March): 1441-1457.

Brännström, T, L Havton, and J O Kellerth. 1992a. "Changes in size and dendritic arborization patterns of adult cat spinal alpha-motoneurons following permanent

axotomy." *The Journal of Comparative Neurology* 318 (4) (April 22): 439-451. 1992b. "Restorative effects of reinnervation on the size and dendritic arborization patterns of axotomized cat spinal alpha-motoneurons." *The Journal of Comparative Neurology* 318 (4) (April 22): 452-461.
Bray, G M, and A J Aguayo. 1974. "Regeneration of peripheral unmyelinated nerves. Fate of the axonal sprouts which develop after injury." *Journal of Anatomy* 117 (Pt 3) (July): 517-529.
Brück, W. 1997. "The role of macrophages in Wallerian degeneration." *Brain Pathology* 7 (2) (April): 741-752.
Brushart, T M. 1993. "Motor axons preferentially reinnervate motor pathways." *The Journal of Neuroscience: The Official Journal of the Society for Neuroscience* 13 (6) (June): 2730-2738.
Burant, C F, S K Lemmon, M K Treutelaar, and M G Buse. 1984. "Insulin resistance of denervated rat muscle: a model for impaired receptor-function coupling." *The American Journal of Physiology* 247 (5 Pt 1) (November): E657-666.
Cajal, S. 1928. *Degeneration and regeneration of the nervous system*. London: Oxford University Press.
Causey, G, and A A Barton. 1959. "The cellular content of the endoneurium of peripheral nerve." *Brain: A Journal of Neurology* 82 (December): 594-598.
Cotman, Carl. 1978. *Neuronal plasticity*. New York: Raven Press.
Cragg, B G, and P K Thomas. 1964. "The conduction velocity of regenerated peripheral nerve fibers." *The Journal of Physiology* 171 (May): 164-175.
Donaldson, D, O B Evans, and R W Harrison. 1986. "Insulin binding in denervated muscle." *Muscle & Nerve* 9 (3) (April): 211-215.
DuBois, D C, and S R Max. 1983. "Effect of denervation and reinnervation on oxidation of [6-14C]glucose by rat skeletal muscle homogenates." *Journal of Neurochemistry* 40 (3) (March): 727-733.
Dubový, P, and H Aldskogius. 1996. "Degeneration and regeneration of cutaneous sensory nerve formations." *Microscopy Research and Technique* 34 (4) (July 1): 362-375.
Duce, I R, and P Keen. 1980. "The formation of axonal sprouts in organ culture and their relationship to sprouting in vivo." *International Review of Cytology* 66: 211-256.
Ehlers, Michael D. 2004. "Deconstructing the axon: Wallerian degeneration and the ubiquitin-proteasome system." *Trends in Neurosciences* 27 (1) (January): 3-6.
Erez, Hadas, Guy Malkinson, Masha Prager-Khoutorsky, Chris I De Zeeuw, Casper C Hoogenraad, and Micha E Spira. 2007. "Formation of microtubule-based traps controls the sorting and concentration of vesicles to restricted sites of regenerating neurons after axotomy." *The Journal of Cell Biology* 176 (4) (February 12): 497-507.
Esper, Raymond M, and Jeffrey A Loeb. 2004. "Rapid axoglial signaling mediated by neuregulin and neurotrophic factors." *The Journal of Neuroscience* 24 (27) (July 7): 6218-6227.
Fawcett, J W, and R J Keynes. 1990. "Peripheral nerve regeneration." *Annual Review of Neuroscience* 13: 43-60.
Friede, R L, and R Bischhausen. 1980. "The fine structure of stumps of transected nerve fibers in subserial sections." *Journal of the Neurological Sciences* 44 (2-3) (January): 181-203.
Fu, S Y, and T Gordon. 1995. "Contributing factors to poor functional recovery after delayed nerve repair: prolonged denervation." *The Journal of Neuroscience: The Official Journal of the Society for Neuroscience* 15 (5 Pt 2) (May): 3886-3895. 1997. "The cellular and molecular basis of peripheral nerve regeneration." *Molecular Neurobiology* 14 (1-2) (April): 67-116.

Funakoshi, H, J Frisén, G Barbany, T Timmusk, O Zachrisson, V M Verge, and H Persson. 1993. "Differential expression of mRNAs for neurotrophins and their receptors after axotomy of the sciatic nerve." *The Journal of Cell Biology* 123 (2) (October): 455-465.

George, E B, J D Glass, and J W Griffin. 1995. "Axotomy-induced axonal degeneration is mediated by calcium influx through ion-specific channels." *The Journal of Neuroscience: The Official Journal of the Society for Neuroscience* 15 (10) (October): 6445-6452.

Geuna, Stefano, Stefania Raimondo, Giulia Ronchi, Federica Di Scipio, Pierluigi Tos, Krzysztof Czaja, and Michele Fornaro. 2009. "Chapter 3: Histology of the peripheral nerve and changes occurring during nerve regeneration." *International Review of Neurobiology* 87: 27-46.

Ghabriel, M N, and G Allt. 1977. "Regeneration of the node of Ranvier: a light and electron microscope study." *Acta Neuropathologica* 37 (2) (February 28): 153-163.

Goldberg, S, B Frank, and S Krayanek. 1983. "Axon end-bulb swellings and rapid retrograde degeneration after retinal lesions in young animals." *Experimental Neurology* 79 (3) (March): 753-762.

Gray, Henry. 1995. *Gray's anatomy : the anatomical basis of medicine and surgery*. 38th ed. New York: Churchill Livingstone.

Groves, M J, T Christopherson, B Giometto, and F Scaravilli. 1997. "Axotomy-induced apoptosis in adult rat primary sensory neurons." *Journal of Neurocytology* 26 (9) (September): 615-624.

Gulati, A K. 1988. "Evaluation of acellular and cellular nerve grafts in repair of rat peripheral nerve." *Journal of Neurosurgery* 68 (1) (January): 117-123.

Haftek, J, and P K Thomas. 1968. "Electron-microscope observations on the effects of localized crush injuries on the connective tissues of peripheral nerve." *Journal of Anatomy* 103 (Pt 2) (September): 233-243.

Hall, S M. 1986a. "Regeneration in cellular and acellular autografts in the peripheral nervous system." *Neuropathology and Applied Neurobiology* 12 (1) (February): 27-46. 1986b. "The effect of inhibiting Schwann cell mitosis on the re-innervation of acellular autografts in the peripheral nervous system of the mouse." *Neuropathology and Applied Neurobiology* 12 (4) (August): 401-414.

Hanz, Shlomit, and Mike Fainzilber. 2006. "Retrograde signaling in injured nerve--the axon reaction revisited." *Journal of Neurochemistry* 99 (1) (October): 13-19.

Heumann, R. 1987. "Regulation of the synthesis of nerve growth factor." *The Journal of Experimental Biology* 132 (September): 133-150.

Hoffman, P N, and D W Cleveland. 1988. "Neurofilament and tubulin expression recapitulates the developmental program during axonal regeneration: induction of a specific beta-tubulin isotype." *Proceedings of the National Academy of Sciences of the United States of America* 85 (12) (June): 4530-4533.

Hoffman, P N, D W Cleveland, J W Griffin, P W Landes, N J Cowan, and D L Price. 1987. "Neurofilament gene expression: a major determinant of axonal caliber." *Proceedings of the National Academy of Sciences of the United States of America* 84 (10) (May): 3472-3476.

Hoffman, S, D R Friedlander, C M Chuong, M Grumet, and G M Edelman. 1986. "Differential contributions of Ng-CAM and N-CAM to cell adhesion in different neural regions." *The Journal of Cell Biology* 103 (1) (July): 145-158.

Jander, S, and G Stoll. 1998. "Differential induction of interleukin-12, interleukin-18, and interleukin-1beta converting enzyme mRNA in experimental autoimmune encephalomyelitis of the Lewis rat." *Journal of Neuroimmunology* 91 (1-2) (November 2): 93-99.

Jander, S, J Pohl, C Gillen, and G Stoll. 1996. "Differential expression of interleukin-10 mRNA in Wallerian degeneration and immune-mediated inflammation of the rat peripheral nervous system." *Journal of Neuroscience Research* 43 (2) (January 15): 254-259.

Jenq, C B, L L Jenq, and R E Coggeshall. 1987. "Numerical patterns of axon regeneration that follow sciatic nerve crush in the neonatal rat." *Experimental Neurology* 95 (2) (February): 492-499.

Kamber, Dotan, Hadas Erez, and Micha E Spira. 2009. "Local calcium-dependent mechanisms determine whether a cut axonal end assembles a retarded endbulb or competent growth cone." *Experimental Neurology* 219 (1) (September): 112-125.

Karns, L R, S C Ng, J A Freeman, and M C Fishman. 1987. "Cloning of complementary DNA for GAP-43, a neuronal growth-related protein." *Science* 236 (4801) (May 1): 597-600.

Koliatsos, V E, W L Price, C A Pardo, and D L Price. 1994. "Ventral root avulsion: an experimental model of death of adult motor neurons." *The Journal of Comparative Neurology* 342 (1) (April 1): 35-44.

Kreutzberg, G. W. 1995. *Reaction of the neuronal cell body to axonal damage.* S. G. Waxman, J. D. Kocsis, and P. K. Stys. The Axon: Structure, Function and Pathophysiology. New York: Oxford University Press.

Kubo, Tateki, Toshihide Yamashita, Atsushi Yamaguchi, Ko Hosokawa, and Masaya Tohyama. 2002. "Analysis of genes induced in peripheral nerve after axotomy using cDNA microarrays." *Journal of Neurochemistry* 82 (5) (September): 1129-1136.

Kurek, J B, L Austin, S S Cheema, P F Bartlett, and M Murphy. 1996. "Up-regulation of leukaemia inhibitory factor and interleukin-6 in transected sciatic nerve and muscle following denervation." *Neuromuscular Disorders* 6 (2) (March): 105-114.

LeBlanc, A C, and J F Poduslo. 1990. "Axonal modulation of myelin gene expression in the peripheral nerve." *Journal of Neuroscience Research* 26 (3) (July): 317-326.

Lindholm, D, R Heumann, M Meyer, and H Thoenen. 1987. "Interleukin-1 regulates synthesis of nerve growth factor in non-neuronal cells of rat sciatic nerve." *Nature* 330 (6149) (December 17): 658-659.

Liu, H M, L H Yang, and Y J Yang. 1995. "Schwann cell properties: 3. C-fos expression, bFGF production, phagocytosis and proliferation during Wallerian degeneration." *Journal of Neuropathology and Experimental Neurology* 54 (4) (July): 487-496.

Lubińska, L. 1982. "Patterns of Wallerian degeneration of myelinated fibres in short and long peripheral stumps and in isolated segments of rat phrenic nerve. Interpretation of the role of axoplasmic flow of the trophic factor." *Brain Research* 233 (2) (February 11): 227-240.

Lundborg, G, L B Dahlin, N Danielsen, H A Hansson, A Johannesson, F M Longo, and S Varon. 1982. "Nerve regeneration across an extended gap: a neurobiological view of nerve repair and the possible involvement of neuronotrophic factors." *The Journal of Hand Surgery* 7 (6) (November): 580-587.

Mackinnon, Susan. 1988. *Surgery of the peripheral nerve.* New York; Stuttgart; New York: Thieme Medical Publishers; G. Thieme Verlag.

Martin, L J, A Kaiser, and A C Price. 1999. "Motor neuron degeneration after sciatic nerve avulsion in adult rat evolves with oxidative stress and is apoptosis." *Journal of Neurobiology* 40 (2) (August): 185-201.

McQuarrie, I G. 1985. "Effect of conditioning lesion on axonal sprout formation at nodes of Ranvier." *The Journal of Comparative Neurology* 231 (2) (January 8): 239-249.

Meller, K. 1987. "Early structural changes in the axoplasmic cytoskeleton after axotomy studied by cryofixation." *Cell and Tissue Research* 250 (3) (December): 663-672.

Midrio, Menotti. 2006. "The denervated muscle: facts and hypotheses. A historical review." *European Journal of Applied Physiology* 98 (1) (September): 1-21.

Miller, F D, W Tetzlaff, M A Bisby, J W Fawcett, and R J Milner. 1989. "Rapid induction of the major embryonic alpha-tubulin mRNA, T alpha 1, during nerve regeneration in adult rats." *The Journal of Neuroscience: The Official Journal of the Society for Neuroscience* 9 (4) (April): 1452-1463.

Minwegen, P, and R L Friede. 1985. "A correlative study of internode proportions and sensitivity to procaine in regenerated frog sciatic nerves." *Experimental Neurology* 87 (1) (January): 147-164.

Mira, J C. 1984. "Effects of repeated denervation on muscle reinnervation." *Clinics in Plastic Surgery* 11 (1) (January): 31-38.

Molander, C, and H Aldskogius. 1992. "Directional specificity of regenerating primary sensory neurons after peripheral nerve crush or transection and epineurial suture A sequential double-labeling study in the rat." *Restorative Neurology and Neuroscience* 4 (5) (January 1): 339-344.

Myers, R R, H C Powell, M L Costello, P W Lampert, and B W Zweifach. 1978. "Endoneurial fluid pressure: direct measurement with micropipettes." *Brain Research* 148 (2) (June 16): 510-515.

Nathaniel, E J, and D C Pease. 1963. "Regenerative changes in rat dorsal roots following Wallerian degeneration." *Journal of Ultrastructure Research* 52 (December): 533-549.

Navarro, Xavier. 2009. "Chapter 27: Neural plasticity after nerve injury and regeneration." *International Review of Neurobiology* 87: 483-505.

Oblinger, M M, and R J Lasek. 1988. "Axotomy-induced alterations in the synthesis and transport of neurofilaments and microtubules in dorsal root ganglion cells." *The Journal of Neuroscience* 8 (5) (May): 1747-1758.

Perry, V H, M C Brown, and S Gordon. 1987. "The macrophage response to central and peripheral nerve injury. A possible role for macrophages in regeneration." *The Journal of Experimental Medicine* 165 (4) (April 1): 1218-1223.

Purves, D. 1975. "Functional and structural changes in mammalian sympathetic neurones following interruption of their axons." *The Journal of Physiology* 252 (2) (November): 429-463.

Rauvala, H, R Pihlaskari, J Laitinen, and J Merenmies. 1989. "Extracellular adhesive molecules in neurite growth." *Bioscience Reports* 9 (1) (February): 1-12.

Robinson, Grant A, and Roger D Madison. 2004. "Motor neurons can preferentially reinnervate cutaneous pathways." *Experimental Neurology* 190 (2) (December): 407-413.

Schlaepfer, W W. 1977. "Structural alterations of peripheral nerve induced by the calcium ionophore A23187." *Brain Research* 136 (1) (November 4): 1-9.

Schlaepfer, W W, and R P Bunge. 1973. "Effects of calcium ion concentration on the degeneration of amputated axons in tissue culture." *The Journal of Cell Biology* 59 (2 Pt 1) (November): 456-470.

Seddon, H. J. 1943. "Three types of nerve injury." *Brain* 66 (4) (December 1): 237 -288.

Seilheimer, B, and M Schachner. 1988. "Studies of adhesion molecules mediating interactions between cells of peripheral nervous system indicate a major role for L1 in mediating sensory neuron growth on Schwann cells in culture." *The Journal of Cell Biology* 107 (1) (July): 341-351.

Selander, D, and J Sjöstrand. 1978. "Longitudinal spread of intraneurally injected local anesthetics. An experimental study of the initial neural distribution following intraneural injections." *Acta Anaesthesiologica Scandinavica* 22 (6): 622-634.

Skene, J H, R D Jacobson, G J Snipes, C B McGuire, J J Norden, and J A Freeman. 1986. "A protein induced during nerve growth (GAP-43) is a major component of growth-cone membranes." *Science* 233 (4765) (August 15): 783-786.

Stoll, G, J W Griffin, C Y Li, and B D Trapp. 1989. "Wallerian degeneration in the peripheral nervous system: participation of both Schwann cells and macrophages in myelin degradation." *Journal of Neurocytology* 18 (5) (October): 671-683.

Sunderland, S, and K C Bradley. 1949. "The cross-sectional area of peripheral nerve trunks devoted to nerve fibers." *Brain: A Journal of Neurology* 72 (3) (September): 428-449.

Sunderland, Sydney. 1978. *Nerves and nerve injuries*. 2nd ed. Edinburgh; New York: Churchill Livingstone; distributed by Longman.

Thomas, P K, and D G Jones. 1967. "The cellular response to nerve injury. II. Regeneration of the perineurium after nerve section." *Journal of Anatomy* 101 (Pt 1) (January): 45-55.

Vanden Noven, S, N Wallace, D Muccio, A Turtz, and M J Pinter. 1993. "Adult spinal motoneurons remain viable despite prolonged absence of functional synaptic contact with muscle." *Experimental Neurology* 123 (1) (September): 147-156.

Vizoso, A D, and J Z Young. 1948. "Internode length and fibre diameter in developing and regenerating nerves." *Journal of Anatomy* 82 (Pt 1-2) (April): 110-134.1.

Waller, Augustus. 1850. "Experiments on the Section of the Glossopharyngeal and Hypoglossal Nerves of the Frog, and Observations of the Alterations Produced Thereby in the Structure of Their Primitive Fibres." *Philosophical Transactions of the Royal Society of London* 140 (January 1): 423-429.

Walsh, F S, and P Doherty. 1996. "Cell adhesion molecules and neuronal regeneration." *Current Opinion in Cell Biology* 8 (5) (October): 707-713.

Watts, Ryan J, Eric D Hoopfer, and Liqun Luo. 2003. "Axon pruning during Drosophila metamorphosis: evidence for local degeneration and requirement of the ubiquitin-proteasome system." *Neuron* 38 (6) (June 19): 871-885.

Waxman, Stephen. 1995. *The axon : structure, function and pathophysiology*. New York; Oxford: Oxford University Press.

Weinberg, H J, and P S Spencer. 1975. "Studies on the control of myelinogenesis. I. Myelination of regenerating axons after entry into a foreign unmyelinated nerve." *Journal of Neurocytology* 4 (4) (August): 395-418.

Witzel, Christian, Charles Rohde, and Thomas M Brushart. 2005. "Pathway sampling by regenerating peripheral axons." *The Journal of Comparative Neurology* 485 (3) (May 9): 183-190.

Ygge, J. 1989. "Neuronal loss in lumbar dorsal root ganglia after proximal compared to distal sciatic nerve resection: a quantitative study in the rat." *Brain Research* 478 (1) (January 23): 193-195.

Zhai, Qiwei, Jing Wang, Anna Kim, Qing Liu, Ryan Watts, Eric Hoopfer, Timothy Mitchison, Liqun Luo, and Zhigang He. 2003. "Involvement of the ubiquitin-proteasome system in the early stages of wallerian degeneration." *Neuron* 39 (2) (July 17): 217-225.

2

Electrodiagnostic Medicine Consultation in Peripheral Nerve Disorders

S. Mansoor Rayegani[1] and R. Salman Roghani[2]
[1]*Shahid Beheshti Medical University, PM&R Research Center,*
[2]*University of Social Welfare and Rehabilitation*
Iran

1. Introduction

Peripheral nerve disorders including entrapment syndromes, nerve lesions and peripheral neuropathic processes are among common disorders that are dealt in routine daily practice of neuromusculoskletal practitioners.

Surgeons, Physiatrists, Rheumatologists, Neurologists and Therapists are involved in this practice. Different fields of practice such as diagnosis, non-surgical management, surgery and rehabilitation medicine are addressed in this era. For proper and effective management, precise and appropriates diagnosis of the disorders is mandatory. In addition to clinical examination i.e, history and physical examination, There are different tools for quantitative assessment and diagnosis of peripheral nerve disorders. Imaging studies such as sonography, MRI and CT-Scan are among such studies.

Electrodiagnostic medicine consultation (EDX) is by far the most routine and precise evaluation methods for peripheral nerve disorders [1]. In fact by EDX study, physiologic aspects of disorders is precisely evaluated.

EDX is a type of medical consultation performed by a qualified physician who has expertise in neuromuscular medicine practice and must be a physician, that can be physiatrist "rehabilitation medicine specialist" and/or trained neurologist [2]. In this chapter basics of EDX, with planned, routine and practical electrodiagnostic medicine evaluation of peripheral nerve disorders are discussed. In addition to EDX studies that are used for physiologic study of peripheral nerve disorders, there is increased tendency to use imaging studies such as sonography for anatomic evaluation of the disorders. Sonography has very significant role as an adjuvant diagnostic method for EDX study and could not be regarded as the alternative to electrodiagnostic medicine consultation a brief discussion about application of sononography in peripheral nerve disorders is also given.

2. Electrodiagnostic medicine consultation

EDX is a specific branch of medicine practiced by a trained physician for diagnosis, treatment and prognostication of neuromuscular disorders. In many instances of peripheral nerve disorders such as entrapment syndromes the only reliable and precise tool to diagnose and differentiate between different types of syndromes is electrodiagnostic medicine studies.(figure 1)

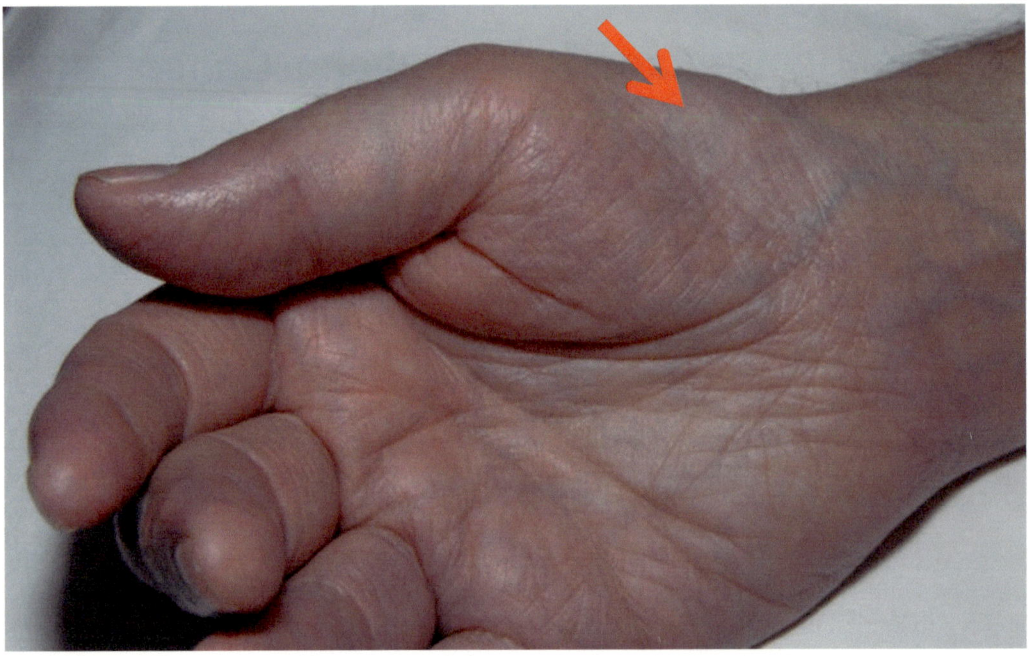

Fig. 1. Thenar atrophy in a 40 Y/O female that could be seen In both CTS and TOS. EDX is unique for differential diagnosis between these 2 entities (From the author personal archive).

There are 2 separate fields of electrodiagnostic medicine study called central and peripheral EDX. In central EDX study by stimulating peripheral sensory systems such as Auditory (cranial nerve VIII) , visual (cranial nerve II) and sensory nerves and recoding from the related cortical and spinal cord areas central nervous disorders are evaluated . These studies that are called auditory brainstem response (ABR), visual evoked potential (VEP) and somatosensory Evoked potentials (SEP) are used mainly for diagnostic evaluation of CNS disorder such as multiple sclerosis, traumatic brain injuries, myelopathic process and other related disorders [3]. There is another type of CNS EDX study called magnetic motor evoked potential "MMEP" that is used for motor stimulation of cortex and spinal cord. MEP is also used for study of deeply seated peripheral nerves such as sciatic, lumbosacral and cervical roots, lumbosacral and brachial plexus. In this study by cortical, spinal cord and/or peripheral nerve stimulation using magnetic coil, proper response is recorded from related limb muscles.

Peripheral EDX study that is used for evaluation of peripheral nervous system disorder i.e motor unit (figure 2) and sensory fibers is composed of nerve conduction studies (NCS) late responses (H-reflex, F-Wave) and needle electromyography (EMG).

The 1st and basic step in performing electrodiagnostic medicine study is pertinent and precise clinical examination including history, physical examination, lab and imaging studies . By Peripheral EDX study, disorders of motor neuron, spinal roots, lumbosacral and brachial plexus, peripheral nerves, neuromuscular junction and muscles are diagnosed and classified according to the site of involvement, type and severity of the disorder.

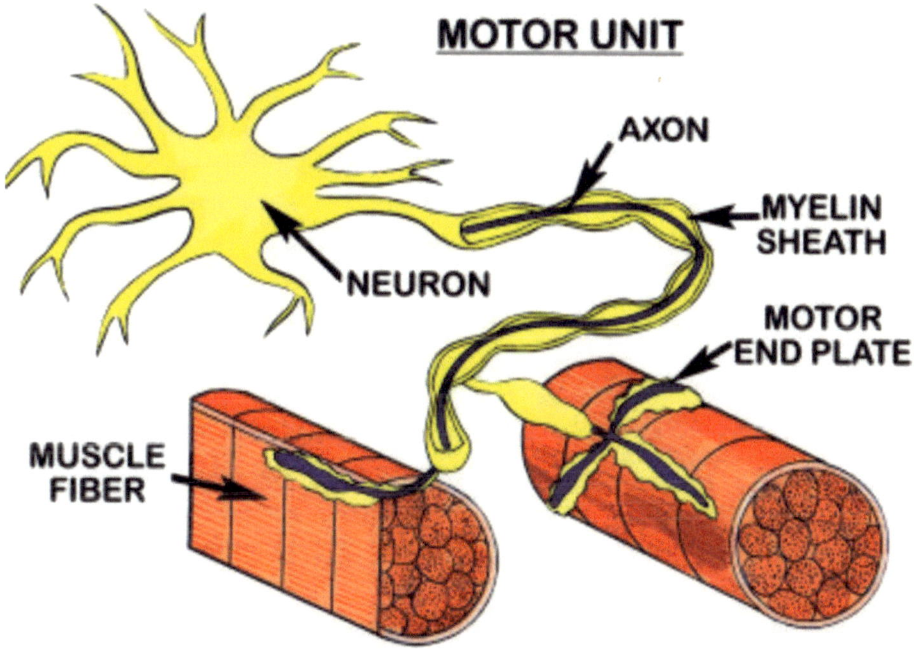

Fig. 2. Typical schematic picture of a motor unit

Taking history and performing physical examination are critical and first step in performing electrodiagnostic medicine consultation. Other items that are critical for EDX evaluation of peripheral nerve disorders include; pathophysiologic types of injuries, timing of study, localization and reinnervation processes that are discussed below [4].

3. History and physical examination

Because in many situations the Electrodiagnostic medicine consultant physician who is performing EDX study, is more familiar and has more experience regarding diagnosis of peripheral nerve disorders and other related musculoskletal disease than the primary referring physician it is mandatory for EDX physician to take a complete pertinent history and perform physical examination to provide related differential diagnosis list.

Deep and precise knowledge of neuromuscular anatomy is needed for clinical evaluation. Distribution of symptoms and weather it is focal or general is critical for establishing the proper plan of study. Whether symptoms are constant or intermittent and changes during day or night time is another important subject to be funded out in history taking. Chronologic status of the symptoms are important for detection of consequent muscular atrophy and/or trophic skin changes.

Past medical history and family history are in many instances pertinent to the patients present symptom and should be addressed.

In addition to history, that is very important for establishing differential diagnosis, precise and detailed pertinent physical examination is very useful for providing clinical diagnosis of peripheral nerve disorders.

There is four basic and mandatory steps in physical examination of peripheral nerve disorders; Manual Muscle Testing (MMT), quantitative sensory testing including deep and superficial, heat and cold, light and pin prick sensation and two point discrimination should be assessed and is useful in some mild lesions, Deep Tendon Reflexes (DTR) should also be evaluated for detecting abnormalities in reflex arc such as roots lesion.

The fourth step in physical examination is performing provocating tests. These tests are used for putting the nerves in such a jeopardized condition to reveal the symptoms. Phalen test is one of the most sensitive and well known prorovacating tests that is used for clinical diagnosis of carpal tunnel syndrome.

4. Pathophysiology of peripheral nerve disorders

Nerve injuries classification is according to completeness and/or pathophysiologic bases.

In complete injuries all of the nerve components at the site of injury are disrupted in contrast to incomplete injuries in which some components of nerves are spared. This classification of complete and incomplete type of injury has very important therapeutic and clinical implications.

Segmental demyelination (ie, neurapraxia) and axonal injury with consequent Wallerian degeneration are the two basic pathophysiologic types of nerve injuries (figure 3). In many instances there is mixed type of neurapraxia and axonal injury involving different nerve fibers at the site of nerve injury.

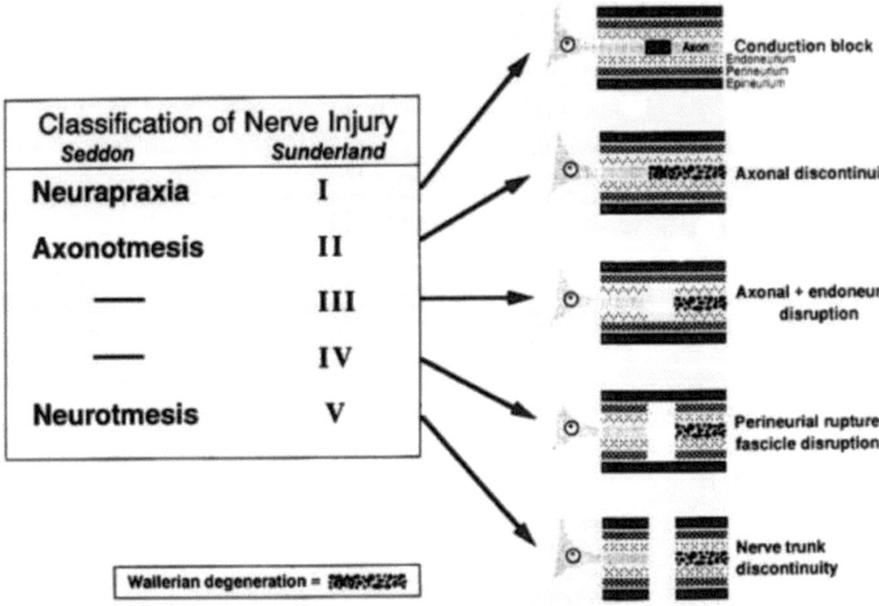

Fig. 3. Pathophysiologic types of nerve injury (from neurosurgery.tv)

Sensory NCS

Nerve / Sites	Rec. Site	Onset ms	Peak ms	NP Amp µV	PP Amp µV
L MEDIAN - Dig III					
1. Wrist	III	3.25	4.15	25.3	38.8
2. Palm	III	1.15	1.55	35.8	64.2

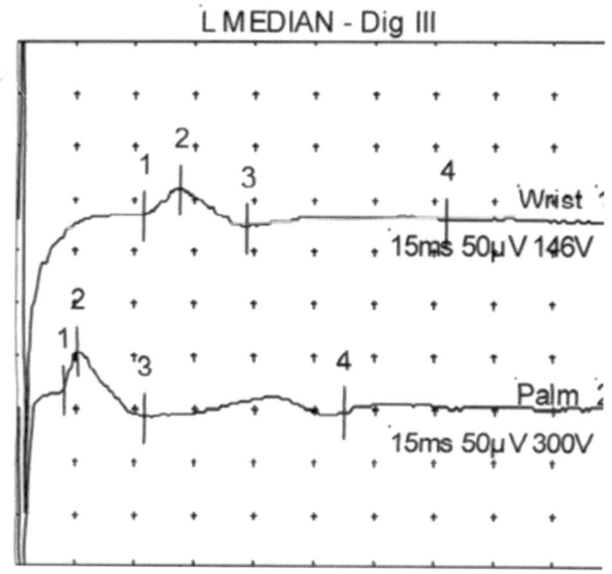

Fig. 4. Mixed type of conduction block and demyelination in a patient with carpal tunnel syndrome(From the author personal archive).

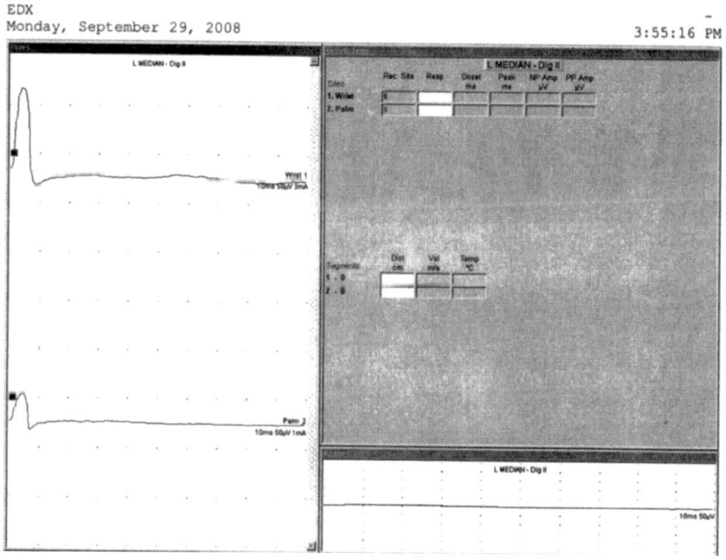

Fig. 5. complete axonal damage with absence of response in distal and proximal stimulation at the site of injury (From the author personal archive) .

In neurapraxia with segmental demyelination the nerve fiber axons are intact and no axonal degeneration and nerve destruction occurs. (figure 4) In axonal injury the injured axons undergo a process known as Wallerian degeneration. Axonal function is disrupted immediately after the injury and although the disconnected distal segment initially survives and conducts the applied stimulus over the course of the next 7 days, finally this segment slowly degenerates in a centrifugal fashion and eventually becomes inexcitable.(figure 5) Axonal injuries that spare the supporting perineural connective tissue sheath are known as axonotmetic injury. The intact perineural connective tissue sheaths provide a conduit for axonal regeneration from the cell body to the target muscle, facilitating recovery. Injuries that disrupt the whole nerve, affecting both the axon and supporting connective tissue, are known as neurotmetic lesions. These injuries are less likely to recover by axonal regeneration and often require surgical repair.

Individual axons can exhibit only one of these types of pathophysiologic change, however an injured nerve is composed of thousands of axons, and a mixed pattern of segmental demyelination and axonal loss is manifested.

A precise and timed electrodiagnostic medicine consultation study is very useful and critical for determining the completeness and pathophysiologic type of all nerve injuries[5].

5. Timing of the EDX study

Timing is an important and critical issue especially regarding acute traumatic nerve injuries. Lack of understanding about influence of timing on EDX studies can result to false negative results. Different pathophysiologic type of injury such as neurapraxia, Demyelination and axonal loss can cause different presentation in EDX findings at different time course of the injury[6]. Following are the electrodiagnostic findings in a defined time course

5.1 Onset to day 7

There is no or small nerve conduction study response with proximal stimulation to the site of lesion depending on the severity of the lesion whether it is partial or complete. However in all types of nerve injuries the distal segment response is elicited. There is no or decreased voluntary motor unit action potentials in EMG study of muscles below lesion in all types of lesion including neurapraxia, demyelination or axonal loss.

5.2 Day 7 to 14

This time window is very important and critical to distinguish between neurapraxia (conduction block/demyelination) and axonal damage. In Axonal damage Wallerian degeneration is progressed toward the muscle end organ and distal stimulation to the site of lesion cause no response in motor nerves at seventh day and sensory nerve at tenth day after injury. Instead in neurapraxic lesion the responses will be elicited by distal stimulation. (figure 6)

In both complete neurapraxia and axonal loss lesions there is no voluntary EMG (MUAPS) activities in muscles distal to the lesion.

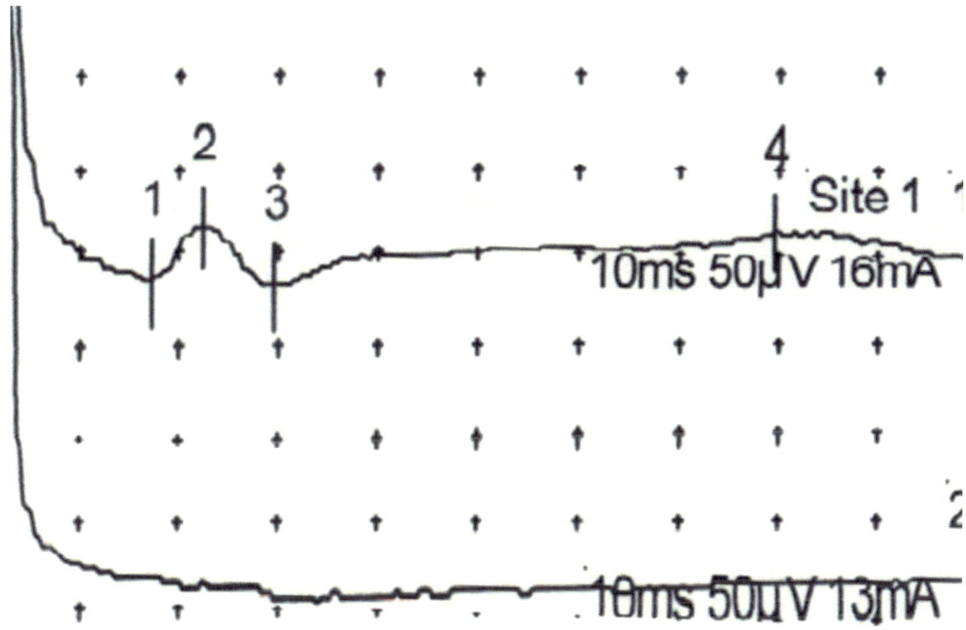

Fig. 6. Pure conduction block with lack of response by proximal stimulation(lower trace) and presence of response by distal stimulation (upper trace) (From the author personal archive).

5.3 Day 14 forward

It takes about 2 to 3 week after onset of injury to see spontaneous EMG potentials. Such as fibrillation and positives sharp waves. These potentials are pathognomonic and specific for detection of axonal loss in peripheral nerve lesions and may persists for a long time(figure7, 8)

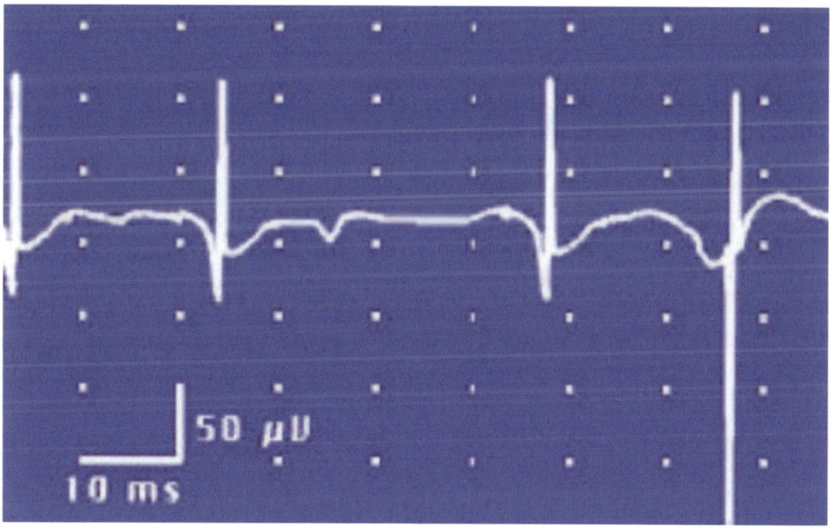

Fig. 7. Fibrillation potentials recorded from denervated muscle 20 days post axonal nerve injury.

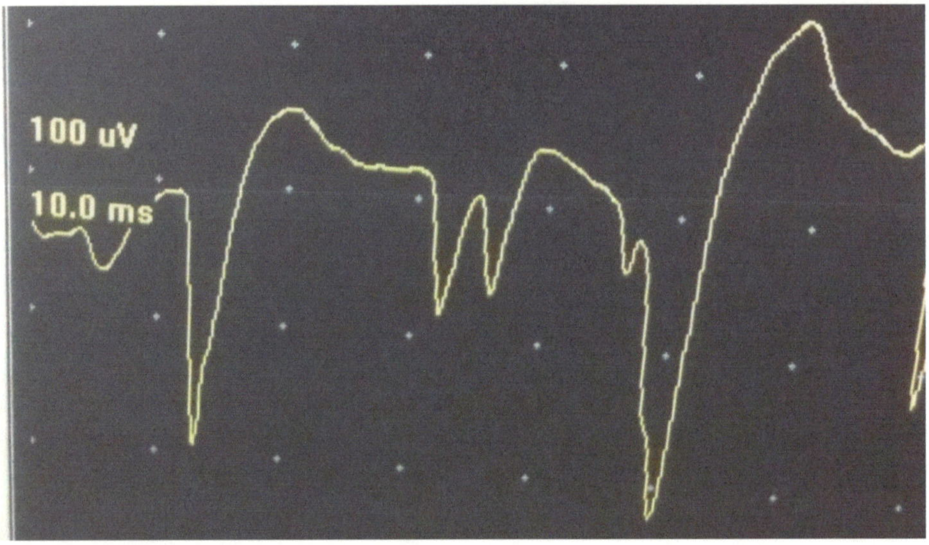

Fig. 8. Positive sharp waves (PSW) recorded from the same muscle at different needle position (The author personal archive).

In contrast to axonal loss, in pure neurapraxic and demyelination it is possible to record the response distal to the site of injury and usually there is no spontaneous activities in needle EMG of distal muscles.

6. Reinnervation process

According to the type of injury; complete or incomplete, there is two main reinnervation process, axonal regrowth and axonal sprouting. Axonal regrowth is occurred in complete axonal injuries proceeding at 1 inch per month and producing short duration and low amplitude motor unit action potentials called nascent MUAPS in needle EMG of involved muscles.

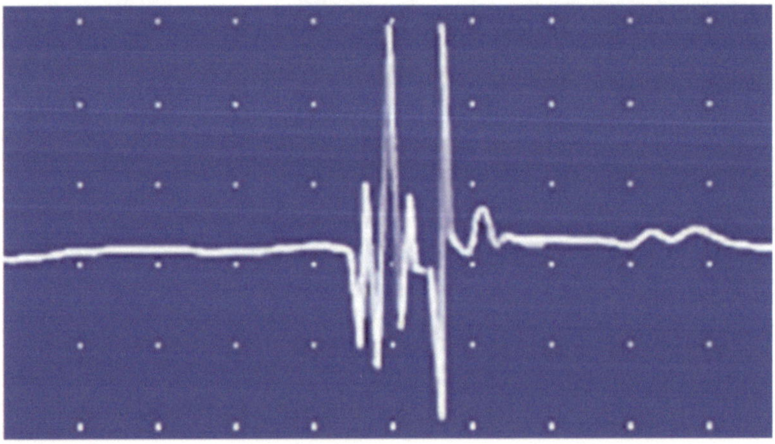

Fig. 9. Polyphasic, long duration, high amplitude MUAPS indicative for reinnervated muscle fibers by axonal sprouting in partial nerve lesion.

In Partial lesions the major process is axonal sprouting that originates from intact axons to innervate orphan muscles fiber cells and producing long duration, high amplitude motor unit action potential in volitional EMC activities (figure 9). In both processes of reinnervation, number of spontaneous activities decreased and distal responses of NCS will be recorded if the reinnervation process continued. Albeit the NCS response nerve reach to the preinjury normal range [7].

7. Localization

One of the most important and key findings in peripheral nerve disorders is localization of the injury site in nerve course. This subject is very important and critical for referring physicians especially surgeons. Both needle EMG and NCS are used for localizing the lesion site. In pure axonal loss with secondary complete Wallerian degeneration, needle EMG of muscles that are located in distal and proximal to the site of presumed injury can localize the injury site.

Knowledge of nerve branching and surface anatomy of peripheral nerve and muscular branching is crucial for the localization .

Nerve conduction studies including distal latency, NCV and amplitude of the recorded responses by proximal and distal stimulation at the presumed site of involvement is more useful in detection of neurapraxia (conduction block) and demyelination types of involvement [8].

8. Prognostication of the injury

There is some factors that are working for prognosis evaluation in peripheral nerve injuries. Pathophysiologic process, i.e axonal loss or demyelination (conduction block), time onset of lesion , severity of the lesion; complete or incomplete and the distance between lesion site and target muscles are the most important determining factors in prognostication of nerve injury [9].

Unfortunately electodiagnostic studies cannot distinguish between complete axonotmetic and neurotmetic lesions. In contrast demyelination and conduction block processes could be easily distinguished.

Serial, periodic and careful EMG follow up examination could be helpful for distinguishing between neurotmesis and axonotmesis. Lack of suspected regeneration in target muscles in estimated time could be attributed to the neurotmetic type of lesion.

Apparently neurapraxic (conduction block) and demyelination type of lesion have better and good prognosis for recovery compared to axonatmesis and neurotmesis.

This is primary and basic role of electrodiagnostic medicine consultant physician to adequately differentiate between complete and incomplete and also axonotmetic and conduction block/ Demyelination types of injury.

Complete nerve injuries that are predominantly neurapraxic can be expected to recover favorably over the course of weeks to months. When such cases do not recover as expected, patients should undergo follow-up electrodiagnostic testing, which may show the presence of significant secondary axonal loss suggesting that the initial testing was done too early, before the electrophysiologic abnormalities had fully evolved. However, if the follow-up study shows persistent conduction block across the injury site, then the patient should be evaluated carefully for an ongoing compressive lesion (eg, hematoma) by appropriate imaging studies.

Complete lesions with electrodiagnostic evidence of axonal loss may be axonotmetic or neurotmetic. Axonotmetic injuries are more likely to recover spontaneously. Neurotmetic injuries often require surgical repair for adequate recovery. The only way to differentiate these injury types noninvasively is to monitor the patient for signs of recovery. However, the chances of successful surgical repair begin to decline by 6 months after the injury. By 18-24 months, the denervated muscles usually are replaced by fatty connective tissue, making functional recovery impossible. In most cases, close clinical observation is warranted for 3-6 months after this type of nerve injury. If no clinical or electrophysiologic evidence of recovery is noted during this period, these patients should be referred for surgical exploration.

Indication for surgical exploration and repair include; complete nerve lesions caused by lacerations or penetrating injuries, significant nerve injuries with no clinical or electrodiagnostic evidence of recovery after 3-6 months of clinical observation are also indications for surgical exploration and intraoperative nerve conduction testing and possible surgical repair.

At the time of surgical exploration, the injured nerve may be obviously severed, in which case the injured segment should be resected and an end-to-end anastomosis (usually with an intervening nerve graft) performed. If the injured nerve segment appears to remain in continuity, intraoperative nerve conduction studies can differentiate axonotmetic from neurotmetic injury[10].

The above discussion is mainly focused on electrodiagnostic evaluation of acute traumatic peripheral nerve injuries in which EDX evaluation and assessment has a crucial role for treatment planning. There are a lot of other types of peripheral nerve disorders such as lumbosacral and cervical radiculopathy, plexopathy, entrapment syndromes and peripheral neuropathic processes in which EDX also is highly applicable and has invaluable diagnostic role. Theses disorders need to be discussed in detail in separate book chapter, however it is worthwhile to mention here that except for time course assessment of the study other issues including localization, prognostication and determining pathophysiologic type of disorders i.e demyelination/axonal involvement are similarly applicable to all types of disorders.

9. Nerve sonography as a complementary method to Electrodiagnostic medicine

High resolution Ultrasonography is a useful method in the evaluation of common neuromuscular disorders as an adjunction to Electrodiagnostic studies (EDX) or independently.[11, 12] Any physician, who is expert in electrodiagnostic medicine, or visits patients with common neuromuscular problems, is likely to improve the care of patients by adding anatomy details of sonography to physiologic data which gathered from EDX. It may confirm Electrodiagnostic findings or find pathologies in case of false negative EDX studies especially in tunnel syndromes[fig10]. [13] Ultrasonography also could identify target muscles more precisely[fig11]; avoid penetrating vasculature [fig12] by EMG needle especially in coagulation disorders and targeting nerves for near nerve conduction studies [fig13]. [14] Risky EMG such as diaphragmatic one could be performed safer under sono guide by real time visualization of diaphragm and lung movements with respiration, which let us accurate estimation and finding optimal needle insertion points and depth . [15]

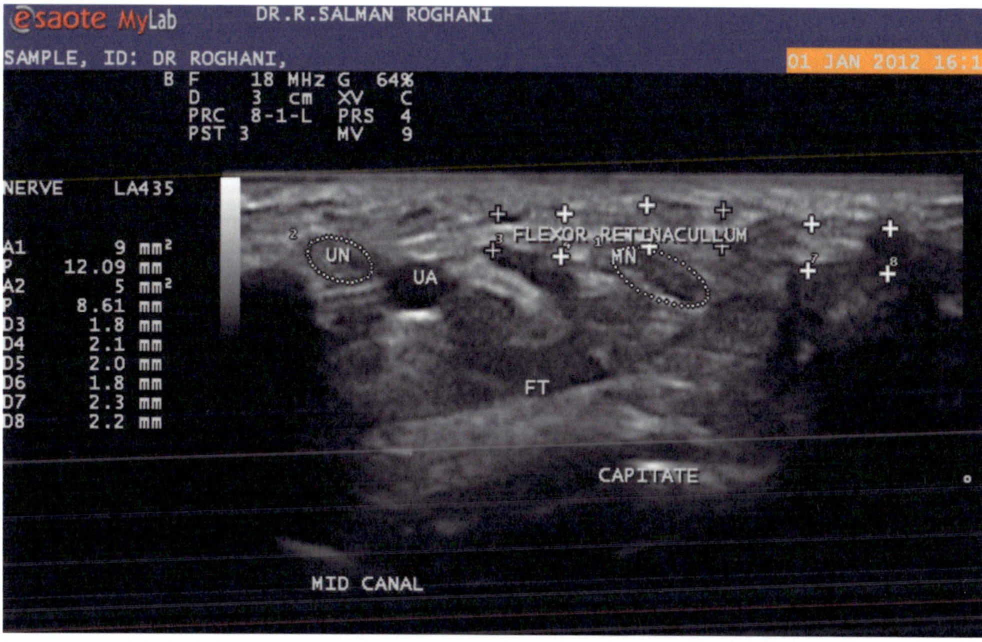

Fig. 10. Ultrasound cross sectional Image at the tunnel of carp with a lot of anatomic information about region(The author[2] personal archive)

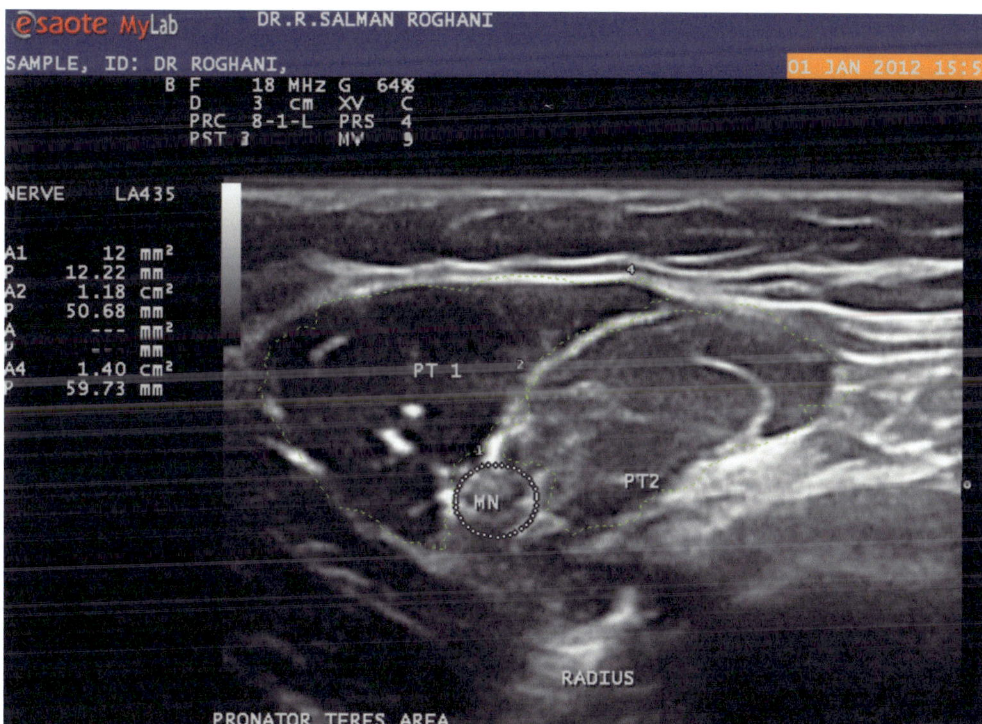

Fig. 11. Precise muscles localization (The author[2] personal archive)

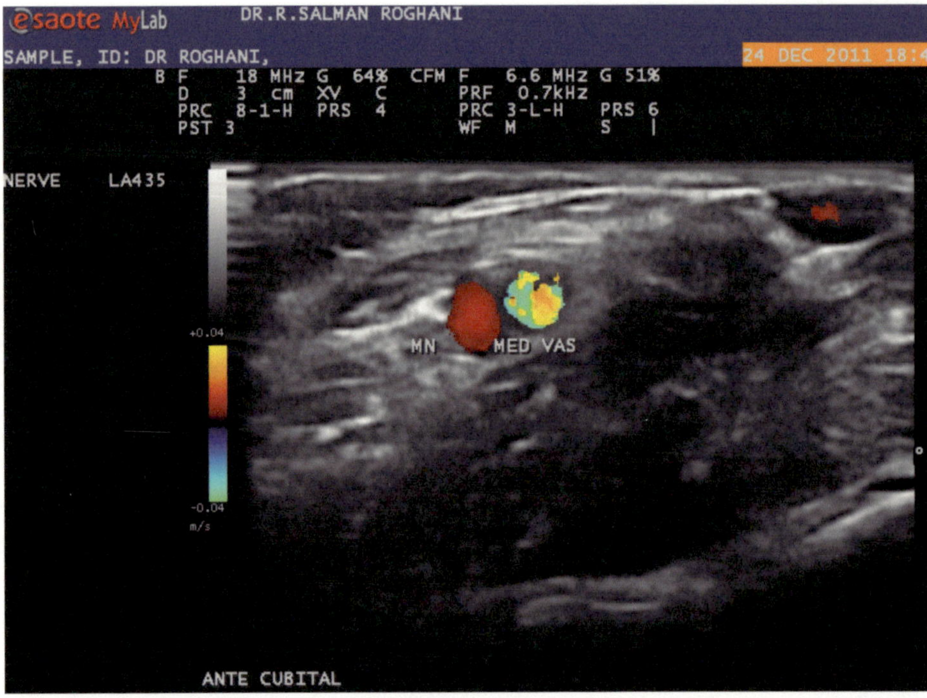

Fig. 12. Doppler Ultrasound image to avoid vasculature penetration (The author[2] personal archive)

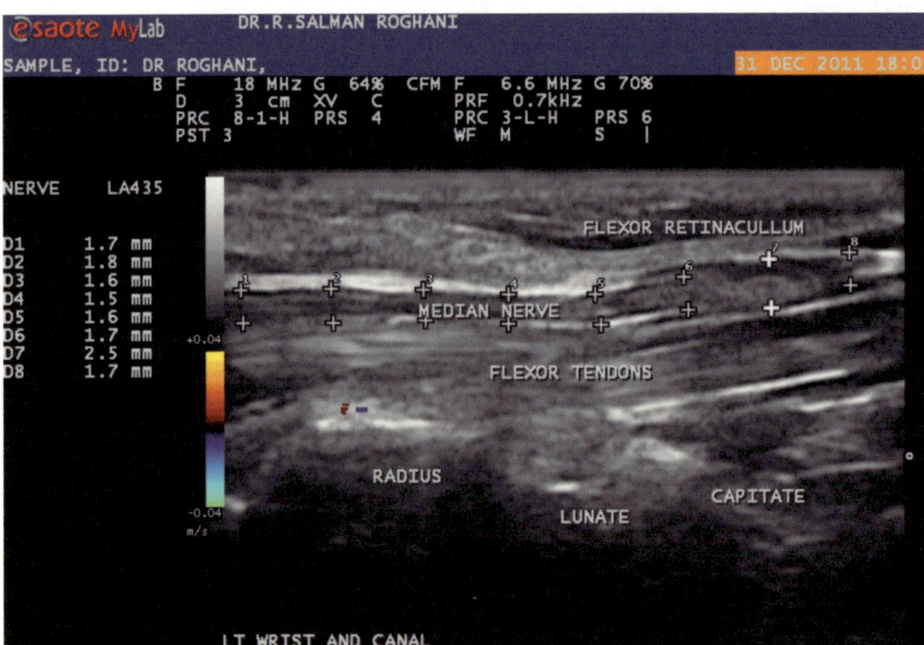

Fig. 13. longitudinal scan of median nerve at wrist which is best for near nerve stimulation or injection. (The author[2] personal archive)

We found that our residents learn nerve, muscle and joints anatomy more accurately with more interest using ultrasonography guide. Selection of muscles for botulinum toxin denervation and tendons for chronic tendinipathies could be done more precisely under sono guide and also injection of these tissue with more confidence. [16] Doppler mode not only could determine main vasculature and avoid them during needling or injection it also could determine inflammation of nerves in inflammatory neuropathies or tendinopathies. [17]

Real time scanning, reasonable price of instrument comparing to other imaging like CT or MRI and relatively short time of scan in a professional hand and also possibility of immediate scan after or during electromyography, make ultrasound a valuable choice in EDX lab for adding anatomic information to physiologic findings.

10. Summary

Electrodiagnostic medicine consultation is highly sensitive indicator of early nerve injury, detects dynamic and functional injury missed by other diagnostic tools such as MRI, provides information regarding chronicity of nerve injury, provides prognostic data, is highly localizing, clarifies clinical scenarios when one disorder mimics another, identifies combined multi-site injury, avoiding missed diagnoses, identifies more global neuromuscular injury with focal onset.

Electrodiagnostic studies are a supplement to, and not a replacement for the history and physical examination.

Results of EDX are often time-dependent and not "standardized" investigations and may be modified by the practitioner to answer the diagnostic question

All results are dependent on a reliable laboratory with full repertoire of techniques and qualified expert consultant Electrodiagnostician physician.

11. Acknowledgement

I wish to thank my wife through her dedication to helping me having a calm environment for editing this chapter and the book, her support in making sure I finally finished this work.

I would also like to thank my daughter, Negar who helped me for arranging the web search and also thanks my son, Hesam for his help in preparing electronic form of my personal archive.

12. References

[1] Van Beek AL.Hand Clin. 1986 Nov;2(4):747-60.

[2] Daniel Dumitru, Anthony A. Amato, Machiel Zwarts. Electrodiagnostic Medicine. Hanley & Belfus (2001).

[3] Physical Medicine and Rehabilitation: Principles and Practice, 4th ed., vol. 1, pp. 105–139. Philadelphia: Lippincott Williams and Wilkins.

[4] Johnson's Practical Electromyography, 4th Edition By William S. Pease, Henry L. Lew, Ernest W. Johnson

[5] Stewart JD. Focal Peripheral Neuropathies. New York: Raven Press;1993
[6] Johnson's Practical Electromyography, 4th Edition pp.259-262 By William S. Pease, Henry L. Lew, Ernest W. Johnson
[7] Korte N, Schenk HC, Grothe C, Tipold A, Haastert-Talini K.Muscle Nerve. 2011 Jul;44(1):63-73
[8] Kimura J: Electrodiagnosis in Diseases of Nerve and Muscle: Principles and Practices (Ed 3), Oxford University Press 2001.
[9] Derr JJ, Micklesen PJ, Robinson LR. Am J Phys Med Rehabil. 2009 Jul;88(7):547-53.
[10] Brown WF, Veitch J. AAEM minimonograph #42: intraoperative monitoring of peripheral and cranial nerves.Muscle Nerve. Apr 1994;17(4):371-7.
[11] Chiou, H.J., et al., Peripheral nerve lesions: role of high-resolution US. Radiographics, 2003. 23(6): p. e15.
[12] Koenig, R.W., et al., High-resolution ultrasonography in evaluating peripheral nerve entrapment and trauma. Neurosurg Focus, 2009. 26(2): p. E13.
[13] Zyluk, A., P. Puchalski, and P. Nawrot, [The usefulness of ultrasonography in the diagnosis of carpal tunnel syndrome--a review]. Chir Narzadow Ruchu Ortop Pol, 2010. 75(6): p. 385-91.
[14] Zheng, H., et al., [Evaluation of safety and anesthetic effect for ultrasound-guided cervical plexus block]. Zhonghua Yi Xue Za Zhi, 2011. 91(27): p. 1909-13.
[15] Boon, A.J., et al., Ultrasound-guided needle EMG of the diaphragm: technique description and case report. Muscle Nerve, 2008. 38(6): p. 1623-6.
[16] Davidson, J. and S. Jayaraman, Guided interventions in musculoskeletal ultrasound: what's the evidence? Clin Radiol, 2011. 66(2): p. 140-52.
[17] Jacob, D., M. Cohen, and S. Bianchi, Ultrasound imaging of non-traumatic lesions of wrist and hand tendons. Eur Radiol, 2007. 17(9): p. 2237-47.

3

Galectin-1 as a Multifunctional Molecule in the Peripheral Nervous System After Injury

Kazunori Sango[1], Hiroko Yanagisawa[1], Kazuhiko Watabe[1], Hidenori Horie[2] and Toshihiko Kadoya[3]
[1]*ALS/Neuropathy Project, Tokyo Metropolitan Institute of Medical Science*
[2]*Research Center of Brain and Oral Science, Kanagawa Dental College*
[3]*Department of Biotechnology, Maebashi Institute of Technology*
Japan

1. Introduction

Restoration from peripheral nerve injury requires both neuronal cell survival and axonal regeneration across the site of injury and along the distal nerve stump as well as functional reconnection with the appropriate targets. It is no doubt that the concerted interplay of regenerating axons, non-neuronal cells (*e.g.* Schwann cells and macrophages), neurotrophic factors and cytokines, cell adhesion molecules, and extracellular matrix components is essential for successful nerve regeneration (Zochodne, 2008). A plenty of molecules have been implicated in the regenerative response to nerve injury (Terenghi, 1999; Yasuda et al., 2003) and the therapeutic approaches using the delivery systems for the target genes have been receiving increasing attention (Mason et al., 2011); however, the signals that prompt neurons to extend processes in peripheral nerves after injury are not fully understood.

We have established three-dimensional collagen gel culture system of ganglion explants, in which adult peripheral ganglia (mainly dorsal root ganglia (DRG)) with nerve fibers are embedded in collagen gel and the number and length of regenerating neurites from nerve-transected terminals are measured under a phase-contrast microscope (Fig.1, right; reproduced from Sango et al., 2006). Since the cell-cell interactions are maintained in the explanted ganglia, it is fair to state that the explant culture system mimics nerve regeneration *in vivo* better than the dissociated cell culture system (Fig.1, left). By employing the explant models, we showed that various kinds of neurotrophic factors (Horie et al., 1991a; Akahori et al., 1997), cytokines (Horie et al., 1997; Shuto et al., 2001), co-cultured tissues (Horie et al., 1991b; Saito et al., 2002) and experimental diabetes (Saito et al., 1999; Sango et al., 2002) enhanced neurite regeneration.

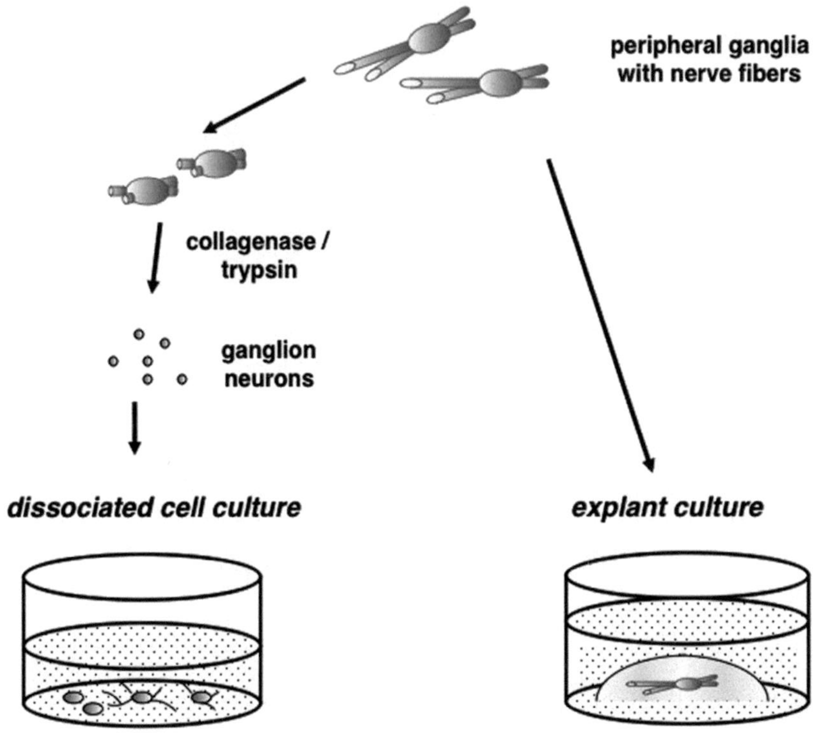

Fig. 1. Schematic representation of the methods for dissociated cell culture and explant culture of peripheral ganglia. In the former, each of the ganglion neurons is mechanically and enzymatically isolated, and seeded onto culture dishes precoated with extracellular substrate(s). In the latter, peripheral ganglia with nerve fibers are embedded in collagen gel. The number and length of regenerating neurites from nerve-transected terminals are measured under a phase-contrast microscope (Reproduced from Sango et al., *Current Diabetes Reviews*, 2006, Vol.2, No.2, pp.169-183, with permission from Bentham Science Publishers Ltd.).

Furthermore, we searched for novel axonal regeneration-promoting factors from the culture supernatants of COS1 cells (a cell line derived from the kidneys), and purified the protein with molecular weight of around 14 kDa. The analysis of the internal amino acid sequences of the active protein indicated that it was identical to galectin-1 (GAL-1) (Horie et al., 1999). GAL-1 is a member of the galectins, a family of β-galactoside binding animal lectin (Barondes et al., 1994) and has been shown to play roles in a wide variety of biological functions such as cell growth and differentiation, apoptosis, cell adhesion, tumor spreading, and inflammatory response (Camby et al., 2006; Rabinovich et al., 2007). Most of the studies on the biological activities of GAL-1 were performed under reducing conditions, and the effects of GAL-1 were inhibited by lactose. However, the 14 kDa protein secreted from COS1 cells exists as an oxidized form of GAL-1 (GAL-1/Ox), containing three intramolecular disulfide bonds (Cys^{2}-Cys^{130}, Cys^{16}-Cys^{88}, and Cys^{42}-Cys^{60}) as shown in Fig. 2. (reproduced from Kadoya & Horie, 2005).

In contrast to the concept that GAL-1 is biologically active only in the reduced form, we introduced GAL-1/Ox as a novel factor enhancing axonal regeneration in peripheral nerves

(Inagaki et al., 2000; Horie et al., 1999, 2004, 2005). The potent activity of recombinant human GAL-1/Ox on axonal regeneration has been confirmed by several *in vivo* experiments (Horie et al., 1999; Fukaya et al., 2003; Kadoya et al., 2005).

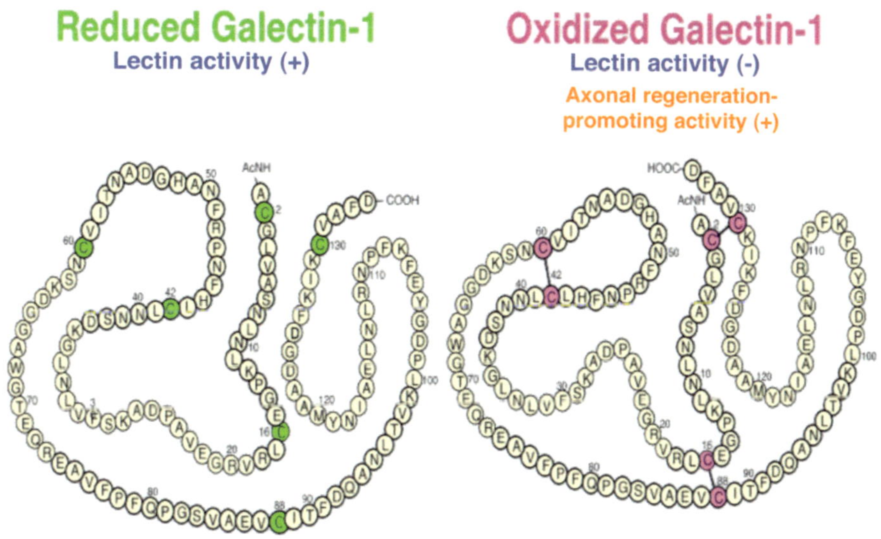

Fig. 2. Bubble map of reduced and oxidized GAL-1. GAL-1 having -galactoside-binding activity exists in a reduced form, whereas oxidized GAL-1 contains three intramolecular disulfide bonds (Reproduced from Kadoya & Horie, *Current Drug Targets,* 2005, Vol.6, No.4, pp. 375-383, with permission from Bentham Science Publishers Ltd.)

The growing evidence suggests that both reduced and oxidized forms of GAL-1 are involved in the repair process after nerve injury (Camby et al., 2006), but there is a marked difference in the structural and functional properties between the two forms; GAL-1 in the reduced form acts on nervous tissue as a lectin (Sasaki et al., 2004; Plachta et al., 2007), whereas GAL-1/Ox lacks lectin activity and acts as a cytokine-like molecule (Horie et al., 1999; Inagaki et al., 2000; Kadoya et al., 2005). In this chapter, we further characterize GAL-1 as a multi-functional molecule in the peripheral nervous system, focusing on its distribution, regulation of synthesis, extracellular release and oxidation, and possible action mechanisms for neuroprotection and axonal regeneration after injury.

2. Localization of GAL-1 in the peripheral nervous system

GAL-1 is encoded by the LGALS1 gene located on the human chromosome 22q13.1. The 0.6 kb transcript results from the splicing of four exons and encodes for a protein of 135 amino acids. It exists as a monomer as well as a non-covalent homodimer with a subunit molecular weight of 14.5 kDa (Barondes et al., 1994; Sango et al., 2004). GAL-1 is highly expressed in peripheral nervous tissues of adult rodents, with immunoreactivity localized to cell bodies of sensory and motoneurons, axons and Schwann cells (Fukaya et al., 2003; Akazawa et al., 2004). GAL-1 mRNA persists in DRG neurons at later developmental stages and is maintained in adult DRG neurons. Using *in situ* hybridization histochemistry, GAL-1 mRNA has been detected in nearly all neurons of the DRG. In general, the staining intensity in smaller diameter (<30 μm) neurons was higher than that in larger diameter neurons (Sango et al., 2004). The small DRG neurons are reported to have small myelinated (Aδ) and unmyelinated (C) fibers, which can play an essential role in thermoreception and nociception; whereas the large neurons have large myelinated (Aβ) fibers and are known to be mostly sensitive mechenoreceptors (Salt & Hill, 1983). Therefore, predominant expression of GAL-1 mRNA/protein in subpopulations of small diameter neurons (Regan et al., 1986, Hynes et al., 1990, Imbe et al., 2003, Sango et al., 2004, McGraw et al., 2005a) suggests that this molecule is involved in the transmission of nociceptive and thermoceptive information. In fact, mice lacking GAL-1 showed reduced sensitivity to noxious thermal stimuli (McGraw et al., 2005b).

2.1 Predominant expression of GAL-1 in small IB4-binding DRG neurons in vivo

Adult DRG neurons can be broadly divided into three principal subgroups by their soma size and characteristic markers (Fig.3; modified from McMahon & Bennett, 2000):

1. large neurons; immunoreactive for 200 kD neurofilaments (NF200),
2. small peptidergic neurons; immunoreactive for calcitonin gene-related peptide (CGRP) and high-affinity NGF receptor (trkA), and
3. small non-peptidergic neurons; immunoreactive for GDNF receptors (Ret, GFRα) and binding to isolectin B4 (IB4).

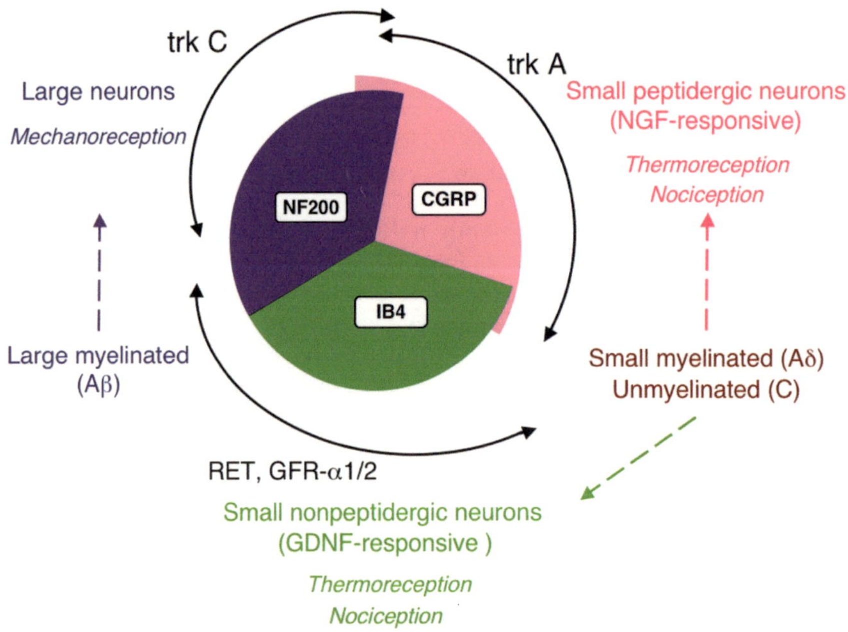

Fig. 3. Three principal subgroups of adult DRG neurons. Large neurons, immunoreactive for 200 kDa neurofilament, are known to possess large myelinated fibers. Small neurons are divided into peptidergic and non-peptidergic neurons; peptidergic neurons are immunoreactive for CGRP and high affinity NGF receptor trkA, whereas non-peptidergic neurons bind the lectin IB4 and express GDNF receptors. Both groups of small neurons are known to possess small myelinated and unmyelinated fibers (modified from McMahon & Benette, *Molecular Basis of Pain Induction*, 2000, pp. 65-86, with permission from John Wiley & Sons, Inc.).

Both small peptidergic and non-peptidergic neurons are responsible for the transmission of nociception and thermoreception, and whether these two groups of neurons have distinct functions has been the subject of controversy (McMahon & Bennett, 2000; Ernsberger, 2009).

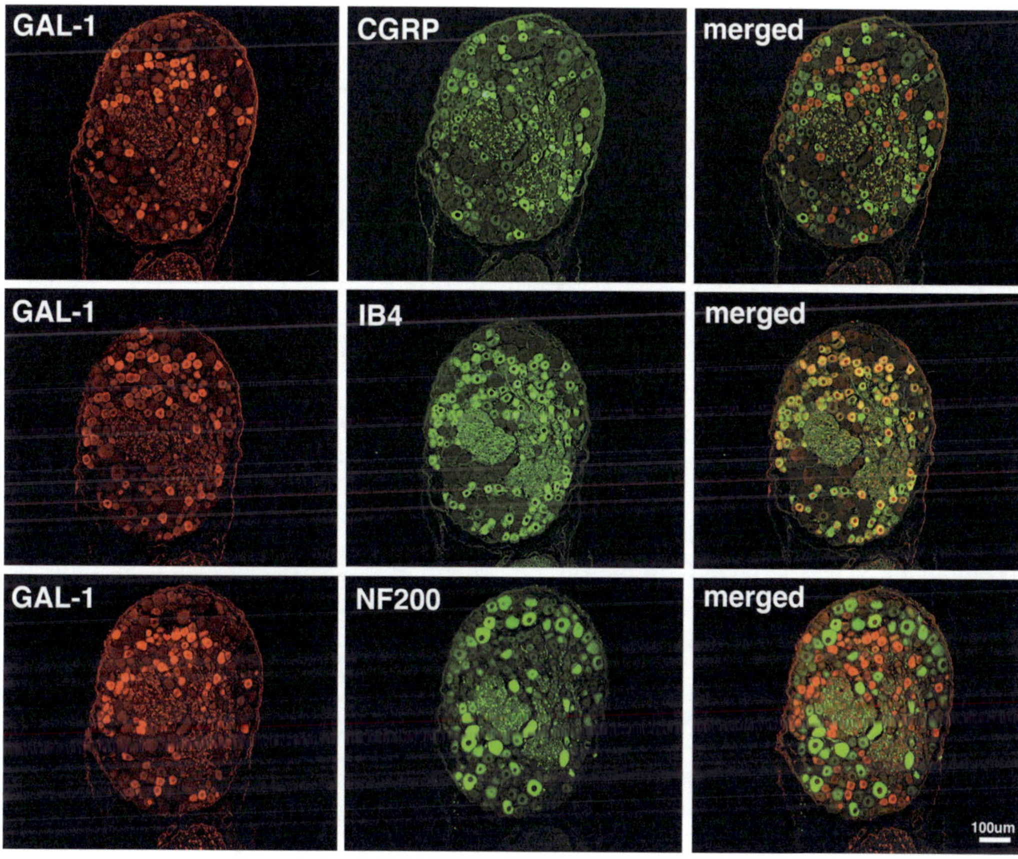

Fig. 4. Predominant expression of GAL-1 in small non-peptidergic neurons of adult rat DRG. Immunofluorescence micrographs of adult rat DRG sections, stained with antibodies to GAL-1 (red) and CGRP, IB4, or NF200 (green). The merged pictures are on the right. Almost all GAL-1 intensely labeled neurons are IB4-binding neurons, and distinguished from CGRP intensely labeled neurons and NF200 intensely labeled neurons.

Our immunohistochemical analysis revealed intense immunoreactivity for GAL-1 in a subset of small diameter neurons in the sections of adult rat lumbar DRG (Fig.4, left). The ratio of GAL-1-immunoreactive (IR) neurons was 31.6±5.4% (mean±SD from nine sections, 1717 neurons from three animals). By double immunofluorescent staining, 96.5±1.3% of the GAL-1-IR neurons were IB4-binding, whereas 3.7±1.2% and 0% were CGRP-IR and NF200-IR, respectively (Fig.4, center and right). These findings agree with the previous study by Imbe et al. (2003); they performed immunohistochemistry and *in situ* hybridization using two pairs of consecutive sections of lumbar DRG, and observed that 93.9% and 6.8% of the intensely GAL-1-IR neurons displayed mRNA for c-RET and trkA, respectively. On the other hand, the double immunofluorescent staining with the sections of cervical DRG (McGraw et al., 2005a) showed that 33% and 28% of the GAL-1-IR neurons were IB4-binding and CGRP-IR. Such differences may arise from variations in the distribution of GAL-1 at different spinal levels and/or different evaluation of the intensity for GAL-1-IR among the investigators. The finding that mice lacking GAL-1 showed reduced proportion of IB4-binding DRG neurons (McGraw et al., 2005b) indicates the involvement of GAL-1 in the proper phenotypic differentiation of the non-peptidergic DRG neurons during development.

2.2 GDNF upregulates protein expression of GAL-1 in cultured DRG cells

Our immunohistochemical analyses revealed that almost all the GAL-1 intensely stained DRG neurons were IB4-binding small non-peptidergic neurons (Figs.3&4). Since NGF and GDNF are likely to exert their major effects on small peptidergic and non-peptidergic neurons, respectively (Molliver et al., 1997), it seems plausible that GDNF regulates synthesis and/or distribution of GAL-1 in non-peptidergic DRG neurons. Following peripheral axotomy, GAL-1 expression was downregulated in small DRG neurons but was upregulated in NF200-IR large neurons (Imbe et al., 2003; McGraw et al., 2005a). These findings imply that retrogradely transported NGF and/or GDNF play a role in the dominant expression of GAL-1 in small DRG neurons (Lindsay & Harmar, 1989; Bennett et al., 1998).

By employing the dissociated cell culture model (Fig.1, left), we examined the effects of recombinant NGF and GDNF on neurite outgrowth and GAL-1 expression in adult rat DRG. As shown in previous studies (Lindsay, 1988; Gavazzi et al., 1999; Sango et al., 2008), both NGF and GDNF promoted neurite outgrowth from small DRG neurons (Fig.5).

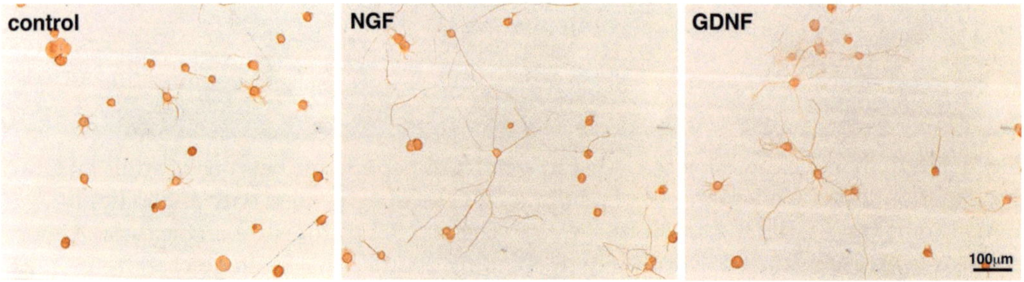

Fig. 5. Adult rat DRG neurons after 2 days in culture were immunostained with anti-βIII tubulin. An application of NGF or GDNF to culture medium (50 ng/ml) enhanced neurite outgrowth, and their effects were small neuron-dominant.

Immunocytochemical analysis showed intense GAL-1-IR in almost all neurons from a very early stage (3 h) to an end of the observation period (> 7 days) in culture in the absence of NGF or GDNF (Fig.6). This finding is in contrast to the predominant expression of GAL-1 in small non-peptidergic neurons *in vivo*. Enzymatic and mechanical treatments for the dissociation of DRG cells, together with disruption of interactions between neurons and non-neuronal cells are detrimental to neurons. Therefore, GAL-1 expressed in cultured neurons may function as a stress marker protein (Iwamoto et al., 2010) and/or a cytoprotective molecule (Lekishvili et al., 2006) during *in vivo-in vitro* replacement.

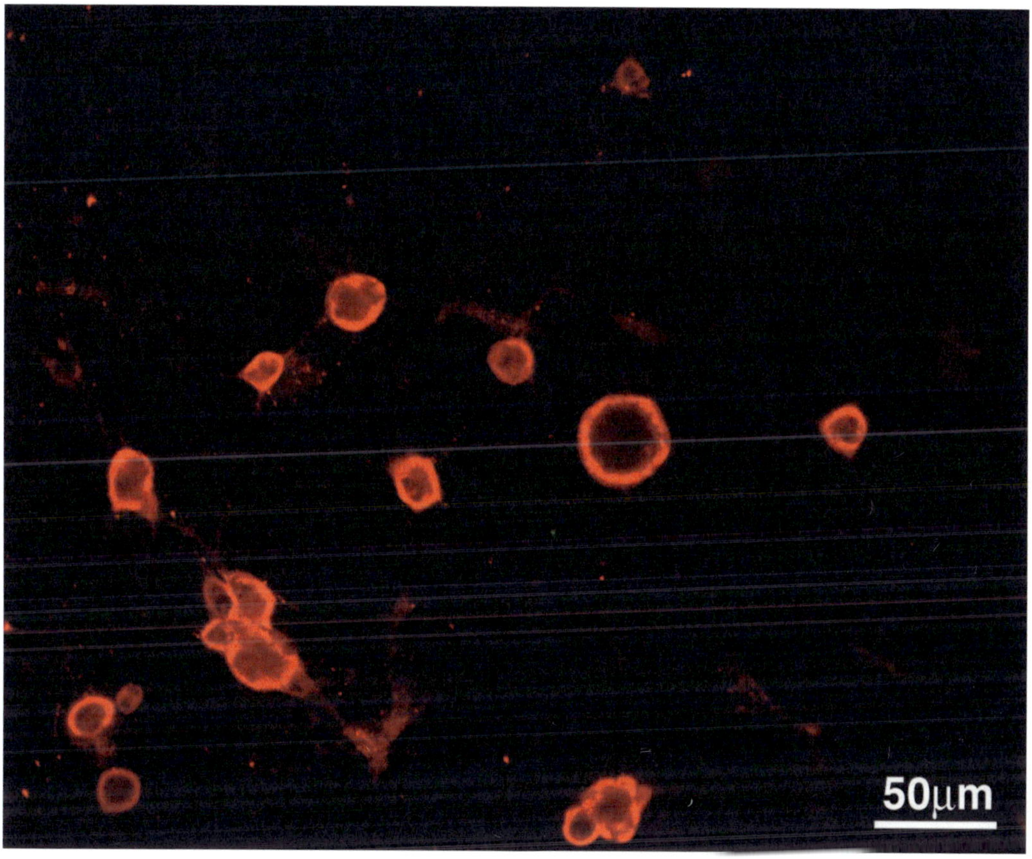

Fig. 6. Immunohistochemical localization of GAL-1 in adult rat DRG neurons after 5 days in culture. Intense GAL-1 immunoreactivity was observed at the surface of almost all neurons.

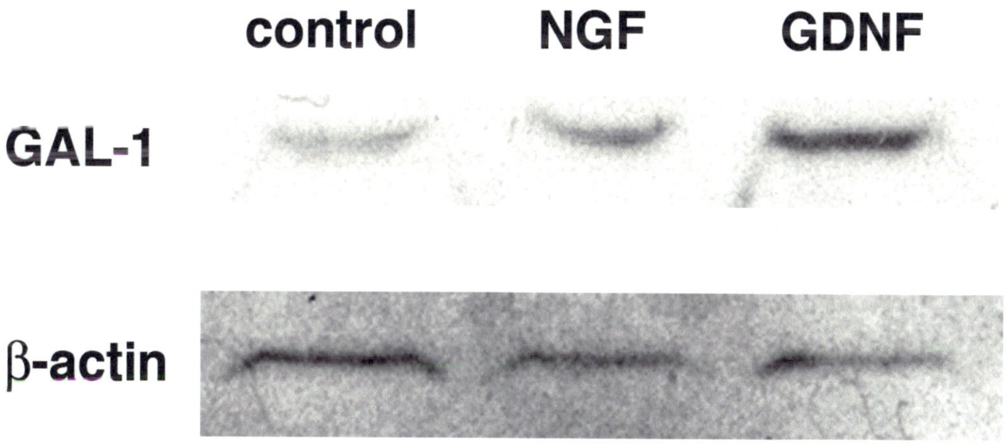

Fig. 7. GDNF, but not NGF, upregulates the expression of GAL-1 in cultured DRG cells: Western blot analysis. The neuron-enriched culture of DRG 12 h after seeding was incubated with serum-free medium containing 50 ng/ml of NGF or GDNF for 36 h.

The abundant expression of GAL-1 in cultured DRG neurons under the basal conditions (Ham's H12 / B27 supplement in the absence of NGF or GDNF) made it difficult to evaluate the effects of NGF or GDNF on the GAL-1-IR by immunocytochemistry. Then we prepared the neuron-enriched DRG culture (>5 × 10^3 cells/cm^2 at seeding) for Western blot analysis as previously described (Sango et al., 2007). The blot showed that GDNF, but not NGF, upregulated protein expression of GAL-1 (Fig.7). This finding suggests that GAL-1 is one of the downstream target molecules of GDNF in cultured DRG neurons. Our current study is aimed at elucidating the signaling molecules and pathways involved in the GDNF-induced neurite outgrowth and upregulation of GAL-1 (Sango et al., in preparation).

3. Externalization of GAL-1 from neurons and Schwann cells

Despite lacking a signal leading peptide, GAL-1 is subject to externalization via non-classical pathway from various kinds of cells (Cooper & Barondes, 1990; Avellana-Adalid et al., 1994; Hughes, 1999). Our immunocytochemical and Western blot analyses showed the externalization of GAL-1 from primary cultured adult rat DRG neurons and Schwann cells, and immortalized adult mouse Schwann cells IMS32 (Watabe et al., 1995; Sango et al., 2004). In addition to these cells, we have recently established spontaneously immortalized Schwann cell lines from long-term cultures of adult Fischer 344 rat DRG and peripheral nerves. One of these cell lines, designated IFRS1, showed distinct Schwann cell phenotypes, such as spindle-shaped morphology under phase-contrast microscopy (Fig.8A), intense immunoreactivity for Schwann cell markers (*e.g.* S100 and p75 low affinity neurotrophin receptor(p75^{NTR})), mRNA expression for neurotrophic factors (NGF, GDNF, CNTF), cell adhesion molecules (L1, NCAM, N-cadherin), transcription factors (Sox10, Oct6, Krox20) and myelin proteins (P0, PMP22, MAG)(Sango et al., 2011). Moreover, IFRS1 cells are capable of myelinating neurites in coculture with adult rat DRG neurons (Sango et al., 2011) and NGF-primed PC12 cells (Sango et al., submitted). We observed the intense immunoreactivity for GAL-1 in the cell bodies and processes of IFRS1 cells (Fig.8B). Further, Western blot analysis revealed the intense immunoreactivity for GAL-1 in both IFRS1 cells and culture medium (supernatant) (Fig.8C). These findings suggest that IFRS1 cells synthesize and secrete GAL-1, in a similar manner to DRG neurons and IMS32 cells (Sango et al., 2004).

Following externalization, some of the galectin molecules are suggested to associate with surface or extracellular matrix glycoconjugates where lectin activity is stabilized, whereas the others free from glycoconjugate ligands are rapidly oxidized in the non-reducing extracellular environment (Tracey et al., 1992).

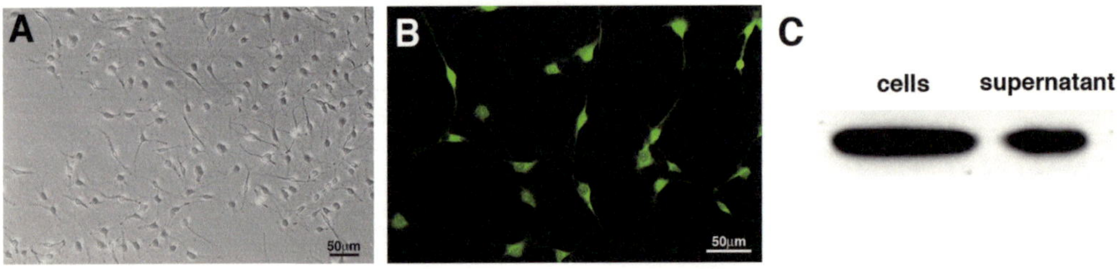

Fig. 8. Localization and externalization of GAL-1 in immortalized adult rat Schwann cells IFRS1. (A) A phase-contrast micrograph of IFRS1 cells. (B) Immunocytochemical localization of GAL-1 in IFRS1 cells. (C) Western blot analysis of IFRS1 cells and supernatant for GAL-1.

4. Biological roles of GAL-1 in the nervous tissue after injury

As described above, GAL-1 exists in both an oxidized and reduced state and only shows the lectin activity in its reduced state. Several studies have been conducted on the bioactivity of the reduced form of GAL-1 on the nervous tissue after injury, whereas we have been focusing on the axonal regeneration-promoting activity of GAL-1/Ox.

4.1 GAL-1 in the reduced form

The bioactivity of recombinant reduced GAL-1 was examined *in vitro*. When used as a coating substrate, it promoted adhesion, aggregation and neurite fasciculation of newborn rat DRG neurons (Outenreath & Jones, 1992) and olfactory neurons (Mahanthappa et al., 1994; Puche et al., 1996). In contrast, however, we saw no significant effects of GAL-1 on adhesion or neurite outgrowth of adult rat DRG neurons (Sango et al., unpublished data). When applied to culture medium, it induced differentiation of primary cultured rat cerebellar astrocytes and production of brain-derived neurotrophic factor (BDNF) (Sasaki et al., 2004; Endo, 2005). Since these changes were inhibited by lactose, the lectin activity of GAL-1 appears to be essential for the induction of astrocyte differentiation. These findings suggest that GAL-1 in the reduced form is involved in the neuroprotective function via acting on astrocytes after brain injury.

Using embryonic stem cell–derived neurons engineered with a $p75^{NTR}$ cDNA, Plachta et al. (2007) identified GAL-1 in the reduced form as an inducible factor for the degeneration of neuronal processes. They also showed the delayed elimination of peripheral nerve endings after sciatic nerve injury in GAL-1 deficient mice. These finding suggest that GAL-1 play a major role in the process of Wallerian degeneration and subsequent functional re-innervation after peripheral nerve injury

4.2 GAL-1 in the oxidized form (GAL-1/Ox)

The bioactivity of recombinant GAL-1/Ox was initially evaluated by DRG explant culture models, as shown in Fig.1. GAL-1/Ox did not show the lectin activity, but enhanced neurite outgrowth from transected nerve terminals of DRG explants in a dose-dependent manner (pg/ml range). We prepared a GAL-1 mutant CSGAL-1, in which all six cysteine residues were replaced by serine. CSGAL-1 did not promote neurite outgrowth, but showed lectin activity even under non-reducing conditions (Inagaki et al., 2000). These findings indicate that the axonal regeneration-promoting activity of GAL-1/Ox is unrelated to its lectin properties.

In stark contrast to the neurotrophic factors (*e.g.* NGF, GDNF, and CNTF), recombinant GAL-1/Ox does not directly work on isolated DRG neurons to promote neurite outgrowth (Horie et al., 1999, 2005; Inagaki et al., 2000). Application of fluorescence-conjugated GAL-1/Ox to DRG neurons, Schwann cells, and peritoneal macrophages, showed that only the surface of macrophages was clearly labeled (Horie et al., 2004). This finding suggests that macrophages are a target cell of GAL-1/Ox. Consistently, recombinant GAL-1/Ox induced tyrosine phosphorylation of proteins in macrophages. Furthermore, conditioned medium from GAL-1/Ox-stimulated macrophages enhanced neurite regeneration and Schwann cell migration from DRG explants greater than that from non-activated macrophages. These findings suggest that GAL-1/Ox binds to macrophages to activate their signal transduction pathways and secrete some neurotrophic molecules. Taking these findings together with those described above, we proposed a possible action mechanism of GAL-1/Ox for the promotion of axonal regeneration after injury (Fig.9). First, cytosolic GAL-1 is released from growing axons and Schwann cells into the extracellular space upon axonal injury. Next, some of the molecules in the extracellular milieu is converted to the oxidized form (GAL-1/Ox). Finally, GAL-1/Ox stimulates macrophages to release some neurotrophic molecules, which in turn enhance neurite regeneration and Schwann cell migration. This hypothesis will be further strengthened by identification of specific receptors for GAL-1/Ox on the macrophages and neurotrophic molecules secreted from macrophages. A recent study by Echigo et al. (2010) showed that GAL-1/Ox acts on the macrophage cell line RAW264.7 to induce phosphorylation of extracellular signal-regulated protein kinase 1/2 (ERK1/2). This cell line can be a valuable tool for the elucidation of the precise mechanisms underlying the promotion of axonal regeneration by GAL-1/Ox.

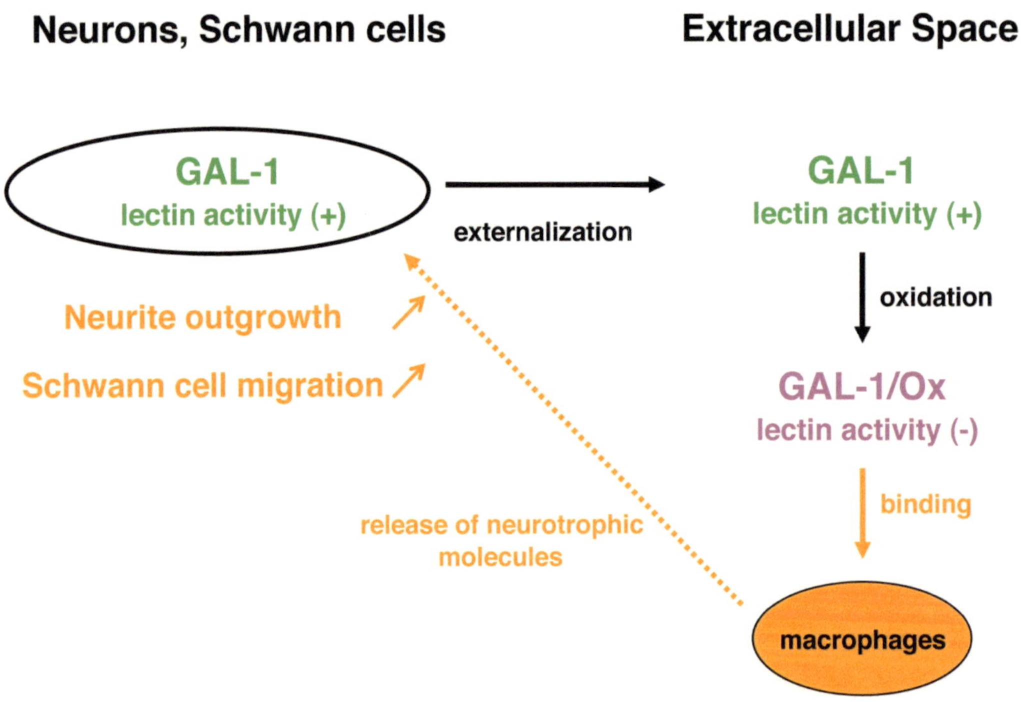

Fig. 9. A possible action mechanism of GAL-1 for the promotion of axonal regeneration. Some of the GAL-1 molecule released from neurons and Schwann cells are converted to the oxidized form with intramolecular disulfide bonds, which lacks lectin activity but could promote axonal regeneration and Schwann cell migration via activating macrophages.

Gaudet et al. (2009) precisely investigated a role for GAL-1 in the accumulation of macrophages following peripheral nerve injury. They observed that the axotomy-induced accumulation of macrophages in normal mouse sciatic nerve distal to ligation was inhibited by injection of anti-GAL-1 antibody. Consistently, mice lacking GAL-1 exhibited delayed and diminished macrophage accumulation by sciatic nerve injury. Further, injection of GAL-1/Ox into uninjured sciatic nerve enhanced the accumulation of macrophages in normal mice. These findings indicate the implication of GAL-1/Ox, as well as GAL-1 in the reduced from (Plachta et al., 2007), in the prompt response of macrophages to nerve injury, which is essential for Wallerian degeneration.

5. Conclusion

Since we introduced GAL-1/Ox as a novel axonal regeneration-promoting factor after injury (Horie et al, 1999), a considerable number of studies have been made on the biological properties of GAL-1 in the nervous system. GAL-1 is a multifunctional protein and plays different roles dependent on whether it is in the reduced or oxidized form. It is noteworthy that both reduced and oxidized forms of GAL-1 participate in the process of Wallerian degeneration (Plachta et al., 2007; Gaudet et al., 2009), although the precise mechanisms underlying it remain unclear. The growing evidence from both *in vivo* and *in vitro* studies suggests that GAL-1/Ox may be useful as a novel therapeutic agent for functional restoration after peripheral nerve injury.

6. Acknowledgement

This study was supported by a Grant-in-aid for Scientific Research, from the Ministry of Education, Science, Sports and Culture, Japan, and by the Umehara Fund, Yokohama, Japan. We thank Drs. Yusaku Nakabeppu, Hitoshi Kawano, Nobuaki Maeda and Shizuka Takaku for helpful suggestions, Hiroko Ueda and the late Kyoko Ajiki for technical assistance, and Bentham Science Publishers Ltd. and John Wiley & Sons, Inc. for permission to reproduce the illustrations.

7. References

Akahori, Y. & Horie, H. (1997). IGF-I enhances neurite regeneration but is not required for its survival in adult DRG explant. *Neuroreport*, Vol.8, No.9-10, (July 1997), pp. 2265-2269, ISSN 0959 4965

Akazawa, C.; Nakamura, Y.; Sango, K.; Horie, H. & Kohsaka, S. (2004). Distribution of the galectin-1 mRNA in the rat nervous system: its transient upregulation in rat facial motor neurons after facial nerve axotomy. *Neuroscience*, Vol.125, No.1, (March 2004), pp. 171-178, ISSN 0306-4522

Avellana-Adalid, V.; Rebel, G.; Caron, M.; Cornillot, J.D.; Bladier, D. & Joubert-Caron, R. (1994). Changes in S-type lectin localization in neuroblastoma cells (N1E115) upon differentiation. *Glycoconjugate Journal*, Vol.11, No.4, (August 1994), pp. 286-291, ISSN 0282-0080

Barondes, S.H.; Castronovo, V.; Cooper, D.N.W.; Cummings, R.D.; Drickamer, K.; Feizi, T.; Gitt, M.A.; Hirabayashi, J.; Hughes, C.; Kasai, K.; Leffler, H.; Liu, F.; Lotan, R.; Mercurio, A.M.; Monsigny, M.; Pillai, S.; Poirer, F.; Raz, A.; Rigby, P.W.J. & Wang, J.L. (1994). Galectins; a family of animal ß-galactoside-binding lectins. *Cell*, Vol.76, No.4, (February 1994), pp.597-598, ISSN 0092-8674

Bennett, D.L.; Michael, G.J.; Ramachandran, N.; Munson, J.B.; Averill, S.; Yan, Q.; McMahon, S.B. & Priestley, J.V. (1998). A distinct subgroup of small DRG cells express GDNF receptor components and GDNF is protective for these neurons after nerve injury. *The Journal of Neuroscience*, Vol.18, No.8, (April 1998), pp. 3059-3072, ISSN 0270-6474

Camby, I.; Le Mercier, M.; Lefranc, F. & Kiss, R. (2006). Galectin-1: a small protein with major functions. *Glycobiology*, Vol.16, No.11, (July 2006), pp. 137R-157R, ISSN 0959-6658

Cooper, D.N. & Barondes, S.H. (1990). Evidence for export of a muscle lectin from cytosol to extracellular matrix and for a novel secretory mechanism. *Journal of Cell Biology*, Vol.110, No.5, (May 1990), pp. 1681-1691, ISSN 0021-9525

Echigo, Y.; Sugiki, H.; Koizumi, Y.; Hikitsuchi, S. & Inoue, H. (2010). Activation of RAW264.7 macrophages by oxidized galectin-1. *Immunology Letters*, Vol.131, No.1, (January 2010), pp. 19-23, ISSN 0165-2478

Endo, T. (2005). Glycans and glycan-binding proteins in brain: galectin-1-induced expression of neurotrophic factors in astrocytes. *Current Drug Targets*, Vol.6, No.4, (June 2005), pp. 427-436, ISSN 1389-4501

Ernsberger, U. (2009). Role of neurotrophin signalling in the differentiation of neurons from dorsal root ganglia and sympathetic ganglia. *Cell and Tissue Research*, Vol.336, No.3, (June 2009), pp. 349-384, ISSN 0302-766X

Fukaya, K.; Hasegawa, M.; Mashitani, T.; Kadoya, T.; Horie, H.; Hayashi, Y.; Fujisawa, H.; Tachibana, O.; Kida, S. & Yamashita, J. (2003). Oxidized galectin-1 advances the functional recovery after peripheral nerve injury. *Journal of Neuropathology & Experimental Neurology*, Vol.62, No.2, (February 2003), pp. 162-172, ISSN 0022-3069

Gaudet, A.D.; Leung, M.; Poirier, F.; Kadoya, T.; Horie, H. & Ramer, M.S. (2009). A role for galectin-1 in the immune response to peripheral nerve injury. *Experimental Neurology*, Vol.220, No.2, (December 2009), pp. 320-327, ISSN 0014-4886

Gavazzi, I.; Kumar, R.D.; McMahon, S.B. & Cohen, J. (1999). Growth responses of different subpopulations of adult sensory neurons to neurotrophic factors in vitro. *European Journal of Neuroscience*, Vol.11, No.10, (October 1999), pp. 3405-3414, ISSN 0953-816X

Horie, H.; Bando, Y.; Chi, H. & Takenaka, T. (1991a). NGF enhances neurite regeneration from nerve-transected terminals of young adult and aged mouse dorsal root ganglia in vitro. *Neuroscience Letters*, Vol.121, No.1-2, (January 1991), pp. 125-128, ISSN 0304-3940

Horie, H.; Fukuda, N. & Bando, Y. (1991b). Hepatocytes enhance neurite regeneration and survival from transected nerve terminals. *Neuroreport*, Vol.2, No.9, (September 1991), pp. 521-524, ISSN 0959-4965

Horie, H.; Sakai, I.; Akahori, Y. & Kadoya, T. (1997). IL-1 beta enhances neurite regeneration from transected-nerve terminals of adult rat DRG. *Neuroreport*, Vol.8, No.8, (May 1997), pp. 1955-1999, ISSN 0959-4965

Horie, H.; Inagaki, Y.; Sohma, Y.; Nozawa, R.; Okawa, K.; Hasegawa, M.; Muramatsu, N.; Kawano, H.; Horie, M.; Koyama, H.; Sakai, I.; Takeshita, K.; Kowada, Y.; Takano, M. & Kadoya, T. (1999). Galectin-1 regulates initial axonal growth in peripheral nerves after axotomy. *The Journal of Neuroscience*, Vol.19, No.22, (November 1999), pp. 9964-9974, ISSN 0270-6474

Horie, H.; Kadoya, T.; Hikawa, N.; Sango, K.; Inoue, H.; Takeshita, K.; Asawa, R.; Hiroi, T.; Sato, M.; Yoshioka, T. & Ishikawa, Y. (2004). Oxidized galectin-1 stimulates macrophages to promote axonal regeneration in peripheral nerves after axotomy. *The Journal of Neuroscience*, Vol.24, No.8, (February 2004), pp. 1873-1880, ISSN 0270-6474

Horie, H.; Kadoya, T.,; Sango, K. & Hasegawa, M. (2005). Oxidized galectin-1 is an essential factor for peripheral nerve regeneration. *Current Drug Targets*, Vol.6, No.4, (June 2005), pp. 385-394, ISSN 1389-4501

Hughes, R.C. (1999). Secretion of the galectin family of mammalian carbohydrate-binding proteins. *Biochimica et Biophysica Acta*, Vol.1473, No.1, (December 1999), pp. 172-185, ISSN 0006-3002

Hynes, M.A.; Gitt, M.; Barondes, S.H.; Jessell, T.M. & Buck, L.B. (1990). Selective expression of an endogenous lactose-binding lectin gene in subsets of central and peripheral neurons. *The Journal of Neuroscience*, Vol.10, No.3, (March 1990), pp. 1004-1013, ISSN 0270-6474

Imbe, H.; Okamoto, K.; Kadoya, T.; Horie, H. & Senba, E. (2003). Galectin-1 is involved in the potentiation of neuropathic pain in the dorsal horn. *Brain Research*, Vol.993, No.1-2, (December 2003), pp. 72-83, ISSN 0006-8993

Inagaki, Y.; Sohma, Y.; Horie, H.; Nozawa, R. & Kadoya, T. (2000). Oxidized galectin-1 promotes axonal regeneration in peripheral nerves but does not possess lectin properties. *European Journal of Biochemistry*, Vol.267, No.10, (May 2000), pp. 2955-2964, ISSN 0014-2956

Iwamoto, M.; Taguchi, C.; Sasaguri, K.; Kubo, K.Y.; Horie, H.; Yamamoto, T.; Onozuka, M.; Sato, S. & Kadoya, T. (2010). The Galectin-1 level in serum as a novel marker for stress. *Glycoconjugate Journal*, Vol.27, No.4, (May 2010), pp. 419-425, ISSN 0282-0080

Kadoya, T. & Horie, H. (2005). Structural and functional studies of Galectin-1: a novel axonal regneration-promoting activity for oxidized Galectin-1. *Current Drug Targets*, Vol.6, No.4, (June 2005), pp. 375-383, ISSN 1389-4501

Kadoya, T.; Oyanagi, K.; Kawakami, E.; Hasegawa, M.; Inagaki, Y.; Sohma, Y. & Horie, H. (2005). Oxidized galectin-1 advances the functional recovery after peripheral nerve injury. *Neuroscience Letters*, Vol.380, No.3, (June 2005), pp.284-288, ISSN 0304-3940

Lekishvili, T.; Hesketh, S.; Brazier, M.W. & Brown, D.R. (2006). Mouse galectin 1 inhibits the toxicity of glutamate by modifying NR1 NMDA receptor expression. *European Journal of Neuroscience*, Vol.24, No.11, (December 2006), pp. 3017-3025, ISSN 0953-816X

Lindsay, R.M. (1988). Nerve growth factors (NGF, BDNF) enhance axonal regeneration but are not required for survival of adult sensory neurons. *The Journal of Neuroscience*, Vol.8, No.7, (July 1988), pp. 2394-2405, ISSN 0270-6474

Lindsay, R.M. & Harmar, A.J. (1989). Nerve growth factor regulates expression of neuropeptide genes in adult sensory neurons. *Nature*, Vol.337, No.6205, (January 1989), pp. 362-364, ISSN 0028-0836

Mahanthappa, N.K.; Cooper, D.N.; Barondes, S.H. & Schwarting, G.A. (1994). Rat olfactory neurons can utilize the endogenous lectin, L-14, in a novel adhesion mechanism. *Development*, Vol.120, No.6, (June 1994), pp. 1373-1384, ISSN 0950-1991

Mason, M.R.; Tannemaat, M.R.; Malessy, M.J. & Verhaagen, J. (2011). Gene therapy for the peripheral nervous system: a strategy to repair the injured nerve? *Current Gene Therapy*, Vol.11, No.2, (April 2011), pp. 75-89, ISSN 1566-5232

McMahon, S.B. & Bennett D.L.H. (2000). Glial cell line-derived neurotrophic factor and nociceptive neurons, In: *Molecular Basis of Pain Induction*, J.N. Wood, (Ed.), 65-86, Wiley-Liss, ISBN 0-471-34607-1, New York, USA

McGraw, J.; Gaudet, A.D.; Oschipok, L.W.; Kadoya, T.; Horie, H.; Steeves, J.D.; Tetzlaff, W. & Ramer, M.S. (2005a). Regulation of neuronal and glial galectin-1 expression by peripheral and central axotomy of rat primary afferent neurons. *Experimental Neurology*, Vol.195, No.1, (September 2005), pp. 103-14, ISSN 0014-4886

McGraw, J.; Gaudet, A.D.; Oschipok, L.W.; Steeves, J.D.; Poirier, F.; Tetzlaff, W. & Ramer, M.S. (2005b). Altered primary afferent anatomy and reduced thermal sensitivity in mice lacking galectin-1. *Pain*, Vol.114, No.1-2, (March 2005), pp. 7-18, ISSN 0304-3959

Molliver, D,C,; Wright, D.E.; Leitner, M.L.; Parsadanian, A.S.; Doster, K.; Wen, D.; Yan, Q. & Snider, W.D. (1997). IB4-binding DRG neurons switch from NGF to GDNF dependence in early postnatal life. *Neuron*, Vol.19, No.4, (October 1997), pp. 849-861, ISSN 0896-6273

Outenreath, R.L. & Jones, A.L. (1992). Influence of an endogenous lectin substrate on cultured dorsal root ganglion cells. *Journal of Neurocytology*, Vol.21, No.11, (November 1992), pp. 788-795, ISSN 0300-4864

Plachta, N.; Annaheim, C.; Bissière, S.; Lin, S.; Rüegg, M.; Hoving, S.; Müller, D.; Poirier, F.; Bibel, M. & Barde, Y.A. (2007). Identification of a lectin causing the degeneration of neuronal processes using engineered embryonic stem cells. *Nature Neuroscience*, Vol.10, No.6, (June 2007), pp. 712-719, ISSN 1097-6256

Puche, A.C.; Poirier, F.; Hair, M.; Bartlett, P.F. & Key, B. (1996). Role of galectin-1 in the developing mouse olfactory system. *Developmental Biology*, Vol.179, No.1, (October 1996), pp. 274-287, ISSN 0012-1606

Rabinovich, G.A.; Toscano, M.A.; Jackson, S.S. & Vasta, G.R. (2007). Functions of cell surface galectin-glycoprotein lattices. *Current Opinion in Structural Biology*, Vol.17, No.5, (October 2007), pp. 513-520, ISSN 0959-440X

Regan, L.J.; Dodd, J.; Barondes, S.H. & Jessell, T.M. (1986). Selective expression of endogenous lactose-binding lectins and lactoseries glycoconjugates in subsets of rat sensory neurons. *Proceedings of the National Academy of Sciences of the United States of America*, Vol.83, No.7, (April 1986), pp. 2248–2252, ISSN 2248-2252

Saito, H.; Sango, K.; Horie, H.; Ikeda, H.; Ishigatsubo, Y.; Ishikawa, Y. & Inoue, S. (1999). Enhanced neural regeneration from transected vagus nerve terminal in diabetic mice in vitro. *Neuroreport*, Vol.10, No.5, (April 1999), pp. 1025-1028, ISSN 0959-4965

Saito, H.; Sango, K.; Horie, H.; Takeshita, K.; Ikeda, H.; Ishigatsubo, Y. & Ishikawa, Y. (2002). Trachea enhances neurite regeneration from adult rat nodose ganglia in vitro. *Life Sciences*, Vol.70, No.16, (March 2002), pp. 1935-1946, ISSN 0024-3205

Salt, T.E. & Hill, R.G. (1983). Neurotransmitter candidates of somatosensory primary afferent fibers. *Neuroscience*, Vol.10, No.4, (December 1983), pp. 1083-1103, ISSN 0306-4522

Sango, K.; Horie, H.; Saito, H.; Ajiki, K.; Tokashiki, A.; Takeshita, K.; Ishigatsubo, Y.; Kawano, H. & Ishikawa, Y. (2002). Diabetes is not a potent inducer of neuronal cell death in mouse sensory ganglia, but it enhances neurite regeneration in vitro. *Life Sciences*, Vol.71, No.20, (Otober 2002), pp. 2351-2368, ISSN 0024-3205

Sango, K.; Tokashiki, A.; Ajiki, K.; Horie, M.; Kawano, H.; Watabe, K.; Horie, H. & Kadoya, T. (2004). Synthesis, localization and externalization of galectin-1 in mature dorsal root ganglion neurons and Schwann cells. *European Journal of Neuroscience*, Vol.19, No.1, (January 2004), pp. 55-64, ISSN 0953-816X

Sango, K.; Saito, H.; Takano, M.; Tokashiki, A.; Inoue, S. & Horie, H. (2006). Cultured adult animal neurons and Schwann cells give us new insights into diabetic neuropathy. *Current Diabetes Reviews*, Vol.2, No.2, (May 2006), pp. 169-183, ISSN 1573-3998

Sango, K.; Yanagisawa, H. & Takaku, S. (2007). Expression and histochemical localization of ciliary neurotrophic factor in cultured adult rat dorsal root ganglion neurons. *Histochemistry and Cell Biology*, Vpl.128, No.1, (July 2007), pp. 35-43, ISSN 0948-6143

Sango, K.; Yanagisawa, H.; Komuta, Y.; Si, Y. & Kawano, H. (2008). Neuroprotective properties of ciliary neurotrophic factor for cultured adult rat dorsal root ganglion neurons. *Histochemistry and Cell Biology*, Vol.130, No.4, (October 2008), pp. 669-679, ISSN 0948-6143

Sango, K.; Yanagisawa, H.; Kawakami, E.; Takaku, S.; Ajiki, K. & Watabe, K. (2011). Spontaneously immortalized Schwann cells from adult Fischer rat as a valuable tool for exploring neuron-Schwann cell interactions. *Journal of Neuroscience Research*, Vol.89, No.6, (March 2011), pp. 898-908, ISSN 0360-4012

Sasaki, T.; Hirabayashi, J.; Manya, H., Kasai, K. & Endo, T. (2004). Galectin-1 induces astrocyte differentiation, which leads to production of brain-derived neurotrophic factor. *Glycobiology*, Vol.14, No.4, (April 2004), pp. 357-363, ISSN 0959-6658

Shuto, T.; Horie, H.; Hikawa, N.; Sango, K.; Tokashiki, A.; Murata, H.; Yamamoto, I. & Ishikawa, Y. (2001). IL-6 up-regulates CNTF mRNA expression and enhances neurite regeneration. *Neuroreport*, Vol.12, No.5, (April 2001), pp. 1081-1085, ISSN 0959-4965

Terenghi, G. (1999). Peripheral nerve regeneration and neurotrophic factors. *Journal of Anatomy*, Vol.194, Part 1, (January 1999), pp. 1-14, ISSN 0021-8782

Tracey, B.M.; Feizi, T.; Abbott, W.M.; Carruthers, R.A.; Green, B.N. & Lawson, A.M. (1992). Subunit molecular mass assignment of 14,654 Da to the soluble beta-galactoside-binding lectin from bovine heart muscle and demonstration of intramolecular disulfide bonding associated with oxidative inactivation. *The Journal of Biological Chemistry*, Vol.267, No.15, (May 1992), pp. 10342-10347, ISSN 0021-9258

Watabe, K.; Fukuda, T.; Tanaka, J.; Honda, H.; Toyohara, K. & Sakai, O. (1995). Spontaneously immortalized adult mouse Schwann cells secrete autocrine and paracrine growth-promoting activities. *Journal of Neuroscience Research*, Vol.41, No.2, (June 1995), pp. 279-290, ISSN 0360-4012

Yasuda, H.; Terada, M.; Maeda, K.; Kogawa, S.; Sanada, M.; Haneda, M.; Kashiwagi, A. & Kikkawa, R. (2003). Diabetic neuropathy and nerve regeneration. *Progress in Neurobiology*, Vol.69, No.4, (March 2003), pp. 229-285, ISSN 0301-0082

Zochodne, D. (2008). *Neurobiology of Peripheral Nerve Regeneration*, Cambridge University Press, ISBN 978-0-521-86717-7, Cambridge, UK

4

Controlled Release Strategy Based on Biodegradable Microspheres for Neurodegenerative Disease Therapy

Haigang Gu[1,3] and Zhilian Yue[2]
[1]Department of Histology and Embryology, Guangzhou Medical College, Guangzhou
[2]Intelligent Polymer Research Institute, AIIM Facility,
Innovation Campus, University of Wollongong
[3]Department of Pharmacology, Vanderbilt University School of Medicine, Nashville
[1]China
[2]Australia
[3]USA

1. Introduction

The past decades have seen considerable advances in our understanding of the developmental mechanisms of neurodegenerative disorders, including Parkinson's, Alzheimer's and Huntington's diseases and spinal cord injury [1-3]. The major neuropathological characteristics of neurodegenerative disorders are atrophy or loss of specific neurons in the specific brain areas, such as cholinergic neuron degeneration observed in the basal forebrain, hippocampus and cortex in Alzheimer's disease (AD) and dopaminergic neuron degeneration observed in the striatum in Parkinson's disease [4-6]. As the life span of human beings increases and more people live beyond the age of 60, the number of people with neurodegenerative disorders is also progressively increased. Contrasting with the enormous toll that these disorders put on patients, their caregivers and the whole society is the lack of effective therapy at present.

Neurotrophic factors (NTFs) are secreted peptides essential for the phenotypic development and maintenance of specific neuronal populations in developing and adult vertebrate nervous system [7-14]. These diffusible proteins act via retrograde signaling from target-neurons and by paracrine and autocrine mechanisms, and regulate many aspects of neuronal and glial structure and function. In addition to playing key roles during development, NTFs are also required in the adult brain for maintaining neuronal function and phenotype. Previous studies of intracerebroventricular (ICV) administration of NTFs have shown to reduce or prevent neuronal atrophy or neuronal loss in neurodegenerative diseases [7-9, 12, 13, 15, 16]. The cholinergic neurons of basal forbrain express both the low affinity receptor (p75NTR) and high affinity receptor (Trk receptor), and respond to neurotrophic factors by increased activity levels of the choline acetyltransferase (ChAT). NTFs exert neurotrophic actions on the cholinergic neurons of the basal forebrain and protect them against neurodegeneration [7, 12, 15, 17]. For example, ICV injection of nerve growth factor (NGF) has shown to improve the learning and memory ability, and the survival of basal forebrain cholinergic neurons in aged or fimbria-fornix lesioned animals. Furthermore, NTFs have been used for the experimental therapies in Parkinson's, Alzheimer's and Huntington's diseases and spinal cord injury [4-14].

Modern biotechnology has enabled the large-scale production of highly purified proteins; therefore, large quantities of growth factors can now be manufactured for clinical use. However, NTFs are large molecular proteins that do not readily cross the blood–brain barrier (BBB), and have short biologic half-life [10-13]. To improve their therapeutic efficacy and patient compliance, local and controlled delivery of NTFs directly to the desired brain area are preferred [3, 18-20]. NGF-releasing and glial cell line-derived neurotrophic factor (GDNF)-releasing microspheres have been developed for the experimental therapy of Alzheimer's and Parkinson's disease (PD) [21-30]. Compared to other exiting approaches, the strategy based on biodegradable microspheres has demonstrated a number of advantages.

- Ease of administration to the targeted area of the brain, thus avoiding open operation and damage to surrounding tissue [31, 32].
- Preservation of drug activity during encapsulation and storage.
- Localized, controlled-release profiles for a desired period, resulting in enhanced therapeutic effect while minimizing side effects.
- Better safety profiles, as compared with gene therapy such as gene delivery and transplantation of genetically modified cells.

In this chapter, to serve as a good example, we presented our previous works focusing on the formulation and characterization of NGF-loaded microspheres. The in vivo efficacy of these microspheres was evaluated in a rat model of AD. The methods described here can be applied broadly to other types of NTF-releasing microspheres.

2. Materials

2.1 Formulation of NGF-releasing microspheres

General regents and instruments for the preparation of NGF-releasing microspheres, the abbreviations and source of these reagents are as follows:

2.1.1 Neurotrophic factors such as human recombinant β-nerve growth factor (NGF) (Calbiochem or Sigma)

2.1.2 Poly(lactide-co-glycolide) (PLGA) (lactic acid/glycolic acid = 75/25) (Birmingham Polymers Inc. or Sigma)

2.1.3 Bovine serum albumin (BSA) or human serum albumin (HSA) (Calbiochem or Sigma).

2.1.4 FITC-labeled BSA (FITC-BSA) (Sigma)

2.1.5 Polyvinyl alcohol (PVA) (Sigma).

2.1.6 Acetone (Sigma)

2.1.7 Methylene chloride (Sigma)

2.1.8 Sonicator (Sonics & materials INC. USA)

2.1.9 Cantilever agitator (IKA. RW20 DZM.n, Guangzhou Scientific Instrument, Ltd Co)

2.2 Characterization of NGF-releasing Microspheres

Instruments for microsphere characterization, the abbreviations and source of these reagents are as follows:

2.2.1 Coulter counter (model ZM, Coulter Electronics Limited, UK)

2.2.2 Scanning electron microscopy (XL30ESEM, Philips, Netherlands)

2.2.3 Rabbit anti-rhNGF-beta polyclonal antibody and CY3-conjugated goat anti-rabbit secondary antibody (Chemicon)

2.2.4 Ultraviolet spectrophotometer (Hach)

2.2.5 Confocal laser scanning microscopy (CLSM; Leica TCS SP5, Leica Mikrosysteme Vertrieb GmbH, Germany)

2.3 Cell culture

General Regents for PC12 cell culture, the abbreviations and source of these reagents are as follows:

2.3.1 Dulbecco Modified Eagle's medium (DMEM) (Invitrogen)

2.3.2 Fetal bovine serum (FBS) (Invitrogen)

2.3.3 Fetal horse serum (FHS) (Invitrogen)

2.3.4 Trypsin-EDTA (1x) (Invitrogen)

2.3.5 Penicillin/Streptomycin (100x) (Invitrogen)

2.3.6 L-glutamine (100x) (Invitrogen)

2.4 Evaluation of in vivo efficacy in a rat model of AD

Normotensive adult male Sprague Dawley (SD) rats weighing 250-300 g are used. The general tools, instruments and reagents for in vivo evaluation in a rat model of AD are as follows:

2.4.1 Narishige stereotaxic instrument (Narishige SR-5, Narishige Scientific Instrument Lab, Tokyo, Japan)

2.4.2 One scalpel size 3 with No. 10 blade

2.4.3 Two small scissors for blunt dissection

2.4.4 One needle holder

2.4.5 One pair of microsurgical scissors

2.4.6 Two pairs of microsurgical forceps

2.4.7 3/0 sutures

2.4.8 Dentistry drill

2.5 Tissue processing

2.5.1 Ice-cold phosphate buffered saline (PBS)

2.5.2 Ice-cold saline.

2.5.3 15% and 30% sucrose in PBS

2.5.4 4% paraformaldehyde

2.5.5 Serum infusion set with a blunted 20-ga needle

2.5.6 OCT Tissue freezing medium

2.5.7 Anti-rhNGF antibody, anti-Choline acetyltransferase (ChAT) antibody and appropriate secondary antibodies

2.5.8 Image J software (National Institutes of Health)

2.6 Assessment of learning and memory impairment

2.6.1 Y-maze test (Chongqing Medical Apparatus Co, China)

3. Methods

3.1 Preparation of NGF-releasing microspheres

NGF-releasing microspheres were formulated using with a modified multiple emulsion solvent extraction-evaporation technique (W/O/W) (see Note 1) [24]. NGF (5-10 mg) (see Note 2) and BSA (1/50-2000, w/w) in 100-200 μL distilled water. The protein solution was emulsified in a solution of PLGA (100-200 mg) (see Note 3) in methylene chloride/acetone (3/1, 4-8 mL) to form the first W/O emulsion (see Note 4), using sonication for 1-2 min at 20-40 W over an ice bath. The first W/O emulsion was then added to 1% PVA aqueous solution (25-50 mL) (see Note 5), and homogenized at 800-2000 rpm for 5-10 min over an ice bath to form W/O/W double emulsion. The W/O/W double emulsion was stirred at room temperature for 3-4 h to allow the evaporation of the organic solvents in the fume hood. The microspheres were collected by centrifugation, and washed three times with distilled water to remove any proteins that were weakly bound onto the surface of microspheres. The harvested microspheres were freeze-dried to obtain a free flowing powder. The NGF/FITC-BSA-releasing microspheres were prepared using in the same way for in vivo release and tracking studies (see Note 6 and 7).

3.2 Characterization of NGF-releasing microspheres

3.2.1 The size distribution of NGF-releasing microspheres was measured using a Coulter counter

3.2.2 The morphology of NGF-releasing microspheres was examined using scanning electron microscopy (SEM)

The freeze-dried NGF-releasing microspheres were mounted on the conductive tap of a metal stub, and sputtered coated with gold before being observed using SEM (Figure 1).

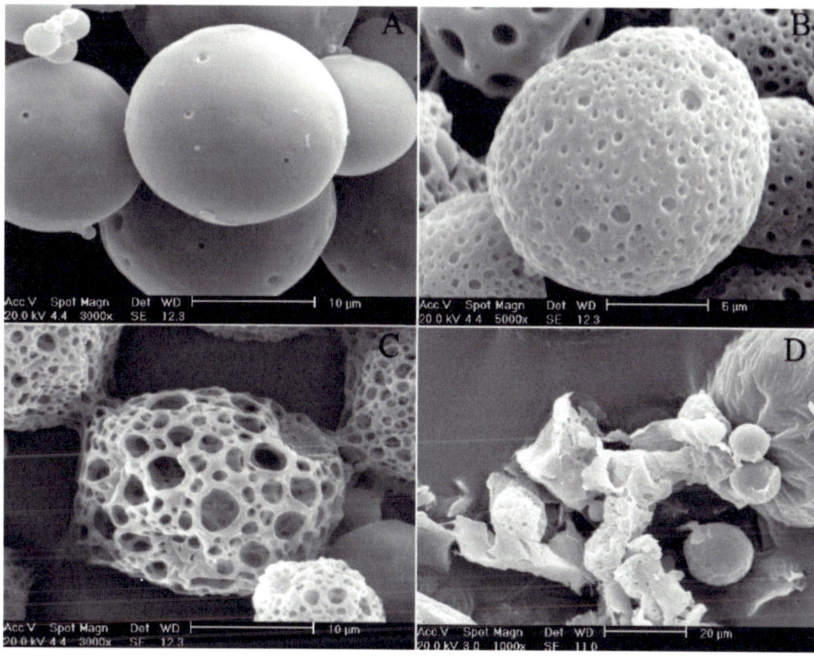

Fig. 1. SEM micrographs of NGF-releasing microspheres after various intervals of incubation in PBS. (A) The microspheres were spherical in shape with smooth surface before incubation with PBS. (B) After 1 week of incubation, shallow pores appeared on the surface of the microspheres that maintained intact spherical shape. (C) After incubation for 3 weeks, the microspheres showed highly porous surfaces and irregular shapes, with eroded inner matrix. (D) After incubation for 5 weeks, most of the microspheres lost their spherical shape and collapsed. This picture was taken from our previous paper and allowed to use here by Polymer International.

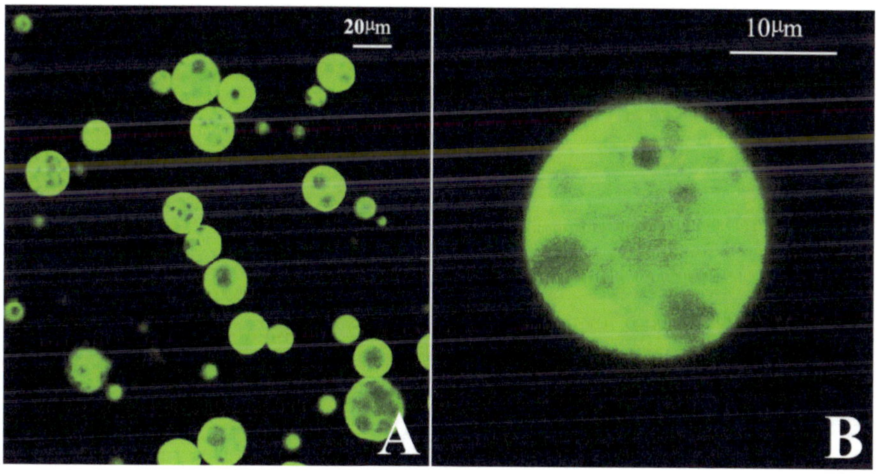

Fig. 2. Confocal Laser Scanning Microscopy (CLSM) micrographs of NGF/FITC-BSA-releasing microspheres at lower magnification (A) and higher magnification (B). This picture was taken from our previous paper and allowed to use here by Polymer International.

3.2.3 The morphology of NGF/FITC-BSA-releasing microspheres was examined by confocal laser scanning microscopy (CLSM)

Freeze-dried NGF/FITC-BSA-releasing microspheres spread on glass coverslips were observed under CLSM (Figure 2).

3.2.4 The amount of the protein encapsulated in the NGF/BSA-releasing microspheres was determined by a protein extraction method described below

Ten to thirty milligrams of microspheres were dissolved in 1-2 mL of chloroform and extracted with 4 mL of deionized water. The mixture was vortex for 5-10 min. The extracted protein in aqueous phase was separated and collected by centrifugation. Three extractions were performed for each sample. The aqueous extracts were pooled together, and the protein concentration was determined by BCA microassay. Experiments were run in triplicate per sample. The protein loading and encapsulation efficiency in microspheres were defined by the following equations:

Protein loading in microspheres (%) = Weight of protein in the aqueous extract/Weight of microspheres extracted × 100

Encapsulation efficiency (%) = Weight of protein in microspheres/Weight of protein in the initial formulation × 100

3.2.5 In vitro release of NGF

In vitro drug release from the NGF-releasing microspheres was monitored in PBS at 37°C, utilizing double-chamber diffusion cells on a shaker stand. Approximately 50 mg of the microspheres were suspended in 4 mL of PBS buffer in the donor chamber. The receiver chamber was filled with 4 mL plain buffer. The donor chamber and receiver chamber were separated with 0.45 μm low-protein absorbable membrane. At predetermined time points, the PBS buffer in the receiver chamber was collected and replaced with same amount of fresh PBS. The protein concentration in the collected buffer solution was analyzed using BCA microassay. The concentration of the released NGF in the buffer solution was measured using ELISA and the amount of released NGF was calculated. Experiments were run in triplicate per sample.

The bioactivity of the released NGF from the microspheres was assessed using PC12 cell culture. PC12 cells were maintained in growth on T-25 cell culture flasks (Corning Inc., Corning, NY) in RPMI 1640 supplemented with 10 wt% horse serum, 5 wt% fetal bovine serum and 50 U mL^{-1} penicillin/streptomycin. For the bioactivity of released NGF testing, PC12 cells were plated on poly (L-lysine) pre-coated 24-well plates. The cells were cultured at 37°C in a 95% water-saturated, 5% CO_2 air atmosphere and plated at a density of approximately 1.0×10^4 cells/cm^2 (in 2 mL). Twenty-four hours, 2 mL solution of in vitro NGF release buffer collected in the first week was sterile-filtered through a 0.22 μm filter (Millipore) and incubated with PC12 cells (30 ng mL^{-1}). Incubating with NGF-supplement medium (30 ng mL^{-1}) alone or with the released buffer from BSA-releasing microspheres (without NGF) served as positive or negative control, separately. To further confirm the bioactivity of the released NGF, anti-NGF antibody was added into the medium to neutralize the bioactivity of the released NGF.

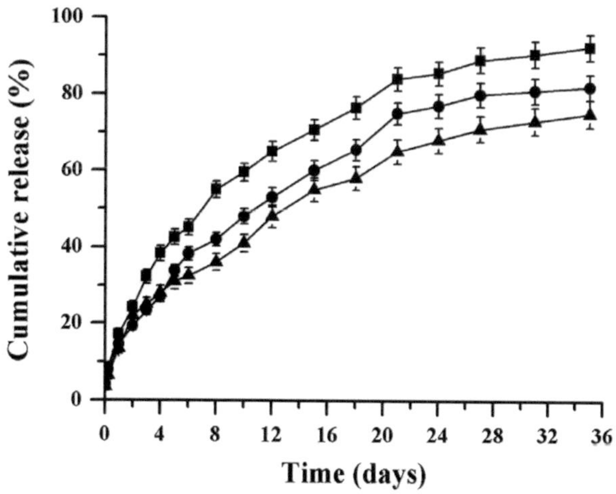

Fig. 3. *In vitro* rhNGF release from rhNGF/BSA-loaded microspheres: with protein/PLGA (w/w) ratio of (▲) 5/100, (●) 10/100, and (■) 15/100. This picture was taken from our previous paper and allowed to use here by Polymer International.

3.2.6 The bioactivity of the released NGF was test using PC 12 cells

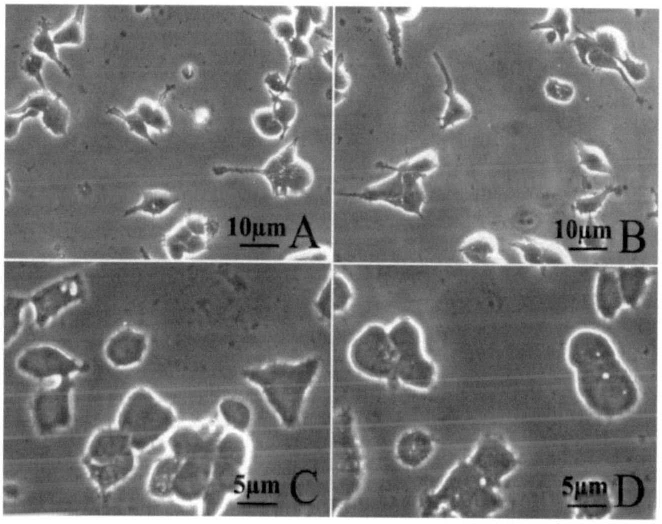

Fig. 4. The bioactivity of the released NGF from the PLGA microspheres as assessed with PC12 cell culture. (A) Positive control cells that were incubated with NGF-supplemented medium at a concentration of 30 ng mL^{-1}; (B) the cells incubated with the released NGF from PLGA microspheres and added to the culture medium at a concentration of 30 ng mL^{-1}; (C) negative control cells incubated with the released BSA from BSA-only PLGA microspheres and added to the culture medium ; (D) cells incubated with the released NGF-supplemented culture medium plus anti-NGF antibody added . The percentage of neurite-bearing cells was determined by counting 100–200 cells in several randomly chosen fields under an optical microscope for each sample after 24 h incubation. This picture was taken from our previous paper and allowed to use here by Polymer International.

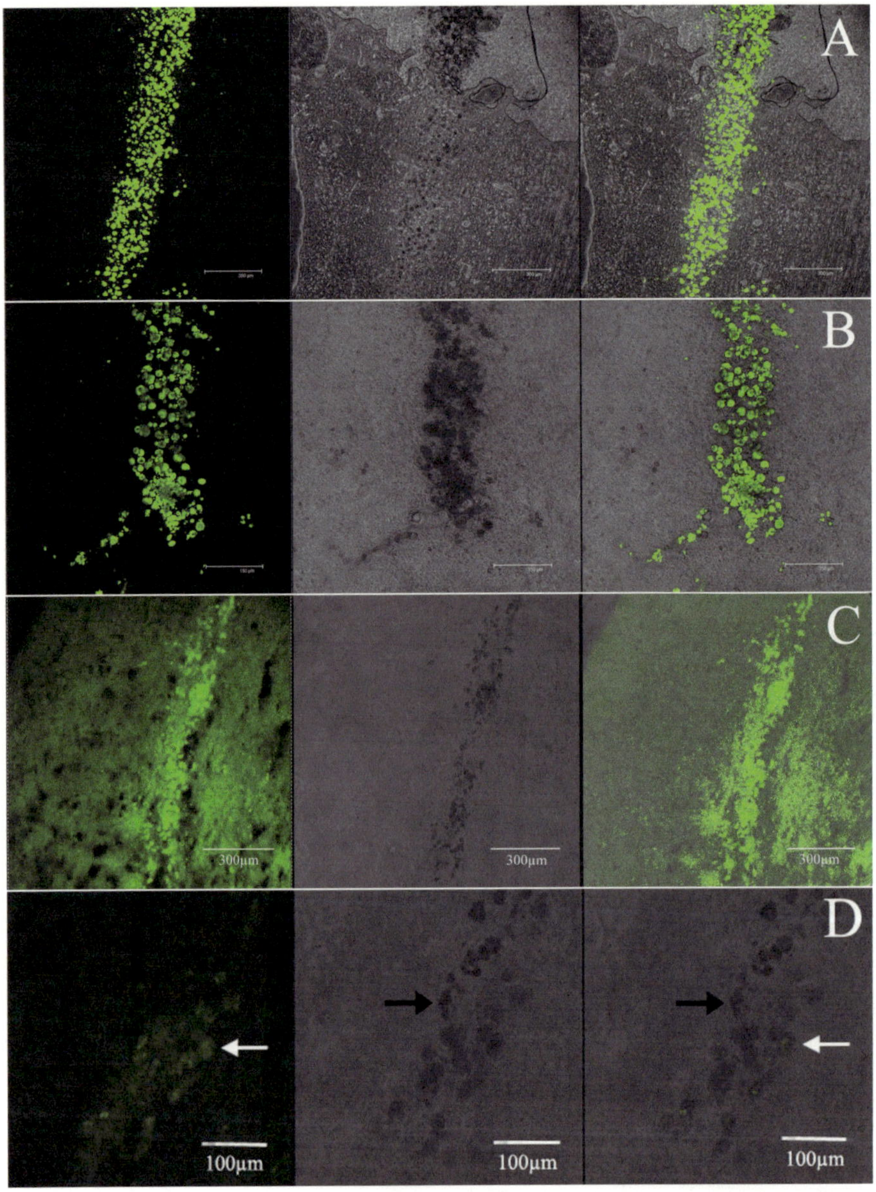

Fig. 5. CLSM micrographs of NGF/FITC-BSA-loaded microspheres implanted in the BF (left column: observed under fluorescent filter; middle column: observed under normal light; right column: merged from left and middle): (A) 1 week after implantation, the fluorescent in implanted NGF/FITC-BSA-loaded microspheres is very strong; (B) 3 weeks after implantation, the fluorescent in implanted NGF/FITC-BSA-loaded microspheres became weak; (C) 4 weeks after implantation, the fluorescent in implanted NGF/FITC-BSA-loaded microspheres was weaker; (D) 5 weeks after implantation; most of the microspheres showed empty microspheres (black and white arrows showing an empty and a still-loaded microsphere, respectively). This picture was taken from our previous paper and allowed to use here by Polymer International.

3.2.7 In vivo tracking and release studies

All experiments were carried out strictly according to the National Institute of Health Guide for the Care and Use of Laboratory Animals (NIH Publications No. 80-23) revised in 1996. All experiments were performed on adult male Sprague-Dawley (SD) rats (250–300 g) (see Note 8). The animals were housed in groups of two or three in macrolon cages; food and water were available ad libitum. All the animals were peritoneally anesthetized with sodium pentobarbital (40 mg kg−1 body weight) by peritoneal injection and positioned in a Narishige stereotaxic instrument (Narishige SR-5, Narishige Scientific Instrument Lab, Tokyo, Japan). An amount of 3 mg of NGF/FITC-BSA-loaded microspheres (suspended in 10 μL of dispersing medium) was implanted into the BF (coordinates: anterior–posterior, +0.6 mm; left lateral, +0.6 mm; dorsal–ventral, −5.5 mm from bregma).

At the predetermined time intervals, animals were perfused via the aorta with PBS (pH = 7.4) 200 ml and fixed with 4 wt% paraformaldehyde for 30 min. The brains were removed and further fixed for 3-6 h at 4°C. The fixed brain was incubated in a 15 wt% sucrose buffer solution overnight and in 30 wt% sucrose buffer solution until it was sunk. Brain sections (20 μm) were cut at the transverse plane on a freezing microtome. These sections were mounted on gelatin-coated slides for directly examining the protein release from the NGF/FITC-BSA-loaded microspheres using CLSM.

3.3 Recombinant human NGF-loaded microspheres implantation promotes survival of basal forebrain cholinergic neurons and improve memory impairments of spatial learning in the rat model of Alzheimer's disease (see Note 9)

Unilateral fimbria-fornix (FF) of SD rats was transected to simulate the impairment of cholinergic neurons of AD by the lesion of the septo-hippocampus pathway. The animals were randomly divided into four groups: (1) normal control group; (2) lesion control group; (3) unloaded microspheres group; (4) rhNGF-loaded microspheres group. At the lesion time, three milligrams of rhNGF-loaded microspheres (corresponding to 5 μg of NGF) (suspended in 10 μl of PBS) were stereotaxically implanted into the basal forbrain.

At the predetermined time points, animals were perfused via the aorta with PBS (pH = 7.4) 200 ml and fixed with 4 wt% paraformaldehyde for 30 min. The brains were removed and further fixed for 3-6 h at 4°C. The fixed brain was incubated in a 15 wt% sucrose buffer solution overnight and in 30 wt% sucrose buffer solution until it was sunk. Brain sections (30 μm) were cut at the transverse plane on a freezing microtome. The cholinergic neurons in medial septum (MS) and vertical diagonal band (VDB) were stained by ChAT immunohistochemistry. In brief, brain sections were incubated with 3% H_2O_2 to block endogenous peroxidase 30 min and then incubated in 10% normal goat serum for 1 h before incubation with rabbit anti-rat ChAT antibodies overnight at 4°C. Following primary antibody incubation, brain sections were washed with 1 × PBS, incubated with secondary antibody HRP-conjugated anti-rabbit IgG 1-2 h at room temperature and washed with 1 × PBS. And then brain sections were incubated with DAB. After incubated with gradient ethanol and xylene, the brain sections were mounted neutral permanent mounting medium.

Y-maze test (see Note 10) was used to evaluate the ability of spatial learning and memory in different trial groups.

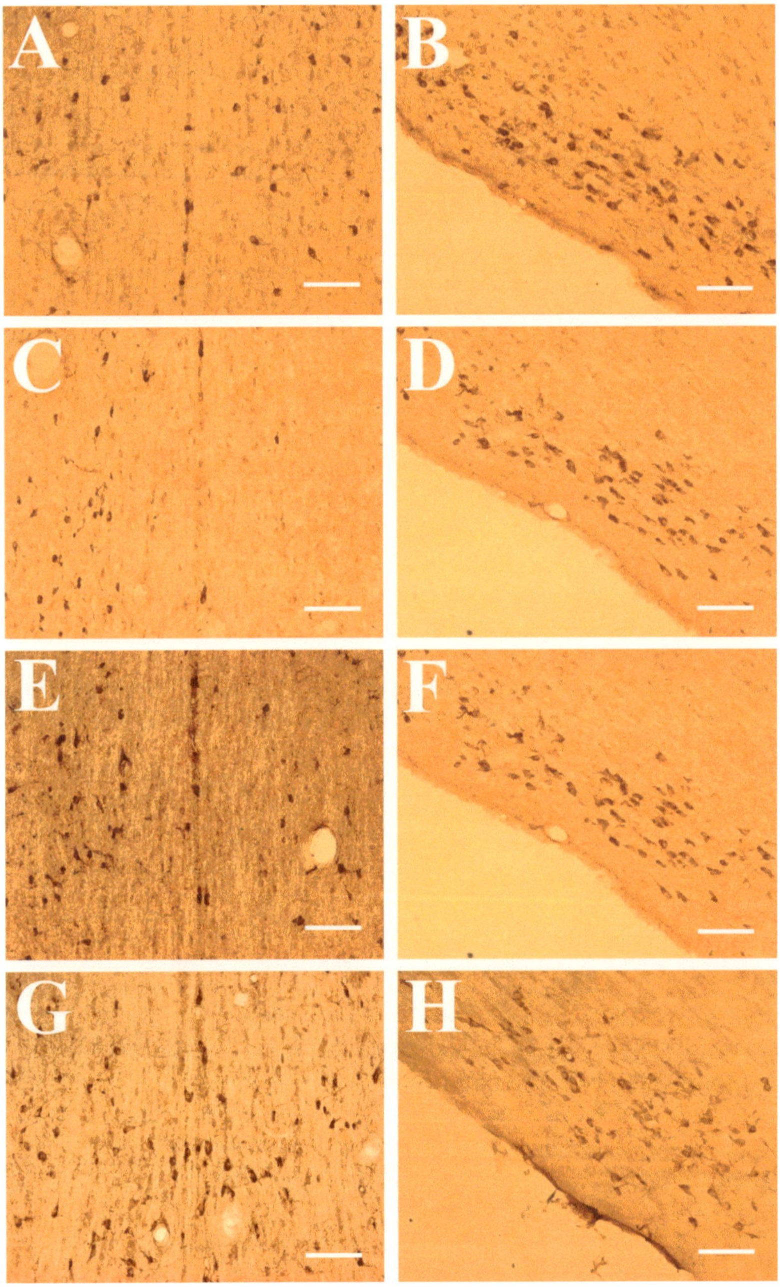

Fig. 6. Immunohistochemistry of cholinergic neurons show ChAT-positive in four groups in basal forebrain 4 weeks after microspheres implantation. (A and B) ChAT-positive in MS and VDB of the normal control group. (C and D) ChAT-positive in MS and VDB of the lesion control group. (E and F) ChAT-positive in MS and VDB of the unloaded microspheres group. (G and H) ChAT-positive in MS and VDB of the rhNGF-loaded microspheres group. Bar = 25 μm. This picture was from our previous paper and allowed to use here by Neuroscience letters.

4. Notes

The protocols given in this chapter are routinely conducted in our laboratory. The following notes may be of interest:

1. Drug-releasing biodegradable polymeric microspheres are commonly prepared by physicochemical processes such as W/O/W emulsion solvent extraction-evaporation method, or mechanical processes such as spray coating, spray drying and spray congealing [33]. It is generally accepted that W/O/W emulsion solvent extraction-evaporation technique is most suitable for encapsulation of proteins and peptides [25].
2. Based on the structure and function, neurotrophic factors (NTFs) are divided into several families: (1) nerve growth factor (NGF)-superfamily, including nerve growth factor (NGF), brain derived neurotrophic factor (BDNF), neurotrophin-3 (NT-3), neurotrophin -4/5 (NT-4/5) and neurotrophin-6 (NT 6); (2) glial cell line-derived neurotrophic factor (GDNF) family, including glial cell line derived neurotrophic factor (GDNF), neurturin (NTN) and persephin (PSP); (3) neurokine superfamily, including ciliary neurotrophic factor (CNTF), leukemia inhibitory factor (LIF), interleukin (IL) and cardiotrophin (CT); (4) non-neuronal growth factor-superfamily, including some members of fibroblast growth factor superfamily, epidermal growth factor (EGF) [10], insulin-like growth factor (IGF) [11, 14], bone morphogenetic protein (BMP) [2, 8, 12]. Furthermore, other growth factors also have neurotrophic function, such as vascular endothelial growth factor (VEGF) and erythropoietin (EPO) [34, 35]. Most of these neurotrophic factors are protein or glycoprotein and are suitable to prepare sustained release microspheres [22, 31, 36-39]. GDNF has been used to prepare sustained release microspheres and to use for the treatment of Parkinson's disease [19, 21, 23, 25, 40]. Basic fibroblast growth factor (bFGF) has been used to formulate bFGF-loaded microshperes and use to treat ischemic hindlimb [27, 41, 42]. In central nervous system, different neurons have express different receptors and react with different neurotrophic factors. For example, cholinergic neurons express low affinity growth factor receptor ($p75^{NGFR}$) and Trk receptor [20, 43].
3. PLGA belongs to a family of polyhydroxyalkanonate that have been extensively used in medical and pharmaceutical fields. It is biodegradable and biocompatible with brain tissue [44]. Drug release in PLGA based microspheres is modulated by both diffusion and degradation of polymer. The degradation process involves hydrolysis of the ester bonds, which is then autocatalyzed by the presence of acidic degradation products. The degradation rate of PLGA microspheres can range from less than one month to a few years, depending on the polymer composition (i.e. the molar ratio of lactic and glycolic acid units). This provides a convenient approach to engineering PLGA microspheres in order to provide a sustained and controlled release profile for a desired period to meet the clinical needs. Thus far, PLGA still remains the most popular polymer for the formulation of NTF-releasing microspheres. Several natural polymers have also been employed for the preparation of NTF-loaded microspheres. These includes hyaluronane derivatives [45], alginate-polylysine [46] and chitosan [47] *etc*. The application of these biomacromolecules needs to pay attention to the purity, batch-to-batch variation, and homogeneity of samples according to their origin.

4. A number of studies have indicated that the methylene chloride/water interface in the first emulsion step is detrimental to the structural integrity of protein, causing substantial conformational changes and protein denaturation [48, 49]. This denature effect could be overcome by optimizing the formulation parameters such as co-encapsulation of BSA [49] and/or PEG 400 [50] as stabilizing agents, the use of low temperatures and short periods of sonication time.
5. PVA has been intensively used as an emulsifier for the formulation of microspheres. Other polymeric surfactants such as polyvinylpyrrolidone (PVP) could serve as alternative emulsifier. Conway *et al* reported that microspheres formulated with PVP exhibited much higher protein loading and pronounced reduction in the "burst" release of protein [51]. However, research activity in this aspect is limited so far, especially in the application for neurodegenerative disease therapy.
6. The formulation of NGF-releasing microspheres must be performed under aseptic conditions and using sterile starting materials. The current available sterilization methods such as autoclaving, γ-ray induced irradiation and ethylene oxide gas can induce protein degradation and/or toxicity.
7. Recently nanospheres have attracted increasing attention in the delivery of growth factors [52]. Their much smaller sizes allow more effective internalization by cells via endocytic pathway, compared to microspheres. In the case of bioactive macromolecules that bind the membrane receptors to exert their functions, microspheres are more advantageous.
8. Anesthesia with sodium pentobarbital is easy to apply by peritoneal injection. This anesthesia method is unexpensive and well tolerated by the animals. This method is simple, repeatable and can provide deep anesthesia more than 1 h that is usually enough for most of surgical procedures. The animals can be applied more this anesthesia chemical if they feel uncomfortable during surgical procedures. Other anesthesia reagents can also be used, such as Ketamine, Medetomidine and so on. If the surgical procedures last more than 2 h, better control of the duration of the anesthesia is required, such as inhalation anesthesia method. Whichever method is used, all the animals should be applied the same anesthetics.
9. Sustained release microspheres are good strategy not only for the treatment of Alzheimer's disease, but also for the other neurodegenerative disorders. As mentioned in Note 2, GDNF-loaded microsphere has been used to treat Parkinson's disease.
10. Learning and memory impairment of Alzheimer's rats can be tested with other mazes, such as Morris water maze and 8-arm maze [53, 54]. Investigators should use different behavioral tests to evaluate different animal models. For Alzheimer's disease animal model, the common behavioral test is maze testing. For Parkinson's disease animal model, rotation, reaching task, forelimb asymmetry test and tactile placing are widely used to evaluate the behavioral changes [55].

5. Acknowledgements

This work was supported by a grant from the National Natural Science Foundation of China (No. 30800345) and Medical Scientific Research Foundation of Guangdong Province, China (No. B2008071).

6. References

[1] Bohn MC, Kozlowski DA, Connor B. (2000). Glial cell line-derived neurotrophic factor (GDNF) as a defensive molecule for neurodegenerative disease: a tribute to the studies of antonia vernadakis on neuronal-glial interactions. *Int J Dev Neurosci*, Vol. 18, No. (7) pp. 679-684, ISSN 0736-5748

[2] Brodski C, Vogt Weisenhorn DM, Dechant G. (2002). Therapy of neurodegenerative diseases using neurotrophic factors: cell biological perspective. *Expert Rev Neurother*, Vol. 2, No. (3) pp. 417-426, ISSN 1744-8360

[3] Popovic N, Brundin P. (2006). Therapeutic potential of controlled drug delivery systems in neurodegenerative diseases. *Int J Pharm*, Vol. 314, No. (2) pp. 120-126, ISSN 0378-5173

[4] Mufson EJ, Bothwell M, Kordower JH. (1989). Loss of nerve growth factor receptor-containing neurons in Alzheimer's disease: a quantitative analysis across subregions of the basal forebrain. *Exp Neurol*, Vol. 105, No. (3) pp. 221-232, ISSN 0014-4886

[5] Fischer W. (1994). Nerve growth factor reverses spatial memory impairments in aged rats. *Neurochem Int*, Vol. 25, No. (1) pp. 47-52, ISSN 0197-0186

[6] Tuszynski MH, Thal L, Pay M *et al.* (2005). A phase 1 clinical trial of nerve growth factor gene therapy for Alzheimer disease. *Nat Med*, Vol. 11, No. (5) pp. 551-555, ISSN 1078-8956

[7] Alberch J. (1997). Neuroprotective effect of neurotrophic factors in experimental models of neurodegenerative disorders. *Methods Find Exp Clin Pharmacol*, Vol. 19 Suppl A, No. pp. 63-64, ISSN 0379-0355

[8] Stahl SM. (1998). When neurotrophic factors get on your nerves: therapy for neurodegenerative disorders. *J Clin Psychiatry*, Vol. 59, No. (6) pp. 277-278, ISSN 0160-6689

[9] Garcia de Yebenes J, Yebenes J, Mena MA. (2000). Neurotrophic factors in neurodegenerative disorders: model of Parkinson's disease. *Neurotox Res*, Vol. 2, No. (2-3) pp. 115-137, ISSN 1029-8428

[10] Siegel GJ, Chauhan NB. (2000). Neurotrophic factors in Alzheimer's and Parkinson's disease brain. *Brain Res Brain Res Rev*, Vol. 33, No. (2-3) pp. 199-227, ISSN 0165-0173

[11] Apfel SC. (2001). Neurotrophic factor therapy--prospects and problems. *Clin Chem Lab Med*, Vol. 39, No. (4) pp. 351-355, ISSN 1434-6621

[12] Fumagalli F, Molteni R, Calabrese F *et al.* (2008). Neurotrophic factors in neurodegenerative disorders : potential for therapy. *CNS Drugs*, Vol. 22, No. (12) pp. 1005-1019, ISSN 1172-7047

[13] Saragovi HU, Hamel E, Di Polo A. (2009). A neurotrophic rationale for the therapy of neurodegenerative disorders. *Curr Alzheimer Res*, Vol. 6, No. (5) pp. 419-423, ISSN 1875-5828

[14] Rangasamy SB, Soderstrom K, Bakay RA *et al.* (2010). Neurotrophic factor therapy for Parkinson's disease. *Prog Brain Res*, Vol. 184, No. pp. 237-264, ISSN 1875-7855

[15] Tuszynski MH, Gage FH. (1990). Potential use of neurotrophic agents in the treatment of neurodegenerative disorders. *Acta Neurobiol Exp (Wars)*, Vol. 50, No. (4-5) pp. 311-322, ISSN 0065-1400

[16] Pardon MC. (2010). Role of neurotrophic factors in behavioral processes: implications for the treatment of psychiatric and neurodegenerative disorders. *Vitam Horm*, Vol. 82, No. pp. 185-200, ISSN 0083-6729

[17] Wuwongse S, Chang RC, Law AC. (2010). The putative neurodegenerative links between depression and Alzheimer's disease. *Prog Neurobiol*, Vol. 91, No. (4) pp. 362-375, ISSN 1873-5118

[18] Camarata PJ, Suryanarayanan R, Turner DA *et al.* (1992). Sustained release of nerve growth factor from biodegradable polymer microspheres. *Neurosurgery*, Vol. 30, No. (3) pp. 313-319, ISSN 0148-396X

[19] Aubert-Pouessel A, Venier-Julienne MC, Clavreul A *et al.* (2004). In vitro study of GDNF release from biodegradable PLGA microspheres. *J Control Release*, Vol. 95, No. (3) pp. 463-475, ISSN 0168-3659

[20] Tamber H, Johansen P, Merkle HP *et al.* (2005). Formulation aspects of biodegradable polymeric microspheres for antigen delivery. *Adv Drug Deliv Rev*, Vol. 57, No. (3) pp. 357-376, ISSN 0169-409X

[21] Gouhier C, Chalon S, Aubert-Pouessel A *et al.* (2002). Protection of dopaminergic nigrostriatal afferents by GDNF delivered by microspheres in a rodent model of Parkinson's disease. *Synapse*, Vol. 44, No. (3) pp. 124-131, ISSN 0887-4476

[22] Carrascosa C, Torres-Aleman I, Lopez-Lopez C *et al.* (2004). Microspheres containing insulin-like growth factor I for treatment of chronic neurodegeneration. *Biomaterials*, Vol. 25, No. (4) pp. 707-714, ISSN 0142-9612

[23] Jollivet C, Aubert-Pouessel A, Clavreul A *et al.* (2004). Striatal implantation of GDNF releasing biodegradable microspheres promotes recovery of motor function in a partial model of Parkinson's disease. *Biomaterials*, Vol. 25, No. (5) pp. 933-942, ISSN 0142-9612

[24] Gu H, Song C, Long D *et al.* (2007). Controlled release of recombinant human nerve growth factor (rhNGF) from poly[(lactic acid)-co-(glycolic acid)] microspheres for the treatment of neurodegenerative disorders. *Polym Int*, Vol. 56, No. pp. 1272-1280, ISSN 0959-8103

[25] Garbayo E, Montero-Menei CN, Ansorena E *et al.* (2009). Effective GDNF brain delivery using microspheres--a promising strategy for Parkinson's disease. *J Control Release*, Vol. 135, No. (2) pp. 119-126, ISSN 1873-4995

[26] Gu H, Long D, Song C *et al.* (2009). Recombinant human NGF-loaded microspheres promote survival of basal forebrain cholinergic neurons and improve memory impairments of spatial learning in the rat model of Alzheimer's disease with fimbria-fornix lesion. *Neurosci Lett*, Vol. 453, No. (3) pp. 204-209, ISSN 1872-7972

[27] Zhao Y, Liu Z, Pan C *et al.* (2011). Preparation of gelatin microspheres encapsulated with bFGF for therapeutic angiogenesis in a canine ischemic hind limb. *J Biomater Sci Polym Ed*, Vol. 22, No. (4-6) pp. 665-682, ISSN 1568-5624

[28] Gu H, Long D, Song C *et al.* (2008). Effect of implantation of rhNGF microspheres on the chat-positive neurons of the basal forebrain after fornix-fimbria transactions. *Anat Res*, Vol. 30, No. (1) pp. 47-51, ISSN 1671-0770

[29] Gu H, Long D, Li X *et al.* (2009). Effects of implantation of neurotrophic factor microspheres on the abilities of learning and memory after fornix-fimbria transections. *Chin J Geront*, Vol. 29, No. (4) pp. 412-414, ISSN 1005-9202

[30] Gu H, Long D, Song C *et al.* (2009). Effect of implantation of neurotrophic factor microspheres on the NGFR-positive neurons of the basal forebrain after fornix-fimbria transections. *J Clin Rehabilit Tiss Eng*, Vol. 13, No. (3) pp. 461-465, ISSN 1673-8225

[31] Lam XM, Duenas ET, Cleland JL. (2001). Encapsulation and stabilization of nerve growth factor into poly(lactic-co-glycolic) acid microspheres. *J Pharm Sci*, Vol. 90, No. (9) pp. 1356-1365, ISSN 0022-3549

[32] Ciofani G, Raffa V, Menciassi A *et al.* (2009). Magnetic alginate microspheres: system for the position controlled delivery of nerve growth factor. *Biomed Microdevices*, Vol. 11, No. (2) pp. 517-527, ISSN 1572-8781

[33] Menei P M-MC, Venier M-C, Benoit J-P. (2005). Drug delivery into the brain using poly(lactide-co-glycolide) microspheres. *Expert Opin Drug Deliv*, Vol. 2, No. (2) pp. 363-376, ISSN 1742-5247

[34] Pereira Lopes FR, Lisboa BC, Frattini F *et al.* (2011). Enhancement of sciatic-nerve regeneration after VEGF gene therapy. *Neuropathol Appl Neurobiol*, Vol. No. pp., ISSN 1365-2990

[35] Xiong N, Zhang Z, Huang J *et al.* (2011). VEGF-expressing human umbilical cord mesenchymal stem cells, an improved therapy strategy for Parkinson's disease. *Gene Ther*, Vol. 18, No. (4) pp. 394-402, ISSN 1476-5462

[36] King TW, Patrick CW, Jr. (2000). Development and in vitro characterization of vascular endothelial growth factor (VEGF)-loaded poly(DL-lactic-co-glycolic acid)/poly(ethylene glycol) microspheres using a solid encapsulation/single emulsion/solvent extraction technique. *J Biomed Mater Res*, Vol. 51, No. (3) pp. 383-390, ISSN 0021-9304

[37] Chung HJ, Kim HK, Yoon JJ *et al.* (2006). Heparin immobilized porous PLGA microspheres for angiogenic growth factor delivery. *Pharm Res*, Vol. 23, No. (8) pp. 1835-1841, ISSN 0724-8741

[38] Tabata Y, Hijikata S, Muniruzzaman M *et al.* (1999). Neovascularization effect of biodegradable gelatin microspheres incorporating basic fibroblast growth factor. *J Biomater Sci Polym Ed*, Vol. 10, No. (1) pp. 79-94, ISSN 0920-5063

[39] Karal-Yilmaz O, Serhatli M, Baysal K *et al.* (2011). Preparation and in vitro characterization of vascular endothelial growth factor (VEGF)-loaded poly(D,L-lactic-co-glycolic acid) microspheres using a double emulsion/solvent evaporation technique. *J Microencapsul*, Vol. 28, No. (1) pp. 46-54, ISSN 1464-5246

[40] Ward MS, Khoobehi A, Lavik EB *et al.* (2007). Neuroprotection of retinal ganglion cells in DBA/2J mice with GDNF-loaded biodegradable microspheres. *J Pharm Sci*, Vol. 96, No. (3) pp. 558-568, ISSN 0022-3549

[41] Hosaka A, Koyama H, Kushibiki T *et al.* (2004). Gelatin hydrogel microspheres enable pinpoint delivery of basic fibroblast growth factor for the development of functional collateral vessels. *Circulation*, Vol. 110, No. (21) pp. 3322-3328, ISSN 1524-4539

[42] Li SH, Cai SX, Liu B *et al.* (2006). In vitro characteristics of poly(lactic-co-glycolic acid) microspheres incorporating gelatin particles loading basic fibroblast growth factor. *Acta Pharmacol Sin*, Vol. 27, No. (6) pp. 754-759, ISSN 1671-4083

[43] Jiang W, Gupta RK, Deshpande MC *et al.* (2005). Biodegradable poly(lactic-co-glycolic acid) microparticles for injectable delivery of vaccine antigens. *Adv Drug Deliv Rev*, Vol. 57, No. (3) pp. 391-410, ISSN 0169-409X

[44] Fournier E, Passirani C, Montero-Menei CN *et al.* (2003). Biocompatibility of implantable synthetic polymeric drug carriers: focus on brain biocompatibility. *Biomaterials*, Vol. 24, No. (19) pp. 3311-3331, ISSN 0142-9612

[45] Ghezzo E, Benedetti M, Rochira M *et al.* (1992). Hyaluronane derivative microspheres as NGF delivery devices: preparation methods and in vitro release characterization. *Int J Pharm*, Vol. 87, No. pp. 21-29, ISSN 0378-5173

[46] Maysinger D, Jalsenjak I, Cuello AC. (1992). Microencapsulated nerve growth factor: Effects on the forebrain neurons following devascularizing cortical lesions. *Neuroscience Letters*, Vol. 140, No. (1) pp. 71-74, ISSN 0304-3940

[47] Mittal S, Cohen A, Maysinger D. (1994). In-vitro effects of brain-derived neurotrophic factor released from microspheres. *Neuroreport*, Vol. 5, No. (18) pp. 2577-2582, ISSN 0959-4965

[48] Benoit J-P, Faisant N, Venier-Julienne M-C *et al.* (2000). Development of microspheres for neurological disorders: From basics to clinical applications. *Journal of Controlled Release*, Vol. 65, No. (1-2) pp. 285-296, ISSN 0168-3659

[49] Sah H. (1999). Stabilization of proteins against methylene chloride/water interface-induced denaturation and aggregation. *Journal of Controlled Release*, Vol. 58, No. (2) pp. 143-151, ISSN 0168-3659

[50] Péan J-M, Boury F, Venier-Julienne M-C *et al.* (1999). Why Does PEG 400 Co-Encapsulation Improve NGF Stability and Release from PLGA Biodegradable Microspheres? *Pharmaceutical Research*, Vol. 16, No. (8) pp. 1294-1299, ISSN 0724-8741

[51] Conway BR, Alpar HO. (1996). Double emulsion microencapsulation of proteins as model antigens using polylactide polymers: Effect of emulsifier on the microsphere characteristics and release kinetics. *European Journal of Pharmaceutics and Biopharmaceutics*, Vol. 42, No. (1) pp. 42-48, ISSN 0939-6411

[52] Gwinn M, Vallyathan V. (2006). Nanoparticles: Health Effects—Pros and Cons. *Environ Health Perspect*, Vol. 114, No. (12) pp. 1818-1825, ISSN 0091-6765

[53] Anger WK. (1991). Animal test systems to study behavioral dysfunctions of neurodegenerative disorders. *Neurotoxicology*, Vol. 12, No. (3) pp. 403-413, ISSN 0161-813X

[54] Ma S, Xu S, Liu B *et al.* (2009). Long-term treatment of l-3-n-butylphthalide attenuated neurodegenerative changes in aged rats. *Naunyn Schmiedebergs Arch Pharmacol*, Vol. 379, No. (6) pp. 565-574, ISSN 1432-1912

[55] Grealish S, Mattsson B, Draxler P et al. (2010). Characterisation of behavioural and neurodegenerative changes induced by intranigral 6-hydroxydopamine lesions in a mouse model of Parkinson's disease. Eur J Neurosci, Vol. 31, No. (12) pp. 2266-2278, ISSN 1460-9568

5

Sensory Nerve Regeneration at the CNS-PNS Interface

Xiaoqing Tang, Andrew Skuba, Seung-Baek Han,
Hyukmin Kim, Toby Ferguson and Young-Jin Son
Shriners Hospitals Pediatric Research Center and Center for Neural Repair and Rehabilitation, Temple University School of Medicine, Philadelphia USA

1. Introduction

Over a century ago, Ramon y Cajal, using the Golgi staining technique to label a subset of dorsal root ganglion (DRG) axons, showed that injured DR axons regenerate within the root but fail to re-enter the adult spinal cord. As shown in his drawing (Fig. 1), DR axons grow away from (arrow), or stop at (arrowheads), the junction between the CNS and PNS, termed the dorsal root entry zone (DREZ). Regeneration of dorsal root (DR) axons into spinal cord is prevented at the dorsal root entry zone (DREZ), the transitional zone between the CNS and PNS. Why regeneration fails at DREZ has remained an interesting issue both because dorsal root injuries are common and because DREZ serves as an excellent model system for studying the reasons for the failure of CNS regeneration.

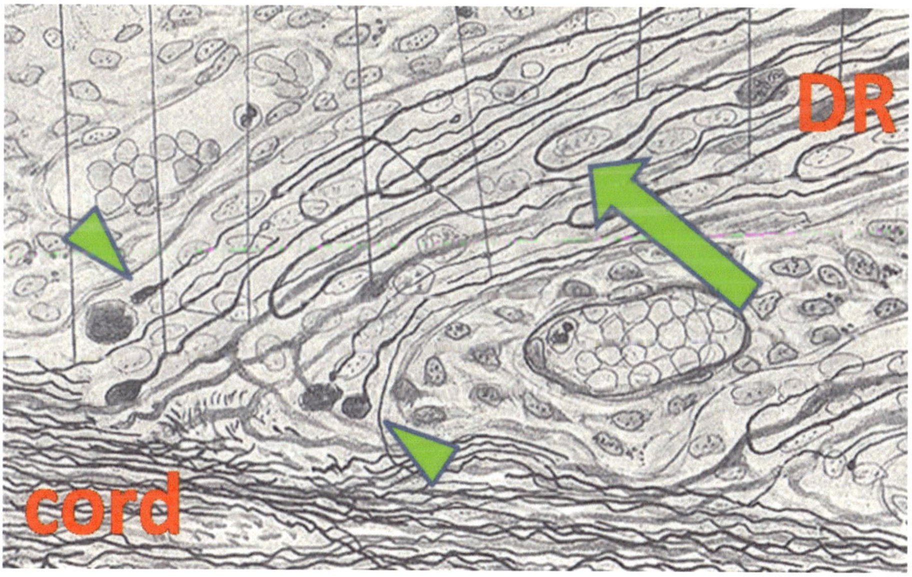

Fig. 1. Cajal's drawing illustrating DR axons growing away from (arrow) or arrested (arrowheads) at the entrance into adult spinal cord.

Spinal root injuries, e.g., brachial plexus, lumbosacral plexus and cauda equina injuries, have profound effects on the spinal cord and evoke chronic, often agonizing, pain and permanent sensory loss. Brachial plexus injury (BPI), the most common form of dorsal root injury, generally results from high-energy traction injuries in which the head and neck are forced away from the shoulder. Obstetrical BPI is a complication in 3/1000 births; in adults, BPI occurs most commonly in high-velocity motor vehicle accidents, particularly involving motorcycles, and in contact sports and falls. Overall, BPI is 10-20 times more common than spinal cord injury (SCI) (Ramer, McMahon, and Priestley 2001; Malessy and Pondaag 2009), and, similar to SCI, produces devastating consequences that include severe, often intractable, pain, and persistent loss of sensation and motor function. There is an urgent need for effective therapies that can reduce the extent of the initial injury acutely or, at a later stage, enhance repair. The need for effective treatment of BPI is increasing due to higher survival rates following severe traumatic injuries and the increasing number of elderly individuals susceptible to BPI because of falls.

2. Dorsal Root Entry Zone (DREZ)

The cell bodies of dorsal root ganglion (DRG) neurons, which relay sensory information into the spinal cord, are located in peripheral ganglia. These cells emit one process that bifurcates into both a peripheral axon branch and a central axon branch that projects into the spinal cord within the dorsal root. DRG neurons mount a robust regenerative response to injury of their peripheral processes, but react much less vigorously to injury of their central processes. Several features make the dorsal root/DREZ system attractive for regeneration studies. First, PNS Schwann cells, which promote regeneration, are immediately juxtaposed to CNS astrocytes, which impede regeneration (Fig. 2).

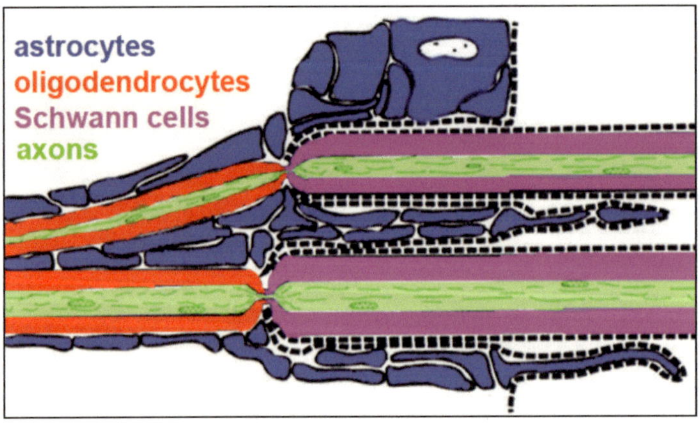

Fig. 2. Glial organization at dorsal root entry zone (DREZ), the interface between CNS and PNS where astrocytes, oligodendrocytes and Schwann cells are juxtaposed in association with DR axons. Central to the interface, myelin sheaths are formed by oligodendrocytes (Red) and the supporting tissue is astrocytic (Blue). Peripheral to it, sheaths are formed by Schwann cells (Pink) enveloped in endoneurial tubes. Adopted and modified from (Fraher 1999).

Because DRG axons must pass through the transitional DREZ to enter the spinal cord, regeneration can be directly contrasted in permissive and non-permissive environments.

Second, the reactions of glial cells at the DREZ closely resemble those within the spinal cord, allowing a major barrier to intraspinal regeneration to be studied without direct injury to spinal cord parenchyma. Lastly, DRG neurons are unique because the regeneration potential of their central processes can be enhanced by a prior injury to their peripheral processes ("conditioning lesion effect"). The model has therefore been extensively used to provide valuable insights into successful and failed CNS regeneration (Ramer, McMahon, and Priestley 2001; Tessler 2004).

3. DREZ after dorsal root injury

Dorsal root (DR) injury (i.e., rhizotomy) in adult mammals evokes complex molecular and cellular changes. On the PNS side, macrophages invade the DR and rapidly phagocytose myelin and degenerating axons (Avellino et al. 1995), while Schwann cells dedifferentiate and occupy axon-free endoneurial tubes, generating a growth-promoting environment. By contrast, on the CNS side, and especially at the DREZ, astrocytes rapidly undergo reactive changes, which include proliferation, hypertrophy and extension of their processes further distally into the DR (i.e., astrogliosis) (Bignami, Chi, and Dahl 1984; Fraher et al. 2002). Microglia/macrophages invade DREZ much more slowly than the PNS (Liu et al. 1998), resulting in markedly delayed elimination of central myelin and axon debris, which likely contributes to the regeneration failure (Ramer et al. 2001).

The extent to which the astrocytic reaction at the DREZ resembles the response to direct CNS lesions remains unclear. Nonetheless, DR axons do contact astrocytes when they have stopped regenerating (Carlstedt 1985; Dockery et al. 2002; Fraher 2000) and reactive astrocytes are thought to form the primary regenerative barrier at the DREZ. In support of this notion, axons grow through the DREZ that has been depleted of astrocytes by X-irradiation (Sims and Gilmore 1994), and, although permissive under some conditions (Golding et al. 1999; Carlstedt, Dalsgaard, and Molander 1987), reactive astrocytes generally inhibit neurite outgrowth (Fawcett and Asher 1999; Silver and Miller 2004). How astrocytes prevent regeneration at the DREZ is uncertain and the molecular basis for astrocytic inhibition is incompletely understood (see below).

Myelin-associated molecules, including Nogo-A, myelin-associated glycoprotein (MAG), and oligodendrocyte myelin glycoprotein, are thought to account for the contribution of oligodendrocytes to regeneration failure at the DREZ (Ramer et al. 2001). If so, their actions seem to be exerted only transiently and during the initial phase of inhibition, because myelin-associated molecules are eventually, although slowly, cleared, while axons that have failed to regenerate remain associated with astrocytes long after injury (Carlstedt 1985; Chong et al. 1999; Fraher et al. 2002). Macrophages are unlikely to directly impede growth at DREZ, because axons grow well in peripheral nerves where macrophages are abundant (Bruck 1997). These considerations highlight our current lack of understanding of the molecular and cellular mechanisms that account for regeneration failure at the DREZ.

Here, we focus our review on intrinsic factors that have been suggested to play a role in preventing axons from regenerating into the DREZ. We then briefly discuss extrinsic factors and treatments reported to promote regeneration at this site. Lastly, we discuss the first *in vivo* imaging study of regenerating dorsal root axons, which was carried out in our laboratory and provides a novel explanation for axon growth cessation at the DREZ.

4. Intrinsic factors preventing regeneration

4.1 Tenascins

Tenascins are a family of extracellular matrix glycoproteins which displays highly dynamic patterns of expression during development and after nervous system injury (Jones and Jones 2000). Members of the tenascin family have been implicated in axon growth and pathfinding during central nervous system development and regeneration. Several reports, however, suggest a role for tenascins as inhibitory molecules preventing axons regenerating into the DREZ. For example, tenascin-C and tenascin-R have been observed within the CNS territory of the DREZ (Golding et al. 1999; Pesheva and Probstmeier 2000). In addition, tenascin-Y, the avian homologue of mammalian tenascin-X, caused rapid collapse of sensory growth cones cultured on fibronectin, and was avoided by growing sensory neurites in microstripe assays (Tucker et al. 2001). It is noteworthy, however, that tenascin-C was highly upregulated along injured dorsal roots, where sensory axons regenerate well, whereas it was only weakly expressed at the DREZ (Zhang et al. 2001). This observation indicates that tenascin-C is unlikely to be the determining factor for regeneration failure at the DREZ.

4.2 Semaphorin3A

Semaphorin3A is a repulsive guidance molecule important for axon pathfinding and targeting during development (Kolodkin et al. 1997; Kolodkin, Matthes, and Goodman 1993; Behar et al. 1996; He and Tessier-Lavigne 1997), and has been implicated as a potential barrier molecule at the DREZ. Semaphorin3A and its receptors, neuropilin-1 and plexin-A1, continue to be expressed in adults (Tanelian et al. 1997; Giger et al. 1998). Injury to the dorsal columns of the spinal cord induced strong expression of semaphorin3A mRNA in fibroblasts associated with the glial scar, and semaphorin3A receptors were present on injured dorsal column axons; dorsal column axons fail to penetrate the semaphorin3A-expressing scar tissue (Pasterkamp, Anderson, and Verhaagen 2001). Increased sensory axon growth was also observed in semaphorin3A knockout mice (Taniguchi et al. 1997). On the other hand, semaphorin3A was absent or greatly downregulated in response to dorsal root injury (Pasterkamp, Anderson, and Verhaagen 2001; Pasterkamp et al. 1999; Pasterkamp, Giger, and Verhaagen 1998). More studies are required to determine the role of Semaphorin3A at the DREZ.

4.3 CSPGs

Several CSPGs in the extracellular matrix are thought to be involved in instructively collapsing or repelling neurite outgrowth (Grimpe et al. 2005; Busch and Silver 2007). CSPGs are also the most prominent growth inhibitory molecules associated with the glial scar, which plays a major role in the regenerative failure after CNS injury (Davies et al. 1999; Rolls, Shechter, and Schwartz 2009). Members of the CSPG family of extracellular matrix (ECM) molecules include neuroglycan 2 (NG2), aggrecan, brevican, neurocan, vesican and phosphacan (Fawcett and Asher 1999). These molecules are expressed by astrocytes and found at the DREZ both during development and after dorsal root injury (Pindzola, Doller, and Silver 1993). The inhibitory properties of CSPGs are primarily due to glycosaminoglycan (GAG) side chains; enzymatic removal of GAG chains by chondroitinase

ABC (ChABC) promotes intraspinal axon regeneration (Bradbury et al. 2002; Grimpe et al. 2005). The differential expression and contribution of individual members of the CSPG family have also been studied. NG2, the most important component, was found to be a major inhibitory proteoglycan for sensory axons (Fidler et al. 1999). NG2 is expressed by oligodendrocyte progenitor cells, which react rapidly following CNS injury, and by some reactive astrocytes. Virus-mediated knockdown or antibody blocking of NG2 has been shown to promote intraspinal sensory axon regeneration (Donnelly et al. 2010). Recently, a transmembrane protein tyrosine phosphatase, PTPσ, was identified as a high affinity receptor of CSPG that mediates its inhibitory effect (Shen et al. 2009). Disruption of the PTPσ gene reduced inhibition by CSPG.

Notably, however, the same CSPG molecules are expressed equally or even more abundantly along the injured dorsal root as at the DREZ or within the spinal cord (Zhang et al. 2001) and degradation of CSPGs by chondroitinase ABC or Pi-PLC, which enhances regeneration after CNS injuries (McKeon, Hoke, and Silver 1995), does not promote regeneration across DREZ (Steinmetz et al. 2005; but see Cafferty et al., 2007).

4.4 Myelin-associated inhibitors

Another group of inhibitory molecules of axon regeneration in the CNS is associated with myelin and includes myelin-associated glycoprotein (MAG), oligodendrocyte-myelin glycoprotein (OMgp), and Nogo (Mukhopadhyay et al. 1994; McKerracher et al. 1994; Kottis et al. 2002; Wang et al. 2002; GrandPre et al. 2000). These molecules are synthesized by oligodendrocytes and distributed in the myelin that ensheathes CNS axons. Their inhibitory role has been demonstrated in tissue culture and *in vivo*. All three myelin inhibitors bind to the glycosylphosphatidylinositol-anchored Nogo-66 receptor (NgR1), which is expressed by many CNS neurons (Hunt, Coffin, and Anderson 2002; Hunt et al. 2002). Treatment with an NgR1 antagonist enhanced neurite outgrowth from DRG neurons in a co-culture model (Hou et al. 2006) but other receptors have also been implicated in the inhibitory effect, including NgR2 and the paired immunoglobulin-like receptor B (PirB) (Venkatesh et al. 2005; Atwal et al. 2008). Blocking both PirB and NgR receptors led to near-complete reversal of myelin inhibition. Harvey et al. reported that a soluble peptide fragment of the NgR (sNgR) which binds and blocks all three inhibitor ligands, elicited extensive ingrowth of myelinated, but not unmyelinated, sensory axons after dorsal root crush (Harvey et al. 2009). Microelectrode recordings from peripheral nerve confirmed that ingrowth was accompanied by gradual restoration of synaptic activities, and paw preference, paw withdrawal and grasping improved in the denervated forelimb.

4.5 Synaptogenic activity

The available evidence suggests that growth inhibitory molecules associated either with astrocytes or oligodendrocytes could account for the turning but not the arrest of DR axons at the DREZ. For example, repellent cues, including CSPGs, Nogo, MAG and OMgp, cause brief growth cone or filopodial collapse and allow axons to turn and grow away without a significant pause or long-term immobilization (Snow et al. 1990; Li et al. 1996; Raper and Kapfhammer 1990; Drescher et al. 1995). Moreover, DRG axons grow despite growth cone collapse (Marsh and Letourneau 1984; Jones, Selzer, and Gallo 2006; Jin et al. 2009) and axons entering the DREZ *in vivo* are accompanied by Schwann cells, which would provide an alternative growth pathway by causing axons to turn around, rather than to stop. These considerations led us to suspect that a novel mechanism plays a more decisive role in preventing regeneration across the DREZ.

Previous studies based on static analyses have provided evidence that is often conflicting or inconclusive. The combination of *in vivo* imaging and fluorescent mouse transgenic technology now allows dynamic processes such as axon regeneration to be studied directly in living spinal cords, providing an unprecedented opportunity to resolve issues that conventional static analyses cannot decipher (Lichtman and Sanes 2003; Bishop et al. 2004; Balice-Gordon and Lichtman 1990; Trachtenberg et al. 2002; Pan and Gan 2008; Grutzendler and Gan 2006; Kerschensteiner et al. 2005; Misgeld, Nikic, and Kerschensteiner 2007). Over the last few years, our laboratory has pioneered in applying *in vivo* imaging to monitor regeneration of DR axons using wide-field microscopy and a line of thy1-YFP mice. Unexpectedly, we observed that > 95% YFP+ axons are immobilized or stabilized surprisingly quickly as they enter the DREZ, even after conditioning lesions that enhanced intrinsic growth potential. Moreover, we have obtained novel evidence that these axons form presynaptic terminals on non-neuronal cells that do not appear to be either astrocytes or oligodendrocytes (Fig. 3; Di Maio et al. 2011).

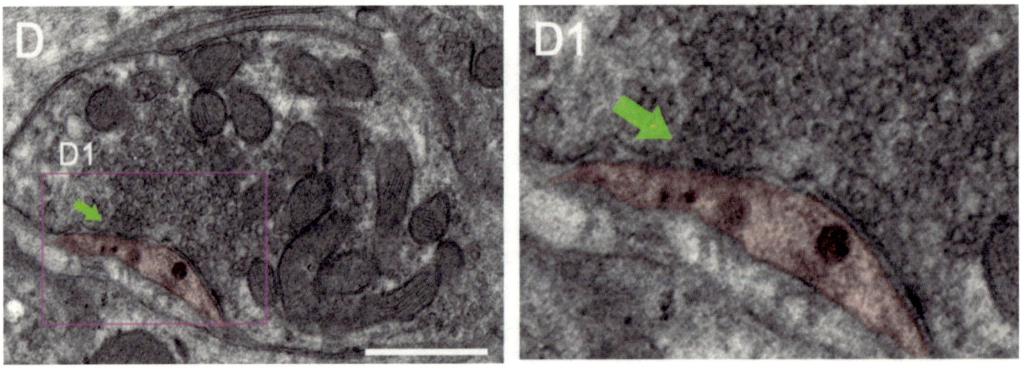

Fig. 3. An electron micrograph of the DREZ 13 days after crush injury showing a presynaptic axonal profile Vesicles are highly clustered and docked at an electron-dense membrane that resembles an active zone (green arrow). D1, an enlarged area of synaptic contact in D. No postsynaptic densities are present on the non-neuronal, postsynaptic cell process. Scale bar, 250nm

The unexpectedly rapid and persistent immobilization of axons entering the DREZ prompted us to determine whether they formed stable structures such as synapses when they arrived. We have found that almost all YFP+ axon tips are intensely immunolabeled with synapse markers such as SV2 and synaptophysin. Notably, in thy1-YFP16 mice, we also observed many additional synapses that did not colocalize with YFP+ axons, and which are presumably associated with YFP negative, small diameter axons. Our ultrastructural analysis of the DREZ demonstrated characteristic features of pre- but not postsynaptic profiles such as vesicles aggregated at the active zone (Fig. 3). Thus, almost all DR axons, including small diameter axons, appear to stop and form presynaptic terminals on non-neuronal cells at the DREZ. These findings thus suggest that axons are neither repelled nor continuously inhibited at the

DREZ by growth inhibitors but are rapidly stabilized after establishing presynaptic terminals on non-neuronal cells. Our findings are in line with an interesting idea raised many years ago and then virtually forgotten, which speculated that regenerating axons stop because they form synapses with non-neuronal cells (Carlstedt 1985; Liuzzi and Lasek 1987).

5. Exogenous factors promoting regeneration

5.1 Neurotrophic factors

During development, neurotrophic factors (NTFs) play a crucial role in axonal growth and pathfinding and neural circuit formation. Therefore, these growth-supportive molecules are excellent candidates to enhance growth-related responses and facilitate CNS regeneration in adults. Several NTFs have been reported to promote sensory axon regeneration across the DREZ and further into spinal cord with functional recovery. Members of the neurotrophin and glial cell line-derived neurotrophic factor (GDNF) families are among the most studied. The neutrophin family consists of nerve growth factor (NGF), brain-derived neurotrophic factor (BDNF), neurotrophin 3 (NT-3) and neurotrophin 4 (NT-4). All neurotrophins bind to low affinity receptor p75, but their specific functions are mediated by distinct high affinity receptors: trkA for NGF, trkB for BDNF/NT-4 and trkC for NT-3. The GDNF family consists of GDNF, neurturin, artemin and persephin. Their function is mediated through a receptor complex, Ret and GFRα1-4, which may be expressed by nociceptive, mechanoreceptive and proprioceptive DRG neurons (Ramer, McMahon, and Priestley 2001).

Ramer et al. conducted a thorough study on the effect of NTFs on dorsal root regeneration (Ramer, Priestley, and McMahon 2000). After cervical dorsal root crushes, continuous intrathecal infusion of NGF, NT-3 or GDNF resulted in regeneration of different subtypes of dorsal root afferent axons, and re-innervation of dorsal horn neurons. Moreover, the trophic effect of these factors corresponded well to the known pattern of receptor distribution on subpopulations of DRG neurons, i.e. NGF led to ingrowth of small unmyelinated nociceptive fibers, NT-3 led to ingrowth of large myelinated fibers, GDNF induced growth of both small and large afferents. Rats treated with NGF and GDNF also showed restoration of nociceptive sensation. Long-term expression of NTFs in dorsal spinal cord by gene therapy techniques has also attracted damaged sensory axons (Romero et al. 2001). This strategy resulted in robust regeneration into both normal and ectopic locations within spinal cord. A combination of NGF and semaphorin3 used to reduce ectopic regrowth, which can potentially cause pain and autonomic dysreflexia, effectively restricted the growth of CGRP positive axons to their normal location within superficial dorsal horn (Tang et al. 2007). More recently, Wang et al. reported almost complete and long-lasting restoration of sensory function after dorsal root injury by systemic artemin, a member of the GDNF family (Wang et al. 2008). Artemin induced multiple classes of dorsal root axons to re-enter correct target layers in the dorsal horn with restoration of complex sensorimotor behavior (Harvey et al. 2010). The caveat of these observations however are the lack of the molecular basis of the non-selective effects of artemin because GFRα3, the major artemin receptors, have been detected primarily in non-myelinated, subclass of the DRG neurons (Orozco et al. 2001).

5.2 Grafts and transplants

After spinal cord injury, peripheral nerve grafts provide neurotrophic support and growth substrate that permit CNS axons to regenerate (Cheng, Cao, and Olson 1996; Fernandez et al. 1985). This strategy has also been applied to promote dorsal root regeneration across the DREZ. Dam-Hieu et al. found that a peripheral nerve autograft (NAG) bridge between the stumps of transected L3 and L4 roots and ipsilateral rostral cord about 10 mm away from DREZ, successfully bypassed the nonpermissive PNS/CNS border, and enabled primary afferents to regenerate through the graft and into the dorsal column over a distance of at least 30 mm (Dam-Hieu et al. 2002). Behavior improvement was also observed. Liu et al. also tested a microsurgical technique that sutured an injured cervical dorsal root to an intact dorsal root via a nerve graft and observed regeneration of dorsal root axons into dorsal horn and functional recovery. Greater recovery occurred when the nerve graft was genetically modified to overexpress neurotrophic factors (Liu et al. 2009).

Embryonic spinal cord transplants have also been used to help injured dorsal root axons to regrow and reconnect with the denervated CNS. For example, after dorsal root injury, embryonic day (E)14 or 15 rat spinal cord transplants were grafted into the dorsolateral quadrant of adult rat spinal cord. Transganglionic labeling and CGRP immunostaining showed regenerated primary sensory fibers within the transplants (Tessler et al. 1988; Itoh, Mizoi, and Tessler 1999). Light and electron microscopy showed that these axons formed synapse-like structures (Itoh and Tessler 1990) and electrophysiological studies demonstrated functional connections between regenerating axons and grafts (Itoh et al. 1996; Houle et al. 1996).

5.3 Olfactory ensheathing cells (OECs)

OECs myelinate olfactory axons and support growth of these axons from PNS to CNS throughout life (Farbman 1990). Transplanted OECs have been reported to promote axon regeneration, remyelination and functional recovery after spinal cord injury (Kato et al. 2000; Pascual et al. 2002; Ramon-Cueto et al. 1998; Ramon-Cueto et al. 2000; Lu et al. 2002; Plant et al. 2003). Corticospinal and noradrenergic axons are among those reported to regenerate but studies of dorsal root afferent regeneration have obtained conflicting results. Pascual et al. transected dorsal roots L6 to S2 bilaterally in rats, which eliminated sensory transmission from the bladder and produced an atonic bladder (Pascual et al. 2002). Transganglionic labeling showed sensory fiber regeneration into dorsal horn and parasympathetic nucleus when OECs were grafted into spinal cord immediately after rhizotomy. Bladder activity was also restored, indicating functional reconnection between the regenerating axons and CNS neurons. Li et al. also found that OECs implanted into the spinal cord and transection site interacted with host astrocytes to promote dorsal root axon regeneration across DREZ into spinal cord grey matter and for long distances in the dorsal columns (Li et al. 2004). Other investigators, however, reported minimal effects of OECs on dorsal root regeneration at the DREZ (Ramer et al. 2004; Riddell et al. 2004). Different sources of OECs and different transplantation techniques may account for these discrepancies.

6. Clinical perspectives

The most common dorsal root injury in adults is caused by traction injury of the brachial plexus (C5-T1), usually from high-speed motor vehicle accidents, particularly motorcycle accidents, in which the head and neck are violently wrenched in the opposite direction from the ipsilateral shoulder and arm (Sherlock and Hems 2004; Yoshikawa et al. 2006). The presenting features of brachial plexus injuries include neck and shoulder pain, and numbness, tingling and weakness of the affected upper limb. In patients whose dorsal roots have been avulsed from the spinal cord numbness is commonly accompanied by severe, often intractable, crushing pain in the hand that intermittently bursts down the arm (Htut et al. 2006).

Brachial plexus injuries are classified by plexus injury location. Most common are C5-6 injuries, which generally have the best prognosis. Also relatively common is involvement of the C5-7 roots. Patients with these types of injury hold the arm internally rotated and adducted. Imbalance of force across the glenohumeral joint also causes abnormal joint development in children (Kozin 2011). More severe injuries involve the entire plexus and may be accompanied by an ipsilateral Horner's syndrome (ptosis, miosis, and anhidrosis). In such severe injury the arm is capable of little movement and long-term prognosis is poor. More severe injuries are also commonly associated with dorsal root avulsions. It is extremely important to distinguish dorsal root injuries (preganglionic) from injuries distal to the dorsal ganglia (postganglionic) because there continues to be no effective therapy for encouraging intraspinal regeneration of the damaged dorsal root whereas postganglionic injuries resemble those of injuries to other peripheral nerves and may be amenable to treatment.

Evaluation of traumatic plexus injury uses nerve conduction studies (NCS), electromyography (EMG), and imaging to classify the pattern of injury and to determine if root avulsions are present. Sensory nerve conduction studies, in particular, can be of great aid in determining if a plexus injury is pre or postganglionic. The DRG cell bodies reside outside of the spinal cord and have both a central process that enters the spinal cord at the dorsal root entry zone (DREZ) and a peripheral process. Root avulsion classically injures the central DRG process but leaves the peripheral process intact. Therefore, sensory NCS, which measure response of the peripheral process, remain normal in root injuries. Thus, normal sensory responses but clinical loss of sensation in a dermatomal pattern suggest preganglionic injury. Motor conduction studies and EMG are most useful in aiding localization and grading motor nerve injury. They cannot, however, help distinguish between root or nerve injury. The EMG is most informative when performed at least fourteen days after injury (Quan D 1999). As NCS/EMG may not detect all root avulsions, brachial plexus imaging is a useful adjunct. Though no imaging modality detects all avulsions, CT myelography is the current accepted standard, with a diagnostic accuracy of 70-95% (Doi et al. 2002). In both conventional and CT myelography, pseudomeningocele formation is a surrogate marker for avulsion.

Treatment of brachial plexus injury is often surgical. In children, ruptured plexus nerve may be repaired with donor nerve (usually the patient's sural nerve) or other graft material including processed cadaveric nerve or extracellular matrix tubes (Waters 2005; Moore et al. 2011). However, in adults the distance required for regeneration is often too lengthy for effective grafting. Nerve anastomosis to a nearby denervated nerve and muscle is useful in both children and adults (Fox and Mackinnon 2011; Pham et al. 2011). However, it must be emphasized that recovery even with these treatments is generally incomplete and that there is no effective therapy for dorsal root avulsions.

7. Summary

Although mechanisms of regeneration failure after direct traumatic lesions to the spinal cord have been explored intensively, regeneration failure at the PNS-CNS interface after damage to the spinal nerve roots has received much less attention. It is largely assumed that inhibitory features of the CNS environment make an important contribution to regeneration failure at DREZ, but the decisive factor(s) and their mechanisms of action remain unclear. Also unknown is whether the growth inhibitory activities at the DREZ are the same or different from those elsewhere within the CNS.

Efforts to overcome regeneration failure at the DREZ have included enhancing the regeneration capacity of sensory axons with neurotrophic factors and neutralizing growth inhibitors. These efforts have been only partially effective, perhaps because they did not treat the stabilizing activity that our laboratory has observed at the DREZ. Continued application of innovative techniques, including *in vivo* imaging, advanced optics, and mouse genetics will be necessary to gain fundamental new insights into why sensory axons stop at the DREZ and fail to regenerate into spinal cord. Of the many possible future directions, we will be particularly interested to learn: 1) the identity of the non-neuronal cells that stabilize regenerating axons at the DREZ; 2) the relative importance of the growth inhibitory cues and the synapse-inducing activity of non-neuronal cells; 3) how this information can be used to optimize recovery of sensory function after spinal cord and root injuries.

8. Acknowledgements

The work conducted in our laboratory has been supported by Craig H. Neilsen Foundation, Jakkal Muscular Dystrophy Foundation, Muscular Dystrophy Association, National Institute of Neurological Disorders and Stroke, Shriners Hospitals for Children. We also thank Srishti Bhagat, Derron Bishop, Alessandro Di Maio, Tim Himes, and Amy Kim for their contributions to the first *in vivo* imaging study of regenerating dorsal roots.

9. References

Atwal, J. K., J. Pinkston-Gosse, J. Syken, S. Stawicki, Y. Wu, C. Shatz, and M. Tessier-Lavigne. 2008. PirB is a functional receptor for myelin inhibitors of axonal regeneration. *Science* 322 (5903):967-70.

Avellino, A. M., D. Hart, A. T. Dailey, M. MacKinnon, D. Ellegala, and M. Kliot. 1995. Differential macrophage responses in the peripheral and central nervous system during wallerian degeneration of axons. *Exp Neurol* 136 (2):183-98.

Balice-Gordon, R. J., and J. W. Lichtman. 1990. In vivo visualization of the growth of pre- and postsynaptic elements of neuromuscular junctions in the mouse. *J Neurosci* 10 (3):894-908.

Behar, O., J. A. Golden, H. Mashimo, F. J. Schoen, and M. C. Fishman. 1996. Semaphorin III is needed for normal patterning and growth of nerves, bones and heart. *Nature* 383 (6600):525-8.

Bignami, A., N. H. Chi, and D. Dahl. 1984. Regenerating dorsal roots and the nerve entry zone: an immunofluorescence study with neurofilament and laminin antisera. *Exp Neurol* 85 (2):426-36.

Bishop, D. L., T. Misgeld, M. K. Walsh, W. B. Gan, and J. W. Lichtman. 2004. Axon branch removal at developing synapses by axosome shedding. *Neuron* 44 (4):651-61.

Bradbury, E. J., L. D. Moon, R. J. Popat, V. R. King, G. S. Bennett, P. N. Patel, J. W. Fawcett, and S. B. McMahon. 2002. Chondroitinase ABC promotes functional recovery after spinal cord injury. *Nature* 416 (6881):636-40.

Bruck, W. 1997. The role of macrophages in Wallerian degeneration. *Brain Pathol* 7 (2):741-52.

Busch, S. A., and J. Silver. 2007. The role of extracellular matrix in CNS regeneration. *Curr Opin Neurobiol* 17 (1):120-7.

Carlstedt, T. 1985. Regenerating axons form nerve terminals at astrocytes. *Brain Res* 347 (1):188-91.

Carlstedt, T., C. J. Dalsgaard, and C. Molander. 1987. Regrowth of lesioned dorsal root nerve fibers into the spinal cord of neonatal rats. *Neurosci Lett* 74 (1):14-8.

Cheng, H., Y. Cao, and L. Olson. 1996. Spinal cord repair in adult paraplegic rats: partial restoration of hind limb function. *Science* 273 (5274):510-3.

Chong, M. S., C. J. Woolf, N. S. Haque, and P. N. Anderson. 1999. Axonal regeneration from injured dorsal roots into the spinal cord of adult rats. *J Comp Neurol* 410 (1):42-54.

Dam-Hieu, P., S. Liu, T. Choudhri, G. Said, and M. Tadie. 2002. Regeneration of primary sensory axons into the adult rat spinal cord via a peripheral nerve graft bridging the lumbar dorsal roots to the dorsal column. *J Neurosci Res* 68 (3):293-304.

Davies, S. J., D. R. Goucher, C. Doller, and J. Silver. 1999. Robust regeneration of adult sensory axons in degenerating white matter of the adult rat spinal cord. *J Neurosci* 19 (14):5810-22.

Di Maio, A., A. Skuba, B. T. Himes, S. L. Bhagat, J. K. Hyun, A. Tessler, D. Bishop, and Y. J. Son. 2011. In vivo imaging of dorsal root regeneration: rapid immobilization and presynaptic differentiation at the CNS/PNS border. *J Neurosci* 31 (12):4569-82.

Dockery, P., J. Fraher, M. Mobarak, D. O'Leary, M. Ramer, T. Bishop, E. Kozlova, H. Aldskogius, J. Priestley, and S. McMahon. 2002. 24: The dorsal root transitional zone model of CNS axon regeneration: morphometric findings. *J Anat* 200 (2):207.

Doi, Kazuteru, Ken Otsuka, Yukinori Okamoto, Hiroshi Fujii, Yasunori Hattori, and Amresh S Baliarsing. 2002. Cervical nerve root avulsion in brachial plexus injuries: magnetic resonance imaging classification and comparison with myelography and computerized tomography myelography. *Journal of neurosurgery* 96 (3 Suppl):277-284.

Donnelly, E. M., P. M. Strappe, L. M. McGinley, N. N. Madigan, E. Geurts, G. E. Rooney, A. J. Windebank, J. Fraher, P. Dockery, T. O'Brien, and S. S. McMahon. 2010. Lentiviral vector-mediated knockdown of the neuroglycan 2 proteoglycan or expression of neurotrophin 3 promotes neurite outgrowth in a cell culture model of the glial scar. *J Gene Med* 12 (11):863-72.

Drescher, U., C. Kremoser, C. Handwerker, J. Loschinger, M. Noda, and F. Bonhoeffer. 1995. In vitro guidance of retinal ganglion cell axons by RAGS, a 25 kDa tectal protein related to ligands for Eph receptor tyrosine kinases. *Cell* 82 (3):359-70.

Farbman, A. I. 1990. Olfactory neurogenesis: genetic or environmental controls? *Trends Neurosci* 13 (9):362-5.

Fawcett, J. W., and R. A. Asher. 1999. The glial scar and central nervous system repair. *Brain Res Bull* 49 (6):377-91.

Fernandez, E., R. Pallini, G. Maira, and G. F. Rossi. 1985. Peripheral nerve autografts to the injured spinal cord of the rat: an experimental model for the study of spinal cord regeneration. *Acta Neurochir (Wien)* 78 (1-2):57-64.

Fidler, P. S., K. Schuette, R. A. Asher, A. Dobbertin, S. R. Thornton, Y. Calle-Patino, E. Muir, J. M. Levine, H. M. Geller, J. H. Rogers, A. Faissner, and J. W. Fawcett. 1999.

Comparing astrocytic cell lines that are inhibitory or permissive for axon growth: the major axon-inhibitory proteoglycan is NG2. *J Neurosci* 19 (20):8778-88.

Fox, Ida K, and Susan E Mackinnon. 2011. Adult peripheral nerve disorders: nerve entrapment, repair, transfer, and brachial plexus disorders. *Plast Reconstr Surg* 127 (5):105e-118e.

Fraher, J., P. Dockery, D. O'Leary, M. Mobarak, M. Ramer, T. Bishop, E. Kozlova, E. Priestley, S. McMahon, and H. Aldskogius. 2002. The dorsal root transitional zone model of CNS axon regeneration: morphological findings. *J Anat* 200 (2):214.

Fraher, J. P. 1999. The transitional zone and CNS regeneration. *J Anat* 194(Pt 2):161-82. 2000. The transitional zone and CNS regeneration. *J Anat* 196 (Pt 1):137-58.

Giger, R. J., R. J. Pasterkamp, S. Heijnen, A. J. Holtmaat, and J. Verhaagen. 1998. Anatomical distribution of the chemorepellent semaphorin III/collapsin-1 in the adult rat and human brain: predominant expression in structures of the olfactory-hippocampal pathway and the motor system. *J Neurosci Res* 52 (1):27-42.

Golding, J. P., C. Bird, S. McMahon, and J. Cohen. 1999. Behaviour of DRG sensory neurites at the intact and injured adult rat dorsal root entry zone: postnatal neurites become paralysed, whilst injury improves the growth of embryonic neurites. *Glia* 26 (4):309-23.

GrandPre, T., F. Nakamura, T. Vartanian, and S. M. Strittmatter. 2000. Identification of the Nogo inhibitor of axon regeneration as a Reticulon protein. *Nature* 403 (6768):439-44.

Grimpe, B., Y. Pressman, M. D. Lupa, K. P. Horn, M. B. Bunge, and J. Silver. 2005. The role of proteoglycans in Schwann cell/astrocyte interactions and in regeneration failure at PNS/CNS interfaces. *Mol Cell Neurosci* 28 (1):18-29.

Grutzendler, J., and W. B. Gan. 2006. Two-photon imaging of synaptic plasticity and pathology in the living mouse brain. *NeuroRx* 3 (4):489-96.

Harvey, P. A., D. H. Lee, F. Qian, P. H. Weinreb, and E. Frank. 2009. Blockade of Nogo receptor ligands promotes functional regeneration of sensory axons after dorsal root crush. *J Neurosci* 29 (19):6285-95.

Harvey, P., B. Gong, A. J. Rossomando, and E. Frank. 2010. Topographically specific regeneration of sensory axons in the spinal cord. *Proc Natl Acad Sci U S A* 107 (25):11585-90.

He, Z., and M. Tessier-Lavigne. 1997. Neuropilin is a receptor for the axonal chemorepellent Semaphorin III. *Cell* 90 (4):739-51.

Hou, S., W. Tian, Q. Xu, F. Cui, J. Zhang, Q. Lu, and C. Zhao. 2006. The enhancement of cell adherence and inducement of neurite outgrowth of dorsal root ganglia co-cultured with hyaluronic acid hydrogels modified with Nogo-66 receptor antagonist in vitro. *Neuroscience* 137 (2):519-29.

Houle, J. D., R. D. Skinner, E. Garcia-Rill, and K. L. Turner. 1996. Synaptic evoked potentials from regenerating dorsal root axons within fetal spinal cord tissue transplants. *Exp Neurol* 139 (2):278-90.

Htut, M., P. Misra, P. Anand, R. Birch, and T. Carlstedt. 2006. Pain phenomena and sensory recovery following brachial plexus avulsion injury and surgical repairs. *J Hand Surg Br* 31 (6):596-605.

Hunt, D., R. S. Coffin, and P. N. Anderson. 2002. The Nogo receptor, its ligands and axonal regeneration in the spinal cord; a review. *J Neurocytol* 31 (2):93-120.

Hunt, D., M. R. Mason, G. Campbell, R. Coffin, and P. N. Anderson. 2002. Nogo receptor mRNA expression in intact and regenerating CNS neurons. *Mol Cell Neurosci* 20 (4):537-52.

Itoh, Y., K. Mizoi, and A. Tessler. 1999. Embryonic central nervous system transplants mediate adult dorsal root regeneration into host spinal cord. *Neurosurgery* 45 (4):849-56; discussion 856-8.

Itoh, Y., and A. Tessler. 1990. Ultrastructural organization of regenerated adult dorsal root axons within transplants of fetal spinal cord. *J Comp Neurol* 292 (3):396-411.

Itoh, Y., R. F. Waldeck, A. Tessler, and M. J. Pinter. 1996. Regenerated dorsal root fibers form functional synapses in embryonic spinal cord transplants. *J Neurophysiol* 76 (2):1236-45.

Jin, L. Q., G. Zhang, C. Jamison, Jr., H. Takano, P. G. Haydon, and M. E. Selzer. 2009. Axon regeneration in the absence of growth cones: acceleration by cyclic AMP. *J Comp Neurol* 515 (3):295-312.

Jones, F. S., and P. L. Jones. 2000. The tenascin family of ECM glycoproteins: structure, function, and regulation during embryonic development and tissue remodeling. *Dev Dyn* 218 (2):235-59.

Jones, S. L., M. E. Selzer, and G. Gallo. 2006. Developmental regulation of sensory axon regeneration in the absence of growth cones. *J Neurobiol* 66 (14):1630-45.

Kato, T., O. Honmou, T. Uede, K. Hashi, and J. D. Kocsis. 2000. Transplantation of human olfactory ensheathing cells elicits remyelination of demyelinated rat spinal cord. *Glia* 30 (3):209-18.

Kerschensteiner, M., M. E. Schwab, J. W. Lichtman, and T. Misgeld. 2005. In vivo imaging of axonal degeneration and regeneration in the injured spinal cord. *Nat Med* 11 (5):572-7.

Kolodkin, A. L., D. V. Levengood, E. G. Rowe, Y. T. Tai, R. J. Giger, and D. D. Ginty. 1997. Neuropilin is a semaphorin III receptor. *Cell* 90 (4):753-62.

Kolodkin, A. L., D. J. Matthes, and C. S. Goodman. 1993. The semaphorin genes encode a family of transmembrane and secreted growth cone guidance molecules. *Cell* 75 (7):1389-99.

Kottis, V., P. Thibault, D. Mikol, Z. C. Xiao, R. Zhang, P. Dergham, and P. E. Braun. 2002. Oligodendrocyte-myelin glycoprotein (OMgp) is an inhibitor of neurite outgrowth. *J Neurochem* 82 (6):1566-9.

Kozin, Scott H. 2011. The evaluation and treatment of children with brachial plexus birth palsy. *The Journal of hand surgery* 36 (8):1360-1369.

Li, M., A. Shibata, C. Li, P. E. Braun, L. McKerracher, J. Roder, S. B. Kater, and S. David. 1996. Myelin-associated glycoprotein inhibits neurite/axon growth and causes growth cone collapse. *J Neurosci Res* 46 (4):404-14.

Li, Y., T. Carlstedt, C. H. Berthold, and G. Raisman. 2004. Interaction of transplanted olfactory-ensheathing cells and host astrocytic processes provides a bridge for axons to regenerate across the dorsal root entry zone. *Exp Neurol* 188 (2):300-8.

Lichtman, J. W., and J. R. Sanes. 2003. Watching the neuromuscular junction. *J Neurocytol* 32 (5-8):767-75.

Liu, L., J. K. Persson, M. Svensson, and H. Aldskogius. 1998. Glial cell responses, complement, and clusterin in the central nervous system following dorsal root transection. *Glia* 23 (3):221-38.

Liu, S., D. Bohl, S. Blanchard, J. Bacci, G. Said, and J. M. Heard. 2009. Combination of microsurgery and gene therapy for spinal dorsal root injury repair. *Mol Ther* 17 (6):992-1002.

Liuzzi, F. J., and R. J. Lasek. 1987. Astrocytes block axonal regeneration in mammals by activating the physiological stop pathway. *Science* 237 (4815):642-5.

Lu, J., F. Feron, A. Mackay-Sim, and P. M. Waite. 2002. Olfactory ensheathing cells promote locomotor recovery after delayed transplantation into transected spinal cord. *Brain* 125 (Pt 1):14-21.

Malessy, M. J., and W. Pondaag. 2009. Obstetric brachial plexus injuries. *Neurosurg Clin N Am* 20 (1):1-14, v.

Marsh, L., and P. C. Letourneau. 1984. Growth of neurites without filopodial or lamellipodial activity in the presence of cytochalasin B. *J Cell Biol* 99 (6):2041-7.

McKeon, R. J., A. Hoke, and J. Silver. 1995. Injury-induced proteoglycans inhibit the potential for laminin-mediated axon growth on astrocytic scars. *Exp Neurol* 136 (1):32-43.

McKerracher, L., S. David, D. L. Jackson, V. Kottis, R. J. Dunn, and P. E. Braun. 1994. Identification of myelin-associated glycoprotein as a major myelin-derived inhibitor of neurite growth. *Neuron* 13 (4):805-11.

Misgeld, T., I. Nikic, and M. Kerschensteiner. 2007. In vivo imaging of single axons in the mouse spinal cord. *Nat Protoc* 2 (2):263-8.

Moore, Amy M, Matthew MacEwan, Katherine B Santosa, Kristofer E Chenard, Wilson Z Ray, Daniel A Hunter, Susan E Mackinnon, and Philip J Johnson. 2011. Acellular nerve allografts in peripheral nerve regeneration: a comparative study. *Muscle & nerve* 44 (2):221-234.

Mukhopadhyay, G., P. Doherty, F. S. Walsh, P. R. Crocker, and M. T. Filbin. 1994. A novel role for myelin-associated glycoprotein as an inhibitor of axonal regeneration. *Neuron* 13 (3):757-67.

Orozco, O. E., L. Walus, D. W. Sah, R. B. Pepinsky, and M. Sanicola. 2001. GFRalpha3 is expressed predominantly in nociceptive sensory neurons. *Eur J Neurosci* 13 (11):2177-82.

Pan, F., and W. B. Gan. 2008. Two-photon imaging of dendritic spine development in the mouse cortex. *Dev Neurobiol* 68 (6):771-8.

Pascual, J. I., G. Gudino-Cabrera, R. Insausti, and M. Nieto-Sampedro. 2002. Spinal implants of olfactory ensheathing cells promote axon regeneration and bladder activity after bilateral lumbosacral dorsal rhizotomy in the adult rat. *J Urol* 167 (3):1522-6.

Pasterkamp, R. J., P. N. Anderson, and J. Verhaagen. 2001. Peripheral nerve injury fails to induce growth of lesioned ascending dorsal column axons into spinal cord scar tissue expressing the axon repellent Semaphorin3A. *Eur J Neurosci* 13 (3):457-71.

Pasterkamp, R. J., R. J. Giger, M. J. Ruitenberg, A. J. Holtmaat, J. De Wit, F. De Winter, and J. Verhaagen. 1999. Expression of the gene encoding the chemorepellent semaphorin III is induced in the fibroblast component of neural scar tissue formed following injuries of adult but not neonatal CNS. *Mol Cell Neurosci* 13 (2):143-66.

Pasterkamp, R. J., R. J. Giger, and J. Verhaagen. 1998. Regulation of semaphorin III/collapsin-1 gene expression during peripheral nerve regeneration. *Exp Neurol* 153 (2):313-27.

Pesheva, P., and R. Probstmeier. 2000. The yin and yang of tenascin-R in CNS development and pathology. *Prog Neurobiol* 61 (5):465-93.

Pham, Christina B, Johannes R Kratz, Angie C Jelin, and Amy A Gelfand. 2011. Child neurology: Brachial plexus birth injury: what every neurologist needs to know. *Neurology* 77 (7):695-697.

Pindzola, R. R., C. Doller, and J. Silver. 1993. Putative inhibitory extracellular matrix molecules at the dorsal root entry zone of the spinal cord during development and after root and sciatic nerve lesions. *Dev Biol* 156 (1):34-48.

Plant, G. W., C. L. Christensen, M. Oudega, and M. B. Bunge. 2003. Delayed transplantation of olfactory ensheathing glia promotes sparing/regeneration of supraspinal axons in the contused adult rat spinal cord. *J Neurotrauma* 20 (1):1-16.

Quan D, Bird SJ 1999. Nerve conduction studies and electromyography in the evaluation of peripheral nerve injuries. . *Univ Penn Ortho J* (12):45-55.

Ramer, L. M., M. W. Richter, A. J. Roskams, W. Tetzlaff, and M. S. Ramer. 2004. Peripherally-derived olfactory ensheathing cells do not promote primary afferent regeneration following dorsal root injury. *Glia* 47 (2):189-206.

Ramer, M. S., I. Duraisingam, J. V. Priestley, and S. B. McMahon. 2001. Two-tiered inhibition of axon regeneration at the dorsal root entry zone. *J Neurosci* 21 (8):2651-60.

Ramer, M. S., S. B. McMahon, and J. V. Priestley. 2001. Axon regeneration across the dorsal root entry zone. *Prog Brain Res* 132:621-39.

Ramer, M. S., J. V. Priestley, and S. B. McMahon. 2000. Functional regeneration of sensory axons into the adult spinal cord. *Nature* 403 (6767):312-6.

Ramon-Cueto, A., M. I. Cordero, F. F. Santos-Benito, and J. Avila. 2000. Functional recovery of paraplegic rats and motor axon regeneration in their spinal cords by olfactory ensheathing glia. *Neuron* 25 (2):425-35.

Ramon-Cueto, A., G. W. Plant, J. Avila, and M. B. Bunge. 1998. Long-distance axonal regeneration in the transected adult rat spinal cord is promoted by olfactory ensheathing glia transplants. *J Neurosci* 18 (10):3803-15.

Raper, J. A., and J. P. Kapfhammer. 1990. The enrichment of a neuronal growth cone collapsing activity from embryonic chick brain. *Neuron* 4 (1):21-9.

Riddell, J. S., M. Enriquez-Denton, A. Toft, R. Fairless, and S. C. Barnett. 2004. Olfactory ensheathing cell grafts have minimal influence on regeneration at the dorsal root entry zone following rhizotomy. *Glia* 47 (2):150-67.

Rolls, A., R. Shechter, and M. Schwartz. 2009. The bright side of the glial scar in CNS repair. *Nat Rev Neurosci* 10 (3):235-41.

Romero, M. I., N. Rangappa, M. G. Garry, and G. M. Smith. 2001. Functional regeneration of chronically injured sensory afferents into adult spinal cord after neurotrophin gene therapy. *J Neurosci* 21 (21):8408-16.

Shen, Y., A. P. Tenney, S. A. Busch, K. P. Horn, F. X. Cuascut, K. Liu, Z. He, J. Silver, and J. G. Flanagan. 2009. PTPsigma is a receptor for chondroitin sulfate proteoglycan, an inhibitor of neural regeneration. *Science* 326 (5952):592-6.

Sherlock, D. A., and T. F. Hems. 2004. Obstetric brachial plexus injuries. *Scott Med J* 49 (4):123-5.

Silver, J., and J. H. Miller. 2004. Regeneration beyond the glial scar. *Nat Rev Neurosci* 5 (2):146-56.

Sims, T. J., and S. A. Gilmore. 1994. Regrowth of dorsal root axons into a radiation-induced glial-deficient environment in the spinal cord. *Brain Res* 634 (1):113-26.

Snow, D. M., V. Lemmon, D. A. Carrino, A. I. Caplan, and J. Silver. 1990. Sulfated proteoglycans in astroglial barriers inhibit neurite outgrowth in vitro. *Exp Neurol* 109 (1):111-30.

Steinmetz, M. P., K. P. Horn, V. J. Tom, J. H. Miller, S. A. Busch, D. Nair, D. J. Silver, and J. Silver. 2005. Chronic enhancement of the intrinsic growth capacity of sensory neurons combined with the degradation of inhibitory proteoglycans allows functional regeneration of sensory axons through the dorsal root entry zone in the mammalian spinal cord. *J Neurosci* 25 (35):8066-76.

Tanelian, D. L., M. A. Barry, S. A. Johnston, T. Le, and G. M. Smith. 1997. Semaphorin III can repulse and inhibit adult sensory afferents in vivo. *Nat Med* 3 (12):1398-401.

Tang, X. Q., P. Heron, C. Mashburn, and G. M. Smith. 2007. Targeting sensory axon regeneration in adult spinal cord. *J Neurosci* 27 (22):6068-78.

Taniguchi, M., S. Yuasa, H. Fujisawa, I. Naruse, S. Saga, M. Mishina, and T. Yagi. 1997. Disruption of semaphorin III/D gene causes severe abnormality in peripheral nerve projection. *Neuron* 19 (3):519-30.

Tessler, A. 2004. Neurotrophic effects on dorsal root regeneration into the spinal cord. *Prog Brain Res* 143:147-54.

Tessler, A., B. T. Himes, J. Houle, and P. J. Reier. 1988. Regeneration of adult dorsal root axons into transplants of embryonic spinal cord. *J Comp Neurol* 270 (4):537-48.

Trachtenberg, J. T., B. E. Chen, G. W. Knott, G. Feng, J. R. Sanes, E. Welker, and K. Svoboda. 2002. Long-term in vivo imaging of experience-dependent synaptic plasticity in adult cortex. *Nature* 420 (6917):788-94.

Tucker, R. P., C. Hagios, A. Santiago, and R. Chiquet-Ehrismann. 2001. Tenascin-Y is concentrated in adult nerve roots and has barrier properties in vitro. *J Neurosci Res* 66 (3):439-47.

Venkatesh, K., O. Chivatakarn, H. Lee, P. S. Joshi, D. B. Kantor, B. A. Newman, R. Mage, C. Rader, and R. J. Giger. 2005. The Nogo-66 receptor homolog NgR2 is a sialic acid-dependent receptor selective for myelin-associated glycoprotein. *J Neurosci* 25 (4):808-22.

Wang, K. C., V. Koprivica, J. A. Kim, R. Sivasankaran, Y. Guo, R. L. Neve, and Z. He. 2002. Oligodendrocyte-myelin glycoprotein is a Nogo receptor ligand that inhibits neurite outgrowth. *Nature* 417 (6892):941-4.

Wang, R., T. King, M. H. Ossipov, A. J. Rossomando, T. W. Vanderah, P. Harvey, P. Cariani, E. Frank, D. W. Sah, and F. Porreca. 2008. Persistent restoration of sensory function by immediate or delayed systemic artemin after dorsal root injury. *Nat Neurosci* 11 (4):488-96.

Waters, Peter M. 2005. Update on management of pediatric brachial plexus palsy. *Journal of pediatric orthopaedics. Part B* 14 (4):233-244.

Yoshikawa, T., N. Hayashi, S. Yamamoto, Y. Tajiri, N. Yoshioka, T. Masumoto, H. Mori, O. Abe, S. Aoki, and K. Ohtomo. 2006. Brachial plexus injury: clinical manifestations, conventional imaging findings, and the latest imaging techniques. *Radiographics* 26 Suppl 1:S133-43.

Zhang, Y., K. Tohyama, J. K. Winterbottom, N. S. Haque, M. Schachner, A. R. Lieberman, and P. N. Anderson. 2001. Correlation between putative inhibitory molecules at the dorsal root entry zone and failure of dorsal root axonal regeneration. *Mol Cell Neurosci* 17 (3):444-59.

6

Peripheral Nerve Reconstruction with Autologous Grafts

Fabrizio Schonauer, Sergio Marlino,
Stefano Avvedimento and Guido Molea
Chair of Plastic Surgery, University "Federico II", Naples
Italy

1. Introduction

A nerve gap is defined as the distance between two ends of a divided nerve. It is caused not just by the nerve tissue lost due to the trauma, or to the following debridement, but also by the actual retraction of the nerve stumps. The retraction is due to the elastic properties of the nerve fibers. Only small nerve gaps, in which minimal tension is required to contrast the elastic properties of the nerve, can be directly repaired (Fig. 1). Any significant tension at the repair site must be managed using other techniques. Peripheral nerve injuries causing gaps larger than 1-2 cm require bridging strategies for repair. Various methods exist to reconstruct nerve lesions with a significant gap: nerve grafts as autologous non-vascularised nerves, vascularised nerve grafts, interposition of venous or arterial segments or interposition of synthetic conduits. Despite the easier availability and execution of these last options, the gold standard, in nerve repair, remains the use of nerve grafts.

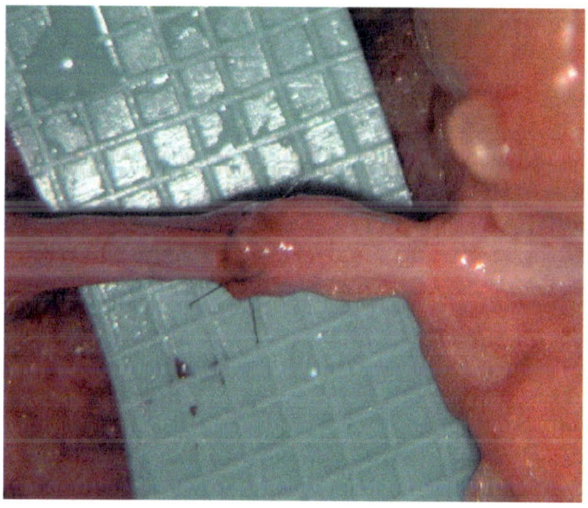

Fig. 1. Magnified view of a directly repaired digital nerve injury.

2. Nerve grafts

Nerve grafts used to be considered less effective than primary repair since the regenerating axons had to cross the gap and two neurorraphies. These impressions were supported by the poor results which normally followed reconstructions using this technique; various factors influenced the results in the early attempts.[1] For a start, it was thought that the longer the nerve graft, the worse the final result would be. This led surgeons to perform all sorts of manoeuvres in order to reduce the distance between the two nerve stumps, including flexing the joints, extensive nerve mobilisations and even bone shortening. The results were disastrous because the disadvantage of the grafts (two anastomosis to cross) was combined with the disadvantage of sutures under tension. We now know that axonal regeneration takes place more easily when crossing two anastomosis sites which are free of tension than across a neurorraphy carried out under unfavourable conditions.

Another point of discussion was the source of the nerve grafts: the harvesting of rather thick segments from nerve trunks of considerable size was thought necessary. However, a nerve graft must first be re-vascularised before being repopulated by fibers. If the nerve graft is too thick, its central part cannot be well re-vascularised and the results of the operation will be poor. The introduction of thin nerve grafts has contributed greatly to the success of this technique. [2]

The principles and techniques for the use of nerve grafts are very similar to those used in primary repair. The proximal and distal ends must be carefully prepared by transverse section. The debate is whether it is better to postpone the graft reconstruction for a few weeks or not. In fact, it may be risky to re-explore the region in complex traumas in which multiple structures such as bone or blood vessels are involved. Under such circumstances, intervention using a primary nerve graft may be justified. Should this be the choice, thorough debridement must be carried out to ensure that the resection is well away from the trauma zone. The dimensions of the defect are then measured with the joints extended to ensure that repair occurs without tension, using a nerve graft of adequate length (Fig. 2 a, b).

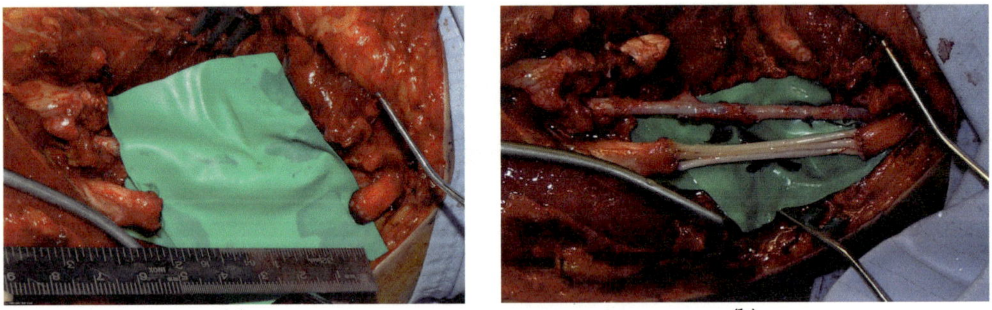

(a) (b)

Fig. 2. (a) Median nerve defect, at the elbow level, with 5 cm nervous gap (b) Use of sural nerve cable grafts to bridge the defect. At the same time brachial artery has been repaired with a vein graft

2.1 Sources of nerve grafts

The selection of the donor nerve depends on the ease of harvesting and on post surgical morbidity. The ideal donor nerve should have the following characteristics: the sensory deficit caused by harvesting should occur in a non-critical cutaneous region; the donor nerve should have sufficiently long segments with no lateral branches; it should be easy to locate and surgically accessible; it should have a small overall diameter and well-developed fascicles.[3]

Donor nerves for peripheral nerve reconstruction include: the medial antebrachial cutaneous nerve (MABCN), the lateral antebrachial cutaneous nerve (LABCN), the terminal sensitive branches of the posterior interosseous nerve and, traditionally, the sural nerve.

The MABCN can provide up to a 10 cm graft. The resultant sensory deficit lies along the medial aspect of the mid-forearm. The MABCN has also been reported as a donor graft for repair of facial nerve defects. Higgins provided criteria for the selection of donor sites for nerve harvest in digital nerve reconstruction.[4] He investigated the cross-sectional area and number of fascicles of both donor nerves and specific digital nerve segments.

The LABCN is the terminal branch of the musculo-cutaneous nerve and provides sensory innervation to the volar forearm. It is easily harvested medial to the cephalic vein, below the elbow (Fig. 3 a, b). Both anterior and posterior divisions can be harvested, obtaining approximately 12 cm of nerve graft.

The LABCN proved to be the most suitable graft for defects at the common digital nerve bifurcation level. In terms of morbidity, the sensory deficit after LABCN harvesting, at the radial aspect of the volar forearm, can be considered negligible due to the overlap in distribution by the radial sensory branch.

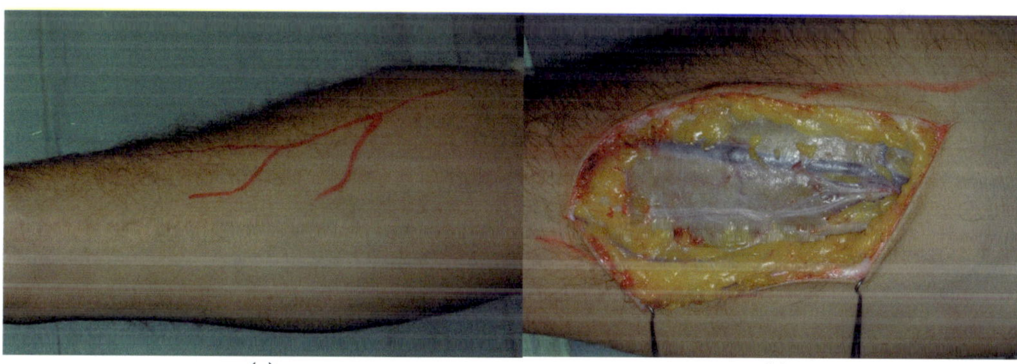

(a) (b)

Fig. 3. (a)Lateral antebrachial cutaneous nerve (LABCN) at the right forearm (b) Harvesting of LABCN at the right forearm

Difficulties can arise when attempting to join the proximal stump of the common digital nerve with two distal stumps of proper digital nerves as in lesions occurring at the web space level. For this clinical condition, we have described the use of the lateral antebrachial cutaneous nerve (LABCN) as donor nerve, by exploiting its natural branching (Fig. 4 a, b, c). When harvested with its branches at the proximal forearm, LABCN can be a valuable alternative to provide Y-shaped nerve grafts.[5]

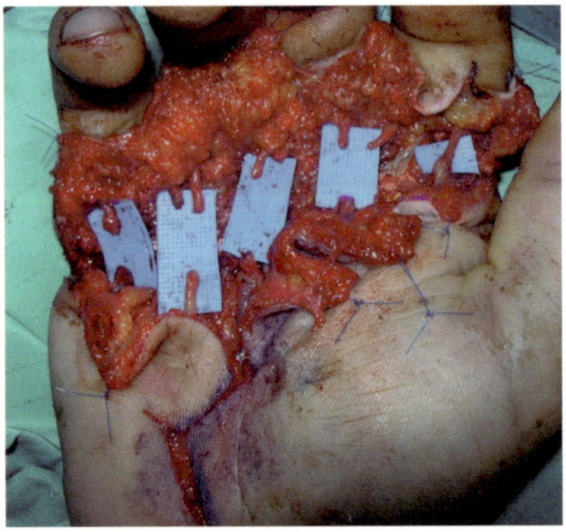

(a)

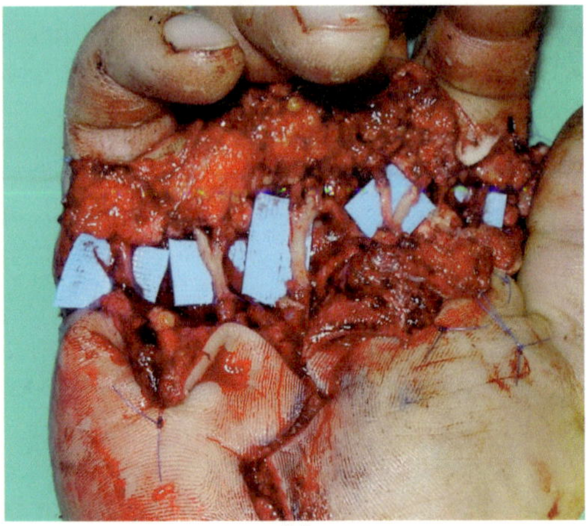

(b)

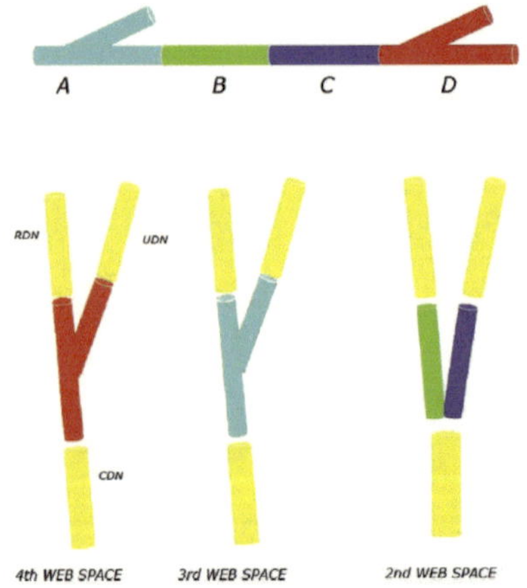

(c)

Fig. 4. (a) Right hand circular saw injury with disruption of all digital nerves in the palm with exception of the digital nerves to the thumb. (b) Use of standard and Y-shaped nerve grafts harvested from the right forearm (c) Use of LABCN and its branchings to mimic common digital nerve bifurcations.

The terminal branch of the posterior interosseus nerve has been used for distal digital nerve graft or as a single fascicular strand that can be used to replace one fascicle of the digital nerve. Today, the posterior interosseus nerve is considered a good choice for digital nerve grafting. The use of this nerve is limited, but there is no functional deficit from harvesting the nerve, as it is an articular branch. The posterior interosseous nerve is found at the wrist level, lying on the interosseous membrane deep to the extensor tendons. As it branches distally, it usually lies just ulnar and deep to the pollicis longus tendon and muscle. This nerve is obtained by a longitudinal dorsal wrist incision. After opening the deep fascia, retraction of the extensor tendons reveals the nerve lying on the interosseous membrane. Care should be taken to preserve the extensor retinaculum. [6]

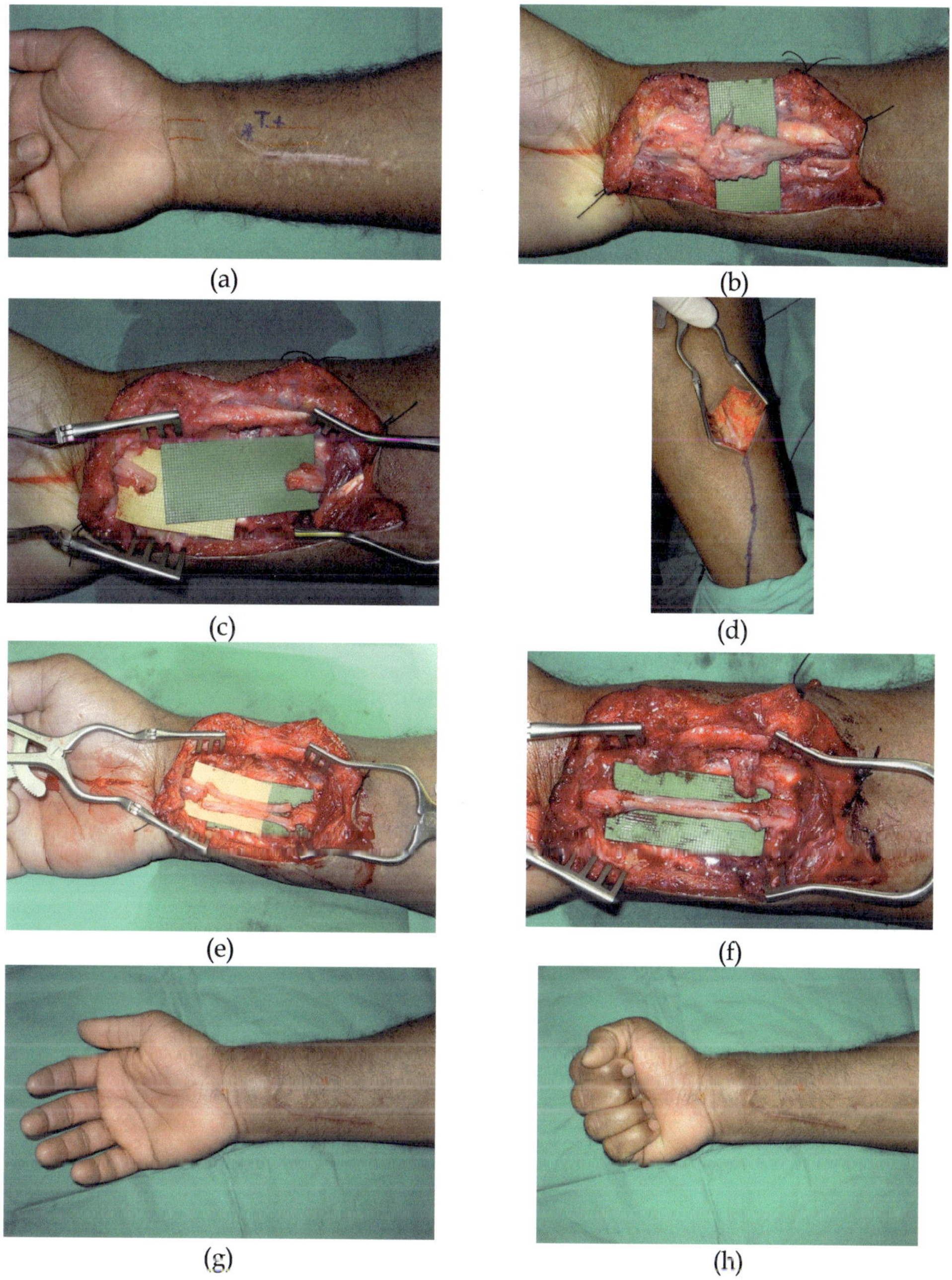

Fig. 5. (a) Right median nerve injury in a 28 years-old 2004 Indian Ocean Tsunami victim. (b) At surgical exploration presence of a large neuroma of the median nerve. (c) After neuroma excision the gap measured 6 cm. (d) Conservative approach for left sural nerve harvesting (e) Reconstruction of median nerve defect with cable grafts. (f) Tailored sural nerve grafts (g) Same patient during the rehabilitation. (h) Same patient showing clinical signs of distal re-innervation (Tinel +).

The sural nerve complex usually consists of three components: the medial sural cutaneous nerve, the peroneal communicating branch and the "proper" sural nerve. In 80% of dissections the sural nerve is formed by the union of the medial cutaneous nerve and the peroneal communicating branch. In 20% of cases the peroneal communicating branch is absent.[7] The nerve is found adjacent to the lesser saphenous vein at the lateral malleolus. When the length of nerve graft need is limited, the peroneal communicating branch can be harvested alone and the medial sural cutaneous nerve can be saved.

Harvest of the sural nerve is usually performed with the patient in a supine position, with the lower extremity flexed and internally rotated at the hip, flexed about 40 degrees at the knee and the ankle dorsiflexed. The sural nerve in the adult can provide 30 to 40 cm of nerve graft. (Fig. 5 a, b, c, d, e, f, g, h)

Sural nerve harvest has traditionally been performed through a "stocking-seam" posterior lower leg incision. This longitudinal approach, that can theoretically extend from the lateral aspect of the ankle to the popliteal fossa, has the advantage of providing excellent visualization of the entire sural nerve anatomy. [8]

The resulting donor-site scar has a tendency to thicken and widen and can be aesthetically unsatisfactory.[9] Alternatively multiple step incisions can be used to harvest the sural nerve.[10] This method yields better donor-site scars, but the limited visualization makes the nerve vulnerable to injury.[11] The use of a tendon stripper with a limited incision at the ankle has also been described.[12-13]

To minimize donor-site scars and maximize visualization, endoscopic harvest of the sural nerve has been proposed by several authors (Kobayashi et al.[14], Capek et al.[9] and Eich and Fix[15]). Endoscopic harvest of the sural nerve offers better results in terms of scars but requires more operating time, familiarity with endoscopic techniques and proper instruments, including long scissors, a nerve retractor and a tendon or nerve stripper device. However, the increase in time as compared with conventional open methods could be counterbalanced by shorted time in suturing the wounds.[16]

3. Vascularized nerve grafts

The theoretical advantage of a vascularized nerve graft (VNG) lies in being able to immediately supply intra-neural perfusion in a poorly vascularized bed in the presence of very wide gaps. Their clinical role has not been well defined despite the fact that they were introduced over two decades ago. Taylor and Ham introduced free vascularized nerve grafts in an attempt to prevent ischemic graft failure.[17] Initial experience with this technique in scarred beds was promising, however results and indications still remain controversial. In general, it may be said that vascularized nerve grafts are indicated when a long graft is required in a poorly vascularized bed, or when a graft with a large diameter is desired, in order to provide it with independent vascularization. Bonney et al [18] reviewed 12 cases of brachial plexus reconstruction with microsurgically revascularization nerve grafts and could only report an "impression" of improved recovery; Gilbert found no superiority of free vascularized grafting over routine sural grafts [19]

More recently VNG have gained a new popularity; clinical studies with VNG of sural nerve have been conducted revealing their usefulness especially in lower limb nerve reconstruction.[20]

4. Nerve conduits

Nerve gaps which are too large to be repaired using tension-free sutures are usually reconstructed using nerve grafts (interpositional nerve grafts). Research on the alternative use of conduits is in continual expansion [21]. The advantage lies in avoiding the donor nerve sacrifice. The first works date back to 1880; since then, nerve conduits have been constructed using biological materials: bone, vein, muscle, artery and synthetic materials (silicon, polyglycolic acid and polyglactin).

For structural reasons, blood vessels were used as an obvious choice, due to the natural presence of a lumen. They were used both to protect the site of nerve anastomoses and as nerve conduits, in a number of modifications. In the past, the use of nerve conduits in nerve reconstruction has provided results inferior to those obtained using nerve grafts; today we see a renewed interest both in venous grafts[22-25] and arterial grafts[26], especially for short gap reconstruction (<3 cm).

4.1 Vein grafts

As we already stated the superior regenerative performance of autologous peripheral nerve grafts has resulted in a wide acceptance as the "gold standard" for peripheral nerve repair. Nevertheless, a number of issues pushed the research towards alternative bridging materials for the repair of peripheral nerve injuries. Such issues included the comorbidity at the site of donor nerve harvesting, the obvious limitations to the amount of donor nerve that can be used and the unsatisfactory functional outcomes in some of the patients receiving nerve autografts.

Vein conduit grafting has not been accepted as an alternative to nerve grafting until 1982, when Chiu et al. proved that it produced regeneration of nerve fascicles and recovery of distal sensation.[27] The vein conduit graft acts as a guide for axonal sprouting and as a barrier against scar tissue ingrowth, maintaining an internal milieu for nerve regeneration.

Vein conduit grafts have two advantages compared to nerve grafts: they are readily accessible and they cause minimal donor-site morbidity.

Walton et al. reported the recovery of two point discrimination in 12 of 18 digital nerves reconstructed with vein conduit grafts.[28]

Chiu and Strauch found that nerve gaps of 3 cm or less could be repaired successfully with vein conduit grafting and demonstrated their efficacy in both acute and delayed digital nerve repair.[22]

Tang et al. repaired nerve defects less then 3 cm long with vein conduit graft and the results were good to excellent in 61.1% of the injured digital nerves.[29]

A potential drawback with vein grafting is that the vein wall may collapse. However, Tseng et al. have demonstrated, in the rat, that hematoma and thrombin within the vein keep the conduit patent. [30]

A limitation of autogenous venous nerve conduit is that its success has only been demonstrated in peripheral sensory nerves with small defects (<3 cm). When nerve defects exceed 3 cm, a vein conduit graft is less effective in maintaining the growth of nerve axons.[31]

In a rabbit model it has been shown that nerve regeneration is enhanced by the distal stump of the transected nerve. This happens mainly because the distal stump of the nerve produces some key factors that promote nerve regeneration as nerve growth factor (NGF). In a rat model, the outcome of an NGF-treated vein graft was better than that of a saline-treated vein graft.[32] Human study also showed good functional recovery in digital, median, ulnar, and superficial radial nerve defects longer than 3 cm with nerve tissue interposed into the vein conduit grafts.[33] Although NGF is present in the intima and adventitia of the femoral veins of rats, the amount of it in a vein graft may be insufficient to promote nerve healing.[34] The 3 cm limit of the vein conduit graft might be overcome by adding NGF to the wound to create a more suitable milieu for nerve regeneration

The technique of repair is based on the classic separate micro sutures (Fig. 6 a, b, c, d) or, alternatively, by a telescoping veno-neurorrhaphy in which the nerve stumps are telescoped into the lumen of the vein conduit and anchored by 9-0 or 10-0 nylon sutures. [35]

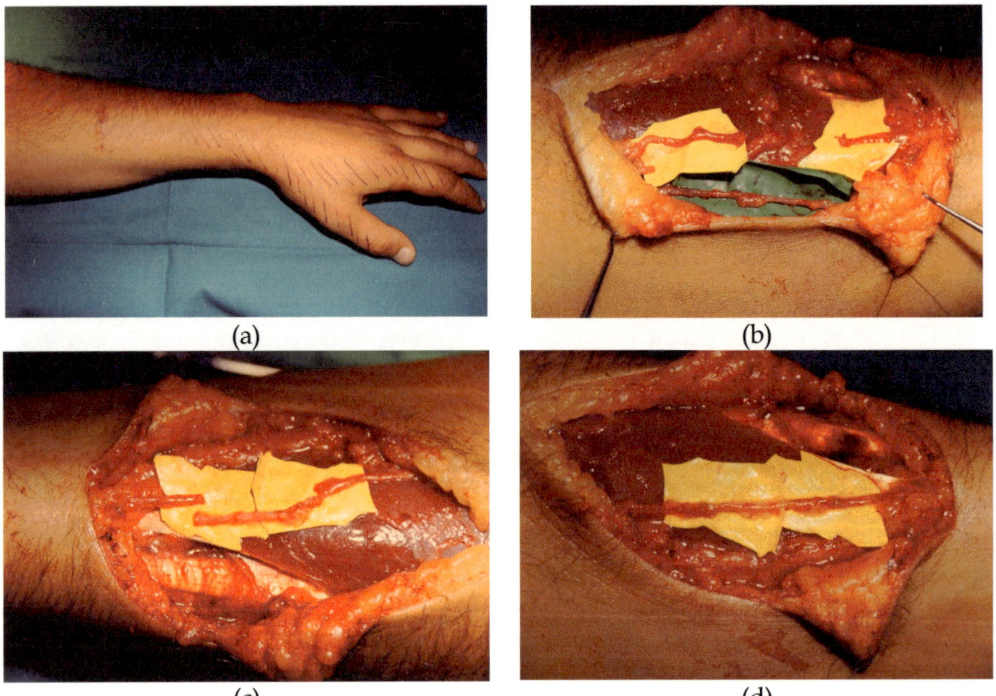

(a) (b) (c) (d)

Fig. 6. (a)Division of the dorsal sensitive branch of the radial nerve at the left forearm. Loss of sensation in the skin area distal to the injury. (b) At surgical exploration the divided dorsal branch of the radial nerve and a donor vein. (c) The nervous gap measured 2,8 cm. The vein was harvested and reversed 180°. (d) Microsurgical reconstruction with the vein graft.

4.2 Arterial grafts

The possibility of using an arterial graft for nerve repair was investigated in rats in the nineties.

Itoh et al. failed to find consistent nerve fiber regeneration with artery graft. They supposed that their failure was caused by a laminin deficiency in the endothelial layer of artery wall.[36] They concluded that arteries should not be used for tubulization.

Many authors reported the beneficial effects of laminin and collagen in the enhancement of peripheral nerve regeneration. The artery wall has three layers: the endothelial layer contains a laminin-rich basal lamina, the media is a muscle layer that is also rich in laminin and the adventitia is rich in collagen. De Castro et al. turned the artery graft inside-out, having these anatomical layers reversed. The resulting conduit exposed regenerating axons directly to the adventitia. De Castro concluded that both the inside-out artery graft and standard artery graft were valuable techniques for the repair of sensory peripheral nerves in rats. [37]

Our group suggested the clinical use of an arterial graft for digital nerve reconstruction: in the presence of an injured digital neurovascular bundle, after the controlateral artery flow has been checked, the use of a digital artery pro nerve graft can be an easy and quick alternative to a standard nerve graft reconstruction (Fig. 7 a, b). [26]

These findings were confirmed by Kosutic at al. in the repair of up to 3 cm digital nerve defects with a segment of digital artery. [38]

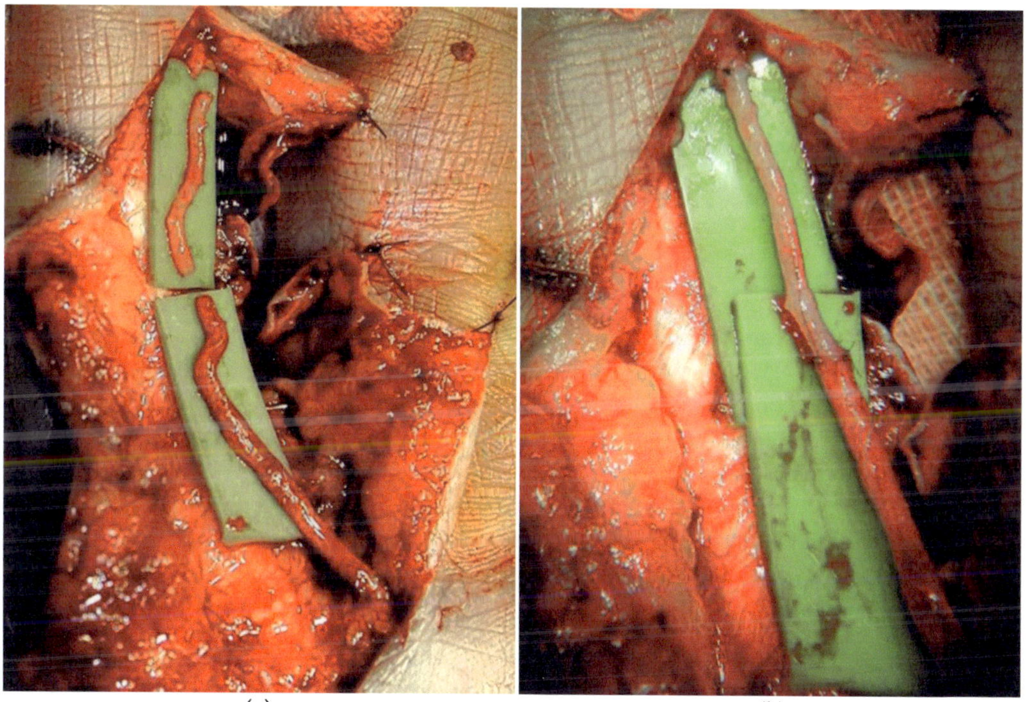

(a) (b)

Fig. 7. (a) Right middle finger circular saw injury with division of the radial neurovascular bundle. The digital artery was used to bridge the nervous gap. (b) Microsurgical sutures at the proximal and distal stumps.

4.3 Muscle grafts

In theory, any biological tissue containing basal lamina may be a candidate to be used as a bridge for nerve regeneration.[35]

The use of muscle conduits has been recorded by multiple authors. The rationale is that the longitudinally oriented basal lamina in skeletal muscle and the extracellular matrix components are sufficient to direct and enhance nerve regeneration. This is based on similarities between the basal lamina of muscle and the endoneural tubes of degenerating nerves.[39-40]

Studies in animals and humans have demonstrated that both fresh and denatured muscle conduits can provide successful regeneration and even lead to superior results when compared with end-to-end sutures.

Skeletal muscle may be pretreated to produce an acute necrosis of myocytes, intramuscular nerves and other cellular components of the skeletal muscle fibers. The cellular debris is removed by macrophages, producing a network of coaxially directed tubes of muscle basal lamina, lowering physical resistance and facilitating nerve regeneration.[41]

Numerous studies have confirmed the efficiency of frozen and thawed muscle grafting in experimental models and animals.[42]

The first clinical trials to repair digital nerves and mixed sensory-motor nerves were encouraging as well. However, motor nerve recovery remained poor in those studies, probably because of considerable delay in repair.

The main concern regarding muscle grafts is the risk that nerve fibers can grow out of the muscle tissue during regeneration, resulting in a decreased number of axons reaching the end organ.[41]

Muscle can be harvested at the time of nerve repair by excising a rectangular muscle block from the inferior border of the great pectoral muscle in the anterior axillary fold. The length of harvested muscle can be approximately twice the nerve gap, to allow for shrinkage during preparation. The block of muscle is frozen in liquid nitrogen until thermal equilibrium has been obtained and then thawed in sterile distilled water. The graft is then trimmed to the appropriate size to bridge the gap, keeping its long axis aligned and leaving it about 2 mm wider in each plane than the diameter of the nerve. The prepared graft is positioned using 4 to 5 monofilament interrupted nylon stitches (Ethilon 8-0) to join the epinevrium of the nerve and the extreme periphery of the muscle graft. [33]

4.3.1 Vein grafts filled with muscle

It is accepted that the use of vein or muscle graft alone is a good solution for nerve reconstruction but suitable only for bridging limited nerve defects (<3 cm). Conversely, these two techniques present important disadvantages for longer distances, such as the collapse of the vein or dispersion of the regenerating axons out of the muscle. To allow for the reconstruction of longer nerve defects and avoid vein collapse, filling of the vein with muscle, or even slices of nerve has been suggested.

In 1993, Brunelli et al. described the use of vein conduits, filled with fresh skeletal muscle, to bridge nerve defects in rats, with functional results better than those obtained with muscle or vein grafts alone and similar to those found with nerve graft.[43] This technique was abandoned for 7 years until Battiston et al. published a clinical report in 2000[44] and a review in 2005.[45] To avoid the dispersion of regenerating axons from the muscle guide, it may be advisable to insert the muscle into the vein or even into artificial conduits.

Even though early experimental and clinical results were good, it is not clear why muscle-in-vein conduit did not convince hand surgeons to proceed with further clinical application of this technique. Perhaps lack of clear indications and limits of use (motor or sensory nerves, or both) or difficulty in assembling the conduit itself could explain the rare application of this technique.

5. Conclusion

It has been clearly demonstrated that the influence of the distal stump can be equally well exerted using a conduit or a nerve graft over short distances less than 3 cm. A vein conduit graft is a good alternative to a nerve graft. Limitations to success are probably due to the medium inside the conduit. Substrates containing components of the extracellular matrix, fibronectin and laminin have been shown to be important as scaffolding for supporting axonal regeneration. Furthermore, several neurotrophic factors and some of their receptors have been shown to be capable of facilitating nerve regeneration. With the advancement of knowledge in the field of neurobiology, researchers are starting to report successes in the progress of regeneration beyond the critical 3 cm gap barrier.

In clinical practice, conduits can be safely used only for gaps of less than 3 cm in reconstructions of exclusively sensory nerves in patients who refuse harvesting of autologous nerve grafts. However, nerve conduits will certainly play a much more important clinical role in the future.

6. References

[1] Bunnell S. Surgery of nerves of the hand. *Gynaecology and Obstetrics, 1927,* 44, 145-152

[2] Beazley WC, Milek MA and Reiss BH. Results of nerve grafting in severe soft tissue injuries. *Clinical Orthopaedics and Related Research 1984 Sep;*(188):208-12.

[3] Sunderland S, Ray L. The selection and use of autografts for bridging gaps in injured nerves. *Brain 1947 Mar;*70(1):75-92.

[4] Higgins JP, Fisher S, Scrletti JM, Orlando GS. Assessment of nerve graft donor sites used for reconstruction of traumatic digital nerve defects. *J Hand Surg Am. 2002 Mar,*27(2):286-92.

[5] Schonauer F., Taglialatela Scafati S., LaRusca I, Molea G. Digital nerve reconstruction by multiple Y-shaped nerve grafts at the metacarpophalangeal joint level. *Plast. Reconstr Surg. 2006 Apr. 15;* 117 (5); 1661-2.

[6] Dellon AL, Seif SS. Anatomic dissections relating the posterior interosseous nerve to the carpus, and the etiology of dorsal wrist ganglion pain. *J Hand Surg Am. 1978 Jul;* 3 (4):326-32.

[7] Ortigüela ME, Wood MB, Cahill DR. Anatomy of the sural nerve complex. *J Hand Surg Am. 1987 Nov;*12 (6):1119-23.
[8] Matsuyama T, Mackay M, Midha R. Peripheral nerve repair and grafting techniques: a review. *Neurol Med Chir (Tokyo). 2000 Apr;* 40(4): 187-99.
[9] Capek L, Clarke HM, Zuker RM. Endoscopic sural nerve harvest in the pediatric patient. *Plast Reconstr Surg. 1996 Oct;* 98(5): 884-8.
[10] Chang DW. Minimal incision technique for sural nerve graft harvest experience with 61 patients. *J Reconstr Microsur. 2002 Nov,* 18(8): 671-6.
[11] Rindell K. and Telaranta T. A new atraumatic and simple method of taking sural nerve grafts. *Ann. Chir. Gynaecol. 1984,* 73:40.
[12] Hill HL, Vasconez LO, and Jurkiewicz MJ. Method for obtaining a sural nerve graft. *Plast. Reconstr. Surg.* 1978, 61:177.
[13] Hankin, F. M., Jaeger, S. H., and Beddings, A. Autogenous sural nerve grafts: A harvesting technique. *Orthopedics 1985,* 8:1160.
[14] Kobayashi, S., Akizuki, T., Sakai, Y., and Ohmori, K. Harvest of sural nerve grafts using the endoscope. *Ann. Plast. Surg. 1995,* 35:249.
[15] Eich, B. S., II, and Fix, R. J. New technique for endoscopic sural nerve graft. *J. Reconstr. Microsurg. 2000,* 16:329.
[16] Lin CH, Mardini S, Levin SL, Lin YT, Yeh JT. Endoscopically assisted sural nerve harvest for upper extremity posttraumatic nerve defects: an evaluation of functional outcomes. *Plast Reconstr Surg. 2007 Feb;* 119(2):616-26.
[17] Taylor G, Ham F. The free vascularized nerve graft. *Plast Reconstr Surg 1976;* 57: 413-26
[18] Bonney G, Birch R, Jamieson AM, Eames RA. Experience with vascularized nerve graft. *Clin Plast Surg. 1984 Jan;*11(1):137-42
[19] Gilbert A. Vascularized sural nerve graft. *Clin Plast Surg. 1984 Jan;*11(1):73-7
[20] Terzis JK, Kostopolous VK. Vascularized nerve grafts for lower extremity nerve reconstruction. *Ann Plast Surg.* 2010 Feb;64(2):169-76
[21] Taras JS, Nanavati V, Steelman P. Nerve conduits. *J Hand Ther 2005* Apr-Jun; 18(2): 191-7.
[22] Suematsu N, Atsuta Y, Hirayama T. Vein graft for repair of peripheral nerve gap. *J Reconstr Microsurg.* 1988;4:313-8.
[23] Chiu DT, Strauch B. A prospective clinical evaluation of autogenous vein grafts used as a nerve conduit for distal sensory nerve defects of 3 cm or less. *Plast Reconstr Surg. 1990 Nov;*86(5):928-34.
[24] Chiu D.T. Autogenous venous nerve conduits. *A review Hand Clinics* 1999 15, 667-71
[25] Risitano G, Cavallaro G, Merrino T, Coppolino S, Ruggeri F. Clinical results and thoughts on sensory nerve repair by autologous vein graft in emergency hand reconstruction. *Chir Main. 2002;* 21: 194-7
[26] Schonauer F, La Rusca I, Molea G. Homolateral digital artery nerve graft. *Plast Reconstr Surg. 2006 Apr 15;*117(5):1661-2.
[27] Chiu DT, Janecka I, Krizek TJ, Wolff M, Lovelace RE. Autogenous vein graft as a conduit for nerve regeneration. *Surgery* 1982;91:226–

[28] Walton RL, Brown RE, Matory WE Jr, Borah GL, Dolph JL. Autogenous vein graft repair of digital nerve defects in the finger: A retrospective clinical study. *Plast Reconstr Surg 1989;*84:944–949

[29] Tang JB, Gu YQ, Song YS. Repair of digital nerve defect with autogenous vein graft during flexor tendon surgery in zone 2. *J Hand Surg B 1993;*18:449–453.

[30] Tseng CY, Hu G, Ambron RT, Chiu DT. Histologic analysis of Schwann cell migration and peripheral nerve regeneration in the autogenous venous nerve conduit (AVNC). *J Reconstr Microsurg.* 2003;19:331–340.

[31] Strauch B, Ferder M, Lovelle-Allen S, Moore K, Kim DJ, Llena J. Determining the maximal length of a vein conduit used as an interposition graft for nerve regeneration. *J Reconstr Microsurg 1996;*12:521–527.

[32] Pu LL, Syed SA, Reid M, Patwa H, Goldstein JM, Forman DL, Thomson JG. Effects of nerve growth factor on nerve regeneration through a vein graft across a gap. *Plast Reconstr Surg 1999;*104: 1379–1385

[33] Tang JB. Vein conduits with interposition of nerve tissue for peripheral nerve defects. *J Reconstr Microsurg 1995;*11:21–26.

[34] Levine MH, Yates KE, Kaban LB. Nerve growth factor is expressed in rat femoral vein. *J Oral Maxillofac Surg 2002;*60:729–733

[35] Dahlin LB, Lundborg G Use of tubes in peripheral nerve repair. *Neurosurg Clin N Am 2001;* 12: 341–352

[36] Itoh S, Shinomiya K, Samejima H, Ohta T, Ishizuki M, Ichinose S. Experimental study on nerve regeneration through the basement membrane tubes of the nerve, muscle, and artery. *Microsurgery 1996;*17: 525–534

[37] Rodrigues Ade C, Silva MD. Inside-out versus standard artery graft to repair a sensory nerve in rats. *Microsurgery 2001;*21(3):102-7.

[38] Kosutic D, Krajnc I, Pejkovic B, Solman L. Autogenous digital artery graft for repair of digital nerve defects in emergency hand reconstruction: two-year follow-up. J *Plast Reconstr Aesthet Surg. 2009* Apr;62(4):553. Epub 2008 Dec 30

[39] Chen LE, Seaber AV, Urbaniak JR, Murrel GA. Denatured muscle as a nerve conduit: a functional, morphologic, and electrophysiologic evaluation. *J Reconstr Microsurg 1994;* 10: 137–144

[40] Roganovic Z., Ilic S, Savic M. Acta Radial nerve repair using an autologous denatured muscle graft: comparison with outcomes of nerve graft repair. *Neurochir (Wien) (2007)* 149: 1033–1039

[41] Meek MF, Varejao AS, Geuna S. Use of skeletal muscle tissue in peripheral nerve repair: review of the literature. *Tissue Eng 2004;* 10: 1027– 1036

[42] Glasby MA, Gschmeissner SE, Huang CL, De Souza BA. Degenerated muscle grafts used for peripheral nerve repair in primates. *J Hand Surg 1986;* 11: 347-351

[43] Brunelli G, Battiston B, Vigasio A, Brunelli G, Marocolo D. Bridging nerve defects with combined skeletal muscle and vein conduits. *Microsurgery 1993;*14:247-251.

[44] Battiston B, Tos P, Cushway TR, Geuna S. Nerve repair by means of vein filled with muscle grafts. I. Clinical results. *Microsurgery 2000;* 20:32–36.

[45] Battiston B, Geuna S, Ferrero M, Tos P. Nerve repair by means of tubulization: literature review and personal clinical experience comparing biological and synthetic conduits for sensory nerve repair. *Microsurgery* 2005;25:258 –267.

7

Surgical Treatment of Peripheral Nerve Injury

Hassan Hamdy Noaman
Sohag University, Sohag, Egypt

1. Introduction

Peripheral nerves were first distinguished from tendons by Herophilus in 300 BC. By meticulous dissection he traced nerves to the spinal cord, demonstrating the continuity of the nervous system[1]. In 900 AD, Rhazes made the first clear reference to nerve repair. However, not until 1795 did Cruikshank demonstrate nerve healing and recovery of distal extremity function after repair. In the early 1900s, Cajal pioneered the concept that axons regenerate from neurons and are guided by chemotrophic substances. In 1945, Sunderland promoted microsurgical techniques to improve nerve repair outcomes [1]. Since that time, there have been a number of advances and new concepts in peripheral nerve reconstruction.

Research regarding the molecular biology of nerve injury has expanded the available strategies for improving results. Some of these strategies involve the use of pharmacologic agents, immune system modulators, enhancing factors, and entubulation chambers. A thorough understanding of the basic concepts of nerve injury and repair is necessary to evaluate the controversies surrounding these innovative new modalities [1,2].

Treatment of peripheral nerve injuries is considered as challenge procedure. In the past there is no definite line of treatment. A lot of cases with peripheral nerve injuries either missed the diagnosis or found no treatment. With the advent of microscope and development of microsurgical instrument, the era of microsurgical nerve reconstruction has been developed. Two lines of treatment for peripheral nerve injuries have been discussed in the literatures and specialized books. The conservative treatment is one line and it was widely used in the past. This line of treatment is mainly described for the non surgical causes of peripheral nerve injuries. There are numerous causes of non surgical peripheral nerve injuries as, metabolic, collagen diseases, malignancies, endogenous or exogenous toxins, thermal, chemical, or nutritional. Surgical causes of peripheral nerve injuries include acute and chronic causes. The acute surgical causes of peripheral nerve injuries mostly due to simple bone fracture, open fracture, cut wound, traction injuries, firearm injuries (either thermal effect or direct injury), crushed injuries, or animal bite injuries. The chronic surgical causes of peripheral nerve injuries include either acute nerve injuries with formation of painful neuroma or entrapment neuropathies.

1.1 Peripheral nerve injury classification

Classification of peripheral nerve injury assists in prognosis and determination of treatment strategy. Classification of nerve injury was described by Seddon in 1943 (3). The classification was based on Neuropraxia

- The lowest degree of nerve injury in which the nerve remains intact but signaling ability is damaged.
- There is physiological loss of nerve conduction. The nerve is temporarily blocked.
- There are sensory-motor problems distal to the site of injury.
- The endoneurium, perineurium, and the epineurium are intact.
- There is no wallerian degeneration.
- In neurapraxia, conduction is intact in the distal segment and proximal segment, but no conduction occurs across the area of injury.
- Common causes are saturday night palsy, honey moon palsy, simple fractures, mild degree of tourniquet paralysis.
- Recovery of nerve conduction deficit is full,and requires days to weeks.
- EMG shows lack of fibrillation potentials (FP) and positive sharp waves.

1.1.1 Axonotmesis

It involves loss of the relative continuity of the axon and its covering of myelin, but preservation of the connective tissue framework of the nerve (the encapsulating tissue, the epineurium and perineurium are preserved).

- Wallerian degeneration occurs below to the site of injury.
- There are sensory and motor deficits distal to the site of lesion.
- There is not nerve conduction distal to the site of injury (3 to 4 days after injury).
- Traction injuries, simple fracture with high energy trauma, severe degree of tourniquet paralysis, are the most common causes.
- EMG shows fibrillation potentials (FP) , and positive sharp waves (2 to 3 weeks postinjury).
- Axonal regeneration occurs and recovery is possible without surgical treatment. Sometimes surgical intervention because of scar tissue formation is required.

1.1.2 Neurotmesis

Neurotmesis is a total severance or disruption of the entire nerve fiber. A peripheral nerve fiber contains an axon (Or long dendrite), myelin sheath (if existence), their schwann cells, and the endoneurium. Neurotmesis may be partial or complete.

Other characteristics:

- Wallerian degeneration occurs below to the site of injury.
- There is connective tissue lesion that may be partial or complete.
- Sensory-motor problems and autonomic function defect are severe.
- There is not nerve conduction distal to the site of injury (3 to 4 days after lesion).
- Cut wounds, crushed injuries, most of open fractures with nerve injuries, iatrogenic nerve injury, gunshot injury, firearm injury are the most common causes.

- EMG and NCV findings are as axonotmesis.
- Because of lack of nerve repair, surgical intervention is necessary.

1.1.3 Sunderland's [1] classification

In 1951, Sunderland[1] expanded Seddon's classification to five degrees of peripheral nerve injury:

First-degree (Class 1): Seddon's neuropraxia and first-degree are the same.

Second-degree (Class 2): Seddon's axonotmesis and second-degree are the same.

Third-degree (Class 3): Sunderland's third-degree is a nerve fiber interruption. In third-degree injury, there is a lesion of the endoneurium, but the epineurium and perineurium remain intact. Recovery from a third-degree injury is possible, but surgical intervention may be required.

Fourth-degree (Class 3): In fourth-degree injury, only the epineurium remains intact. In this case, surgical repair is required

Fifth-degree (Class 3): Fifth-degree lesion is a complete transection of the peripheral nerve. Recovery is not possible without an appropriate surgical treatment.

Although Sunderland's classification provides a concise and anatomic description of nerve injury, the clinical utility of this system is debatable. Many injuries cannot be classified into a single grade. Mixed nerve injuries, in which all fibers are affected but to varying degrees, are common among peripheral nerve injuries. Furthermore, although Sunderland's classification accurately describes the pathoanatomy of nerve injury, it is seldom possible to accurately subclassify an axonotemetic nerve injury on the basis of preoperative clinical and electromyographic data. The subtype is usually discernible only by histologic examination of the injured nerve [2].

Non Degenerative

1. neuropraxia

Degenerative nerve injury

2. axonotmesis
3. neurotmesis

1.2 Manifestations of peripheral nerve injury

1.2.1 Motor

1. Muscle wasting, muscle atrophy and even muscle paralysis
2. Loss of reflex according to the affected muscle e.g. loss of biceps reflex in case of musculocutaneous nerve injury, loss of triceps reflex in case of radial nerve injury, loss of knee reflex in case of femoral nerve injury and loss of ankle reflex in case of posterior nerve injury.
3. Joint contracture and fixed deformity, this can be happened in longstanding nerve injury due to muscle imbalance.

1.2.2 Sensory

1. Loss of superficial sensation including pain (anesthesia, hyposthesia, parathesia), touch, temperature.
2. Loss of deep sensation including sense of position, sense of movement and sterognosis (identification of object by touch with closed eyes).

1.2.3 Vasomotor

The skin supplied by the injured nerve become pale and dry (anhydrosis) with crust formation.

1.3 Indications for nerve surgery

1. Cases with neuropraxia that failed to recover within the first 3 months.
2. Cases with definite nerve injuries as, open fracture, crushed injuries, firearm and gunshot injuries, cut wounds, iatrogenic nerve injuries, postreduction injuries, animal bite injuries.
3. Chronic nerve lesions with painful neuroma.
4. Entrapment neuropathies.

There is a lot of debate for surgical treatment of nerve injuries especially those associated with simple fracture. One school of surgeons prefers treatment of fracture and wait for months to give chance for nerve to be recovered spontaneously. The other school advises to explore the nerve and treat both the fracture and injured nerve simultaneously. Actually I prefer early surgical exploration and surgical treatment of the fracture at the same time. The chance of simultaneously nerve recovery is decreased with surgical maneuver around the injured nerve, the time elapsed between nerve injury and exploration is sufficient enough for nerve regeneration after surgical treatment even after nerve repair, to explore the injured nerve acutely passed the chance for nerve graft which is more complex of course than neurolysis or nerve repair.

1.4 Timing of nerve surgery

It has been the time-honored policy to advise primary suture when possible. This recommendation is logical when one considers what happens to the distal end of the nerve, motor end plates, sensory nerve endings, muscles, joints, and other tissues of the denervated extremity. The controversy concerning whether primary or secondary nerve repair is better is unresolved. Primary repair done in the first 6 to 8 hours or delayed primary repair done in the first 7 to 18 days is appropriate when the injury is caused by a sharp object, the wound is clean, and there are no other major complicating injuries. Ideally, such repairs should be performed by an experienced surgeon in an institution where adequate equipment and personnel are available. The development of magnification devices, new instruments, and new techniques and the modification of a variety of small instruments for use in nerve surgery have improved the technique of early repair. Primary repair should shorten the time of denervation of the end organs, and fascicular alignment should be improved because minimal excision of the nerve ends is required. For several reasons a primary peripheral nerve repair is favourable. Technically, a primary repair of a sharp injury is easier. The rotation of the nerve segment can be easily judged since the epineurial blood vessels can be identified on the surface of the nerve trunk. The nerve stumps can also easily be cleaned, i.e. excision of nonviable tissue, to help coaptation [4].

When the diagnosis of division of a peripheral nerve has been made, if conditions are suitable and repair is indicated, one should not delay repair in anticipation of spontaneous regeneration. Only if the patient's life or limb is seriously endangered should the operation be long postponed. However, an important part of nerve repair is to judge the extent of necrotic tissue in specific injuries. In severe cases, caused by for example a gun shot wound, there may be widespread injury to the peripheral nerve components. It can be difficult in the fresh case to evaluate how much of the nerve ends needs to be resected. In such injuries it is of extreme importance to tidy up the wound and remove all other necrotic tissues to avoid infection. In some cases with severe nerve injuries it may be advisable to delay the nerve reconstruction until all other tissues, such as muscle, have healed properly. However, this is not the case in a sharp transection injury where a primary suture is the best alternative. A fracture is not a contraindication for operation. Operation before the fracture becomes united may be advantageous for two reasons: (1) If bone shortening is necessary, resection of an ununited or partially united fracture is a much less formidable procedure than resection of a fully united bone; and (2) restriction of joint motion is minimal if the nerve is repaired soon after the injury; later, motion would be more limited, perhaps so severely as to prevent flexing the joint enough to overcome a gap between the nerve ends.

Another interesting issue is exploration of the radial nerve in patients with radial nerve dysfunction in connection with a humeral shaft fracture. The radial nerve can in such cases be injured or even ruptured. If the humeral shaft fracture is to be repaired with plates and screws one may consider exploring the dysfunctional radial nerve at the same time. In case one is convinced that the radial nerve is severely lacerated an early repair should be considered based on the neurobiological alterations and impaired axonal outgrowth with time described earlier. However, one can not as a general rule recommend a generous exploration of all radial nerves that may have some dysfunction after humeral shaft fracture [5].

1.5 Author preferred method

A radial nerve injury associated with a humeral shaft fracture is an important injury pattern among trauma patients [6]. It is the most common peripheral nerve injury associated with fracture of long bones [7-10]. As our understanding of the pathoanatomy of the humerus and surrounding neurovascular structures has evolved, surgeons have adapted their strategies to improve outcome. There are differences in opinion regarding the treatment of choice. Early exploration of the radial nerve claims a variety of advantages. It is technically easier and safer than the delayed procedure. Direct examination of the nerve clarifies the diagnosis and the extent of the lesion. Early stabilization of the fracture reduces the chance of the nerve being enveloped by scar tissue and callus. Reduction of the open fracture helps lessen the risk of further neural damage from mobile bone ends. Shortening of the humerus to facilitate nerve repair is better done before healing of the fracture is complete [11-13]. However, opponents of early exploration have observed high rate of spontaneous recovery and have advised a policy of expectancy, [14-21] believing that this approach mitigates an unnecessary complications attendant upon exploration. Thickening of the neurilemmal sheath during waiting helps to define the extent of nerve damage and facilitates repair. It is easier to treat the nerve when the fracture is healed. Most of these papers describe small numbers of patients and all are uncontrolled retrospective case series. Although treatment for this injury pattern is a controversial subject among upper-extremity surgeons, certain principles of management need to be applied in all cases. We limited our analysis to post-humeral fracture radial nerve palsies, which were operated due to the presence of neurological deficits after the fracture. We recorded the type of fracture, treatment used to achieve bone healing, surgical approach, and type of radial nerve surgery. Between April 2001 and April 2007, 36 patients with fractures of the shaft of the humerus with palsy of the radial nerve were treated by early exploration of the radial nerve and internal fixation by narrow DCP plate. Twenty four were male and 14 female, with a mean age of 30.3 years (8-53 years). The most common cause of injury was motor car accident in 25 patients, falling from height in 5 patients, fire arm injury in 4 patients, and machine injury in 2 cases. A lesion of the radial nerve had occurred at the time of injury in 27 patients, 7 of these patients had open fracture, and post reduction injury occurred in 9 cases. The fracture patterns were varied. The most common pattern of fracture was transverse pattern involved the distal third occurred in 16 cases, oblique fracture in the distal third (Holstein-Lewis fracture) in 7 cases, spiral fracture involved the middle third in 8 cases, transverse fracture involved the middle third in 3 cases and fracture involved the junction of middle and upper third of the humerus in 2 cases. Twelve patients had surgery on the day of injury and the other 26 at a mean of 8 days later (3 to 14). The mean follow up was 28 months (9 to 72). The anesthesia was general, the position was laterally and the approach was posterior approach. Exploration of the radial nerve demonstrated compression at the lateral intermuscular septum in 19 cases, entrapment in the fracture site in 9 cases and loss of its continuity in 8 cases. Neurolysis was required in 20 cases, epineurorrhaphy in 9 cases, nerve grafts in five, and first-intention tendon transfer in two. Plate fixation was generally used for fixation. Results of nerve surgery were assessed used the MRC (Medical Research Council) at a mean follow-up of 8.2 years. Outcome was rated good to excellent in 28 patients, fair in one and poor (failure) in three. First-intention tendon transfers were performed in two patients and two patients were lost to follow-up. Mean delay to recovery was five months after neurolysis, eight months after nerve repair and fifteen months after nerve grafts. The fracture was united in all cases. The mean time of union was 5 months.

2. The technique of nerve repair

The anaethesia have to be tailored according to the site, the affected nerve, the age and the need of the patient. The operation is performed under tourniquet, and wide exposure is used. Dissection is carried out from normal to abnormal tissue, with an attempt not to disturb the local blood supply (Fig. 1a). The procedure of repairing a nerve trunk can be divided into four steps. Initially the nerve ends are prepared to get a viable nerve end without necrotic tissue (preparation) (Fig. 1b). The nerve ends are handled with care using microsurgical instruments. A pair of sharp micro scissors or a surgical blade can be used to remove the necrotic part of the nerve ends. The extent of resection can be difficult to judge if there is a laceration or a contusion by for example a gun shot. After the nerve ends are prepared, they should be approximated keeping in mind the importance of adjusting the length of the gap and the tension of the nerve segments (approximation). During the approximation the nerve ends can be slightly mobilised by dissection but one should avoid extensive intrafascicular dissection. The nerve ends are coaptated. The nerve repair is maintained by stitches (maintenance) (Fig. 1c); 9–0 or 10–0 nylon (sometimes thicker suture materials can be suitable in specific cases) is inserted into the epineurium.

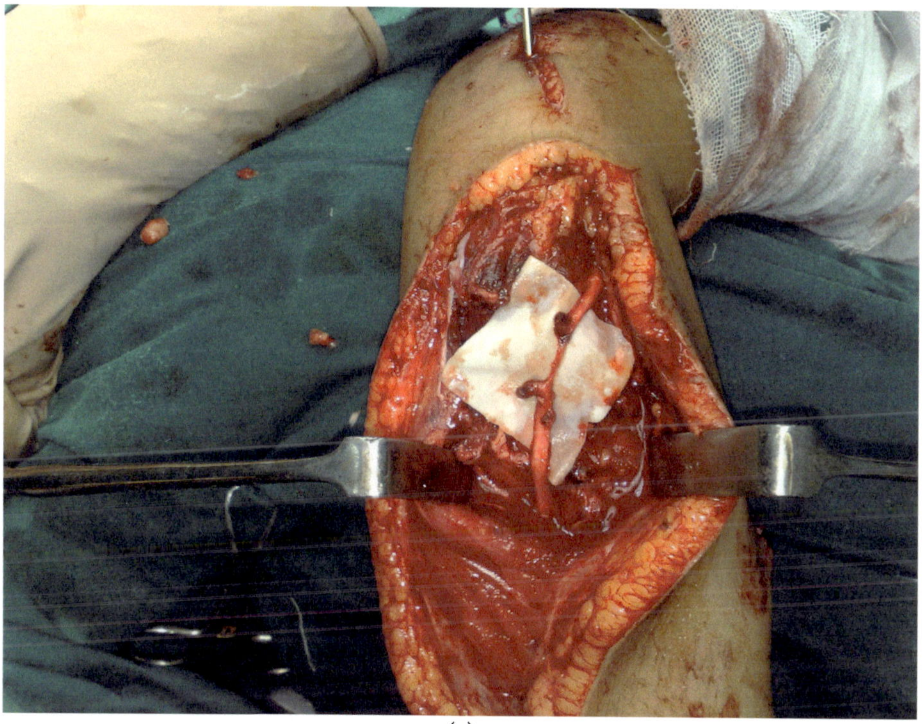

(a)

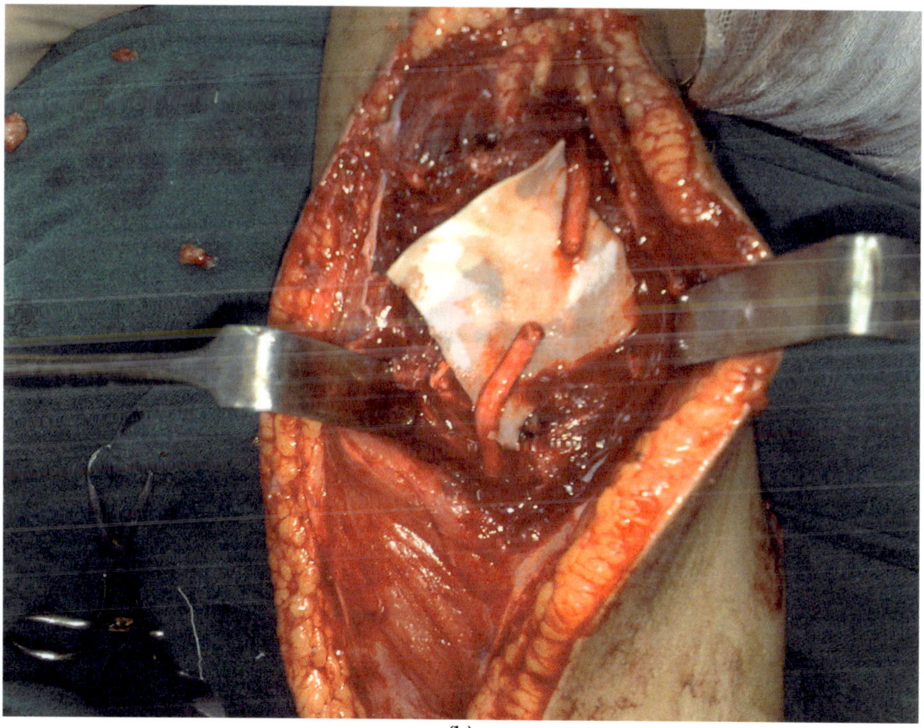

(b)

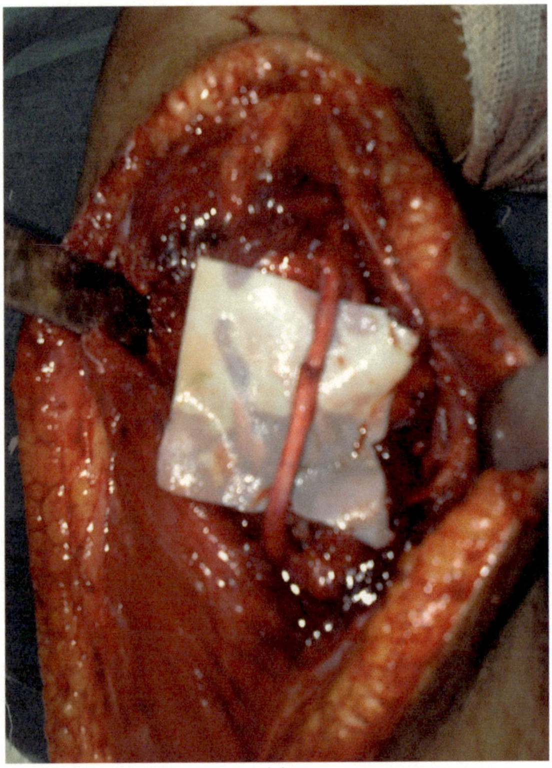

(c)

Fig. 1. Male patient 9 years old subjected to firearm injury caused open fracture humerus with radial nerve injury, (a) Intraoperative photo showing laceration of both ends of the radial nerve. (b) Intraoperative photo after preparation of both stumps. (c) Intraoperative photo after maintenance of the repair by 10/0 Nylon.

Thus, interrupted epineurial sutures maintain the repair. In a digital nerve it may be enough with three 9–0 sutures, while in a larger ulnar or median nerve several interrupted sutures are applied, sometimes with thicker suture material. When the sutures are placed one should try to avoid malrotation of the nerve ends. Identification of the longitudinal intraneural blood vessels may help in this. In specific cases it is possible to identify individual fascicular groups for attachment (group fascicular nerve repair), predominantly at a distal level where fascicles with specific targets are well defined. The ulnar nerve at wrist level is one nerve where such a repair technique can be used since it contains two separate motor and sensory components. All nerve repairs are explored by the use of surgical loupe (magnification × 3.5), but a microscope is routinely used during repair. Nerve suturing is the key of success for nerve surgery. The aim is to convert the distal nerve stump into patent tube to receive the growth cone of the axons. The regenerating nerve axons have to cross smoothly through the site of nerve anastomosis (neurorrhaphy).

3. Neurorrhaphy (direct nerve repair)

Historically, it was thought best to wait 3 weeks before repair to allow the conclusion of wallerian degeneration. However, Mackinnon (22) and other authors have shown that immediate primary repair is associated with better results. Prerequisites are a clean wound, good vascular supply, no crush component of the injury, and adequate soft-tissue coverage. Skeletal stability is paramount, and there should be minimal tension on the nerve repair. Although the classic technique of neurorrhaphy is devoid of tension, Hentz et al (23) studied a primate model and showed that a direct repair under modest tension actually does better than a tension-free nerve graft over the same regenerating distance. With the advent of microsurgical instrumentation and technique, attempts at group fascicular repair, rather than simple epineurial coaptation, have been attempted. Proponents argue that group fascicular repair is better because axonal realignment is more accurate with this technique. However, others have shown that there is no functional difference in outcome between epineurial and group fascicular repair. Furthermore, group fascicular repair has the potential disadvantage of increased scarring and damage to the blood supply as a result of the additional dissection. Lundborg et al (24) concluded that although this technique purportedly ensures correct orientation of regenerating axons, there is little evidence that it is superior to the less exact but simpler epineurial repair.

Monofilament nylon suture is the preferred suture type because of its ease of use and minimal foreign body reactivity. Using a cadaveric median nerve model, Giddins et al (25) demonstrated that 10-0 nylon failed under tension, that 9-0 nylon withstood the greatest distractive force before repair gapping; and that 8-0 nylon had a tendency to pull out of the repaired nerve ending.

A number of techniques are available to facilitate fascicular matching. Visual alignment may be aided by topographic sketches of both cut ends. With this method, it can be determined which fascicular group of the proximal stump corresponds to the fascicular group of the distal stump. Electrical stimulation can be used to identify sensory fascicles in the proximal stump in an awake patient, but because wallerian degeneration of the distal axon begins within 2 to 4 days after transection, motor fascicles can be identified reliably only by direct nerve stimulation in fresh injuries. Nerve ends can also be stained to differentiate between motor and sensory axons. Initially, staining was too time-consuming to be clinically useful, but recent advances have been made. Gu et al (26) reported on a 30-minute technique for blue- SAb staining of sensory fascicles and showed that staining does not affect the growth and metabolism of neurons. Sanger et al (27) have reported on carbonic anhydrase staining and cholinesterase staining of sensory and motor neurons, respectively. Carbonic anhydrase staining took 12 minutes, and cholinesterase staining took 1 hour. The stain persisted for 35 days in the proximal stump and 9 days in the distal stump. These techniques may aid in both immediate and delayed primary nerve repair. Direct nerve repair (neurorrhaphy) can be performed in different ways:

1. Epineurorrhaphy this means the stitches passed through the epineurium. This is the most common types of nerve suturing. Its main drawback is malalignment of the different nerve fascicles. The incidence of mismatching is higher than the other types of nerve suturing. Its advantages are less time consuming, avoid intraneural dissection and intraneural fibrosis. There is significant difference in the results when compared by other types of nerve suturing.
2. Perineurorrhaphy, this is means the suturing is passed through the perineurium. It decreases the incidence of the mismatching of nerve fascicles. It gives good nerve alignment. It is used in cases with deficient nerve sheath (epineurium).
3. Epiperineurorrhaphy, the needle passed through both the epineurium and perineurium. It gives strong coaptation. It provides better nerve alignment. It can be widely used in frersh cases (primary nerve repair).

3.1 Author preferred method

There is no significant difference in the result of nerve repair when the principles of neuromicrsurgery have been taken. The above 3 types of nerve repair can be used in one nerve repair. I prefer to do epineurorrhaphy in primary nerve repair, specially if the epineurium is intact (Fig 2). In cases with injured epineurium and the nerve is divided into group of fascicles, perineurorrhaphy is the good solution. In cases with delayed primary or even secondary nerve repair, the use of epiperineurorrhapy is the method of choice to have good suturing strength because of the fragility of nerve sheath.

4. Specific nerve repair

4.1 Radial nerve repair

The radial nerve arises from the posterior cord of the brachial plexus. It receives contributions from C5-8 spinal roots. It runs medial to the axillary artery. At the level of the coracobrachialis, it courses posteriorly to lie in the spiral groove of the humerus. In the lower arm, it pierces the lateral intermuscular septum to run between the brachialis and the brachioradialis. It divides 2 cm distal to the elbow into a superficial sensory branch and a deep motor branch, the PIN. The radial nerve gives off branches to the extensor carpi radialis longus and brevis, brachioradialis, and anconeus before giving off the PIN branch. The PIN continues on between the superficial and deep head of the supinator muscle, to exit on the dorsal forearm. After it emerges from the distal border of the supinator, the PIN sends branches to the extensor digitorum communis, extensor carpi ulnaris, extensor digiti quinti, extensor pollicis longus and brevis, and extensor indicis proprius in descending order, although there may be considerable variation.

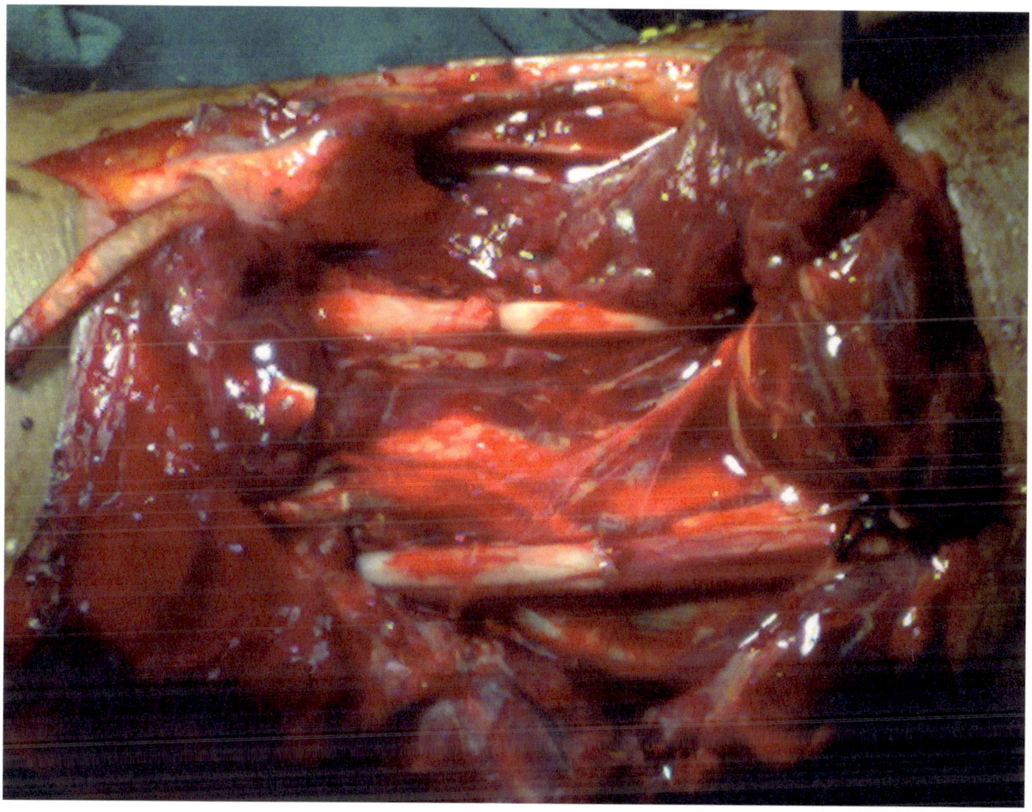

Fig. 2. Intraoperative photo showing epi-neurorrhaphy of both median and ulnar nerves at the musculotendinous junction of the forearm with cut of all the flexor tendons.

Radial nerve is the most common peripheral nerve to be injured. It travels for long distance so different levels of injuries are well known. It may vulnerable for injury in the axilla, along the arm, spiral groove posteriorly, lateral intermuscular septum laterally, between brachioradialis and brachialis anterioly, opposite to the radial head laterally, in the proximal forearm posteriorly and finally its sensory part in the forearm anteriorly. In this study, we present 62 patients who had radial nerve injuries. Forty eight were male and 14 were females. The average age of the patient was 26 years (ranged between 6-42 years). The right side was involved in 37 cases while 25 cases had left radial nerve injury. Motor car accident was responsible for the majority of lesion (32 patients), fire arm injuries was the next common cause of injury (15 patients), cut wound caused injury of 8 cases, while machine injury of the radial nerve occurred in 7 cases. Radial nerve injuries associated with fracture humerus occurred in 42 patients while isolated radial nerve injuries happened in 20 cases. The indication for radial nerve exploration were cut wound, firearm injuries, open fracture, postreduction injuries and cases with transverse fracture of the distal humerus. The mean time elapsed between injury and exploration was 12 hours (ranged between 2- 76 hours). The average surgical time 2.5 hours (ranged between 2-6 hours). The surgical procedures were neurolysis in 16 patients, epineurorraphy in 33 patients and nerve graft in 13 patients. We used nylon 10/0 for suturing under microscope in all cases of repair or graft. We used Medical research council grading for evaluation of wrist and finger extensors and sensation along the radial nerve sensory supply. Motor recovery of wrist and finger extensors was M5 in 60 patients (97%), M4 in one case and M3 in one patient. Sensory recovery was S3+ in 52 Patients, S3 in 7 patients and S2+ in 3 patients. The hand grip, hand pinch were the same as the non injured side. All the patients returned to their original activities. The time of recovery after surgery depend on the level of injury, the age of the patient and the type of surgical treatment. The average time of recovery was 7 month (ranged from 4 to 24 month). The average follow up was 12 years (Fig. 3,4).

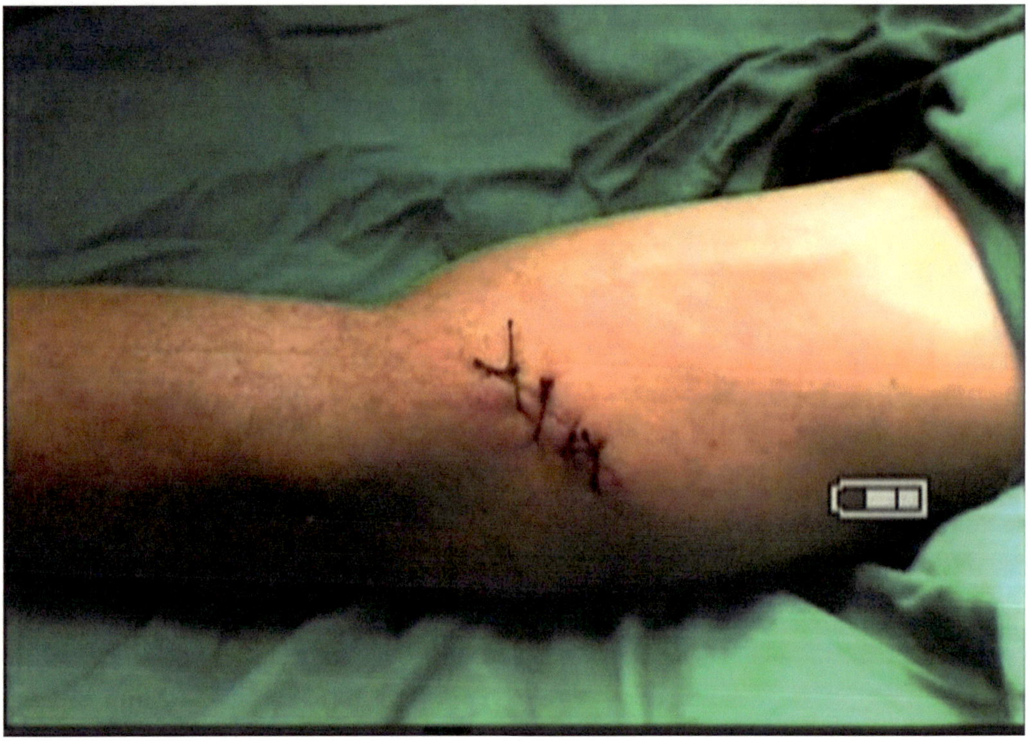

(a)

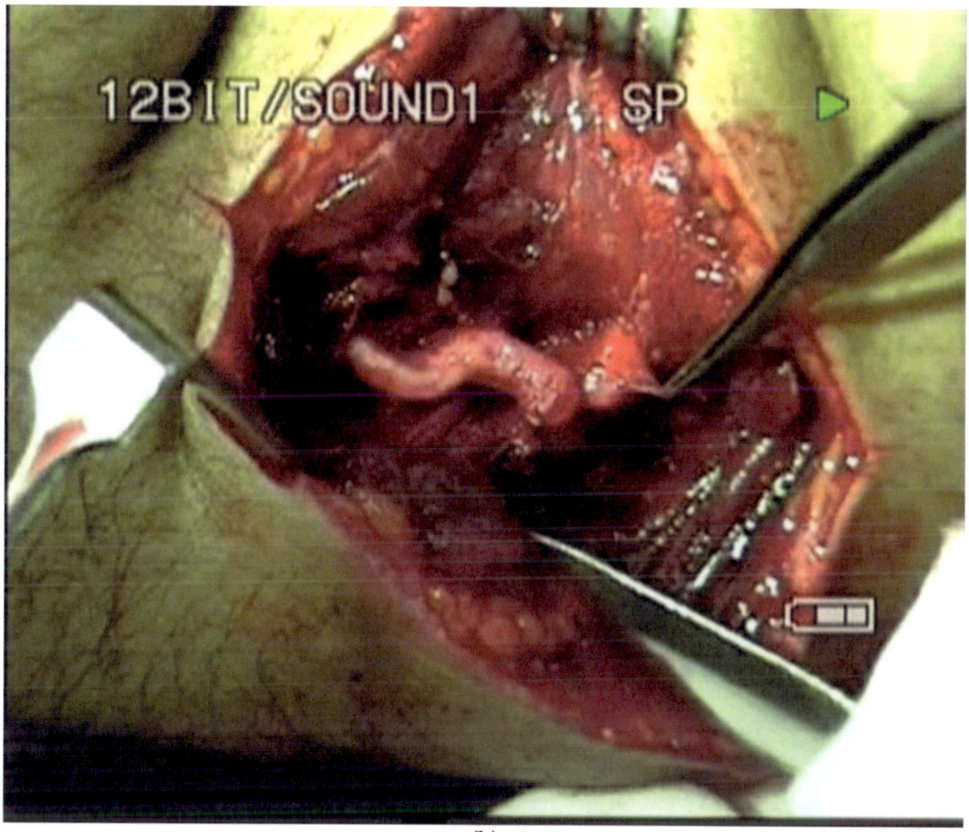

(b)

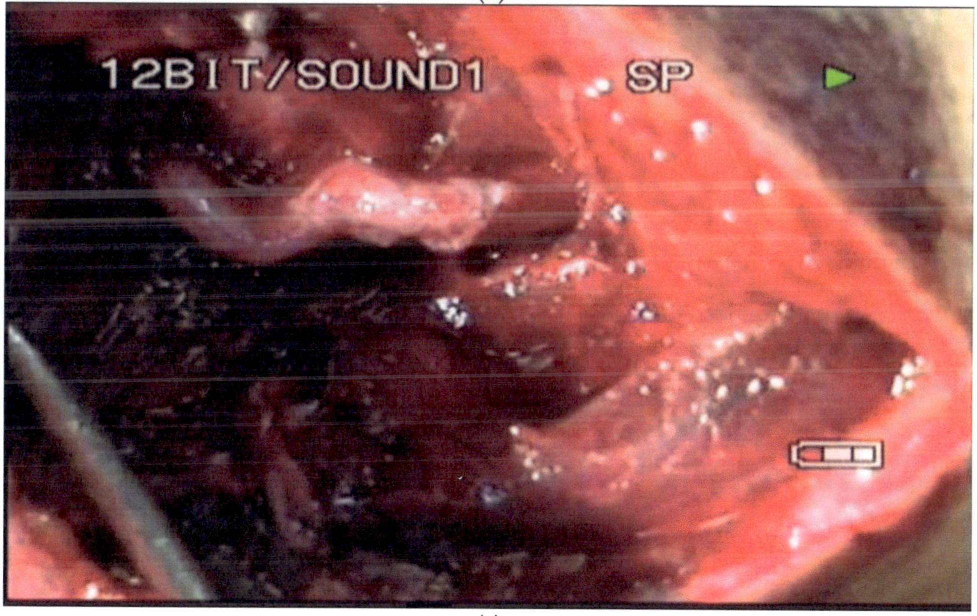

(c)

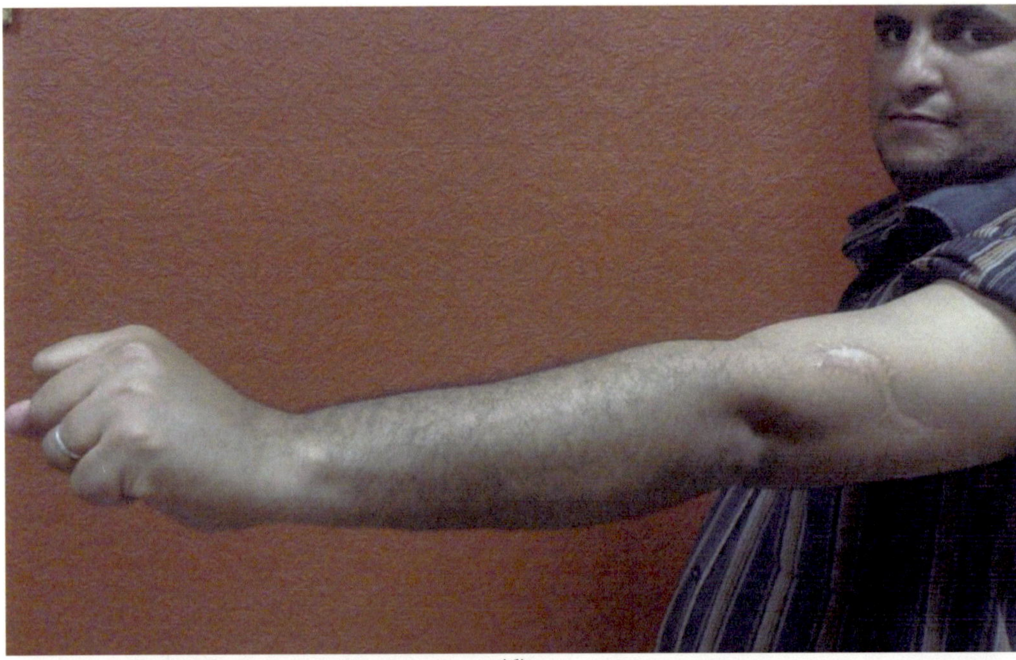

(d)

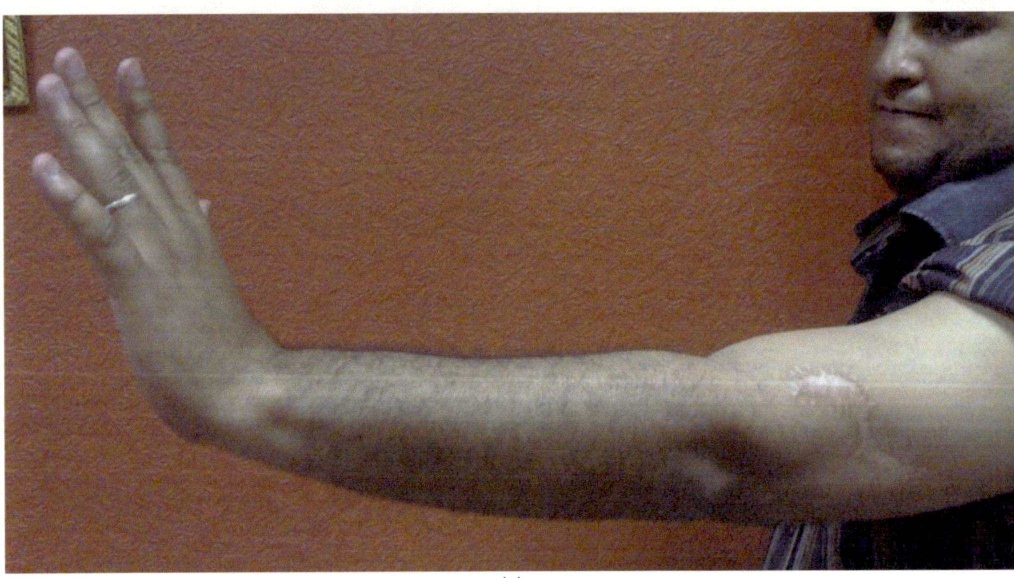

(e)

Fig. 3. Male patient 28 years old subjected to stab wound at distal left arm caused radial nerve injury, (a) Site of the stab wound with stitches. (b) Intraoperative photo showing complete transaction of the radial nerve. (c) Micro-epi-neurorrhaphy of he nerve. (d) 12 months of follow up with complete wrist extension. (e) 12 months of follow up with complete finger extension.

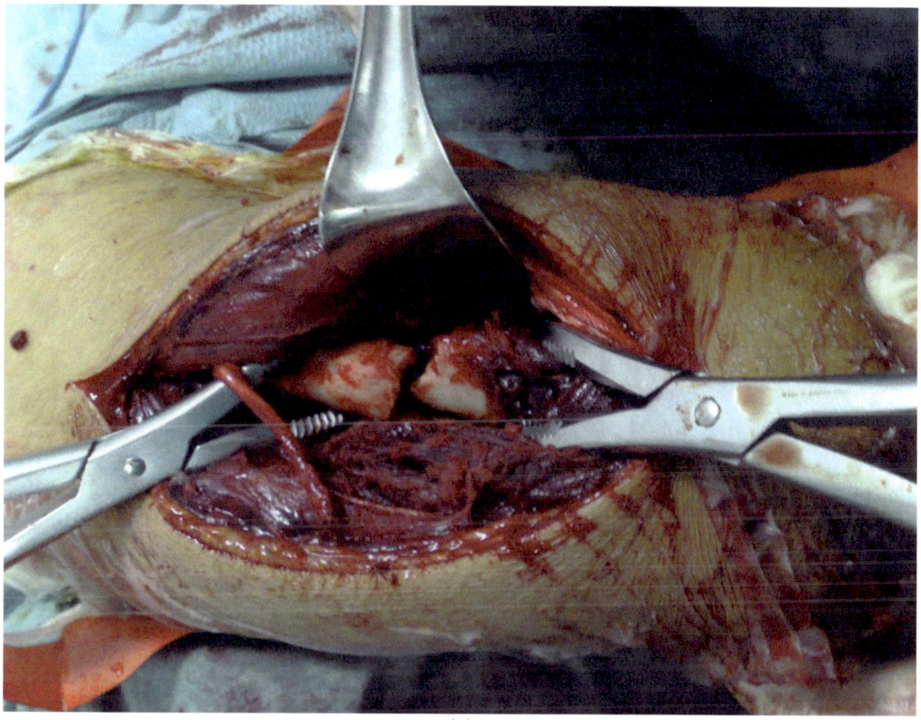

(a)

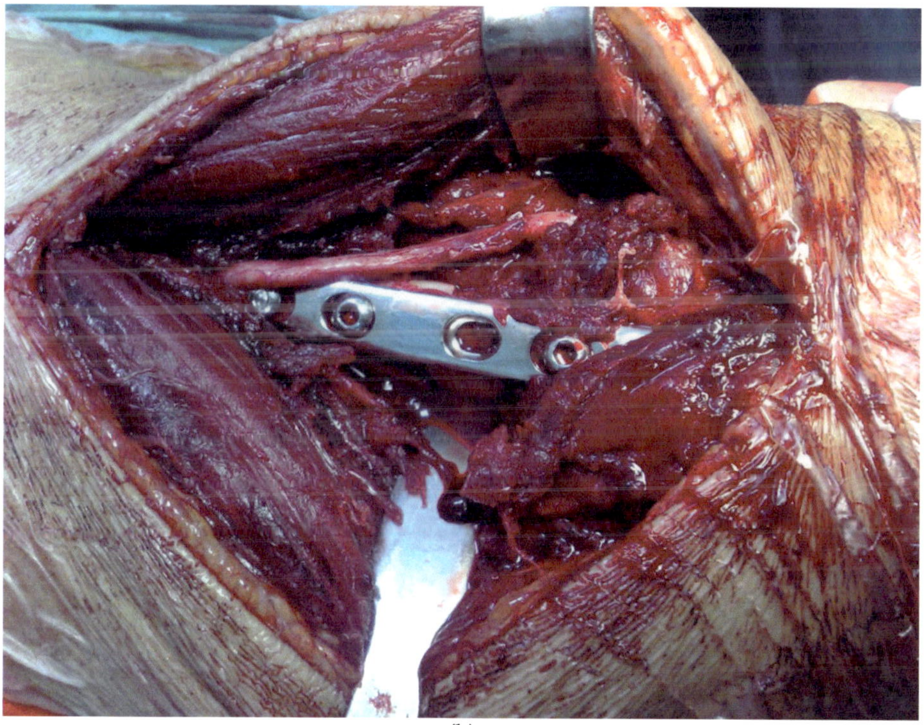

(b)

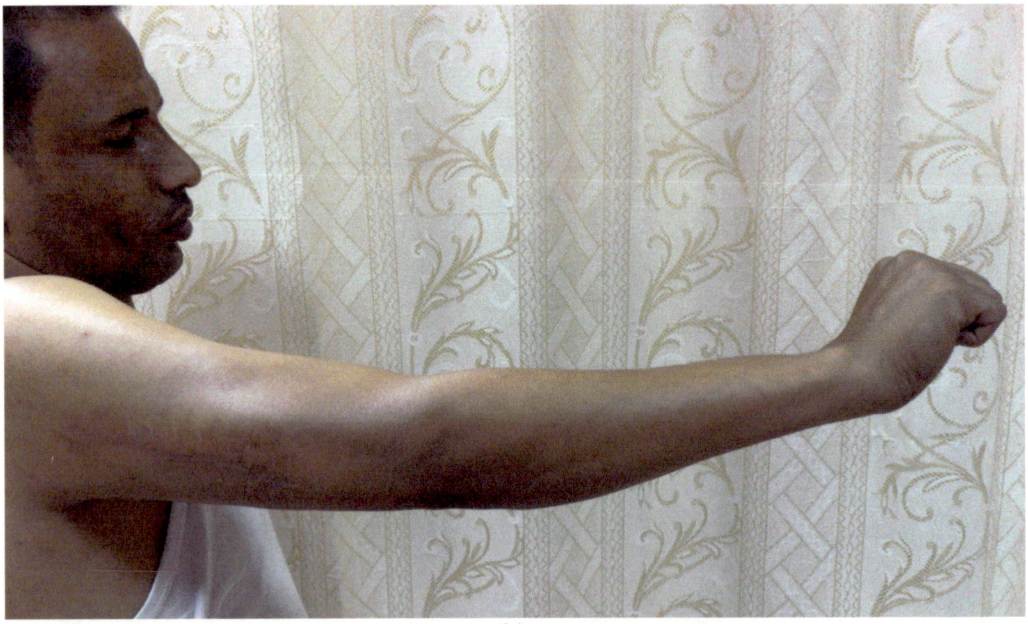

(c)

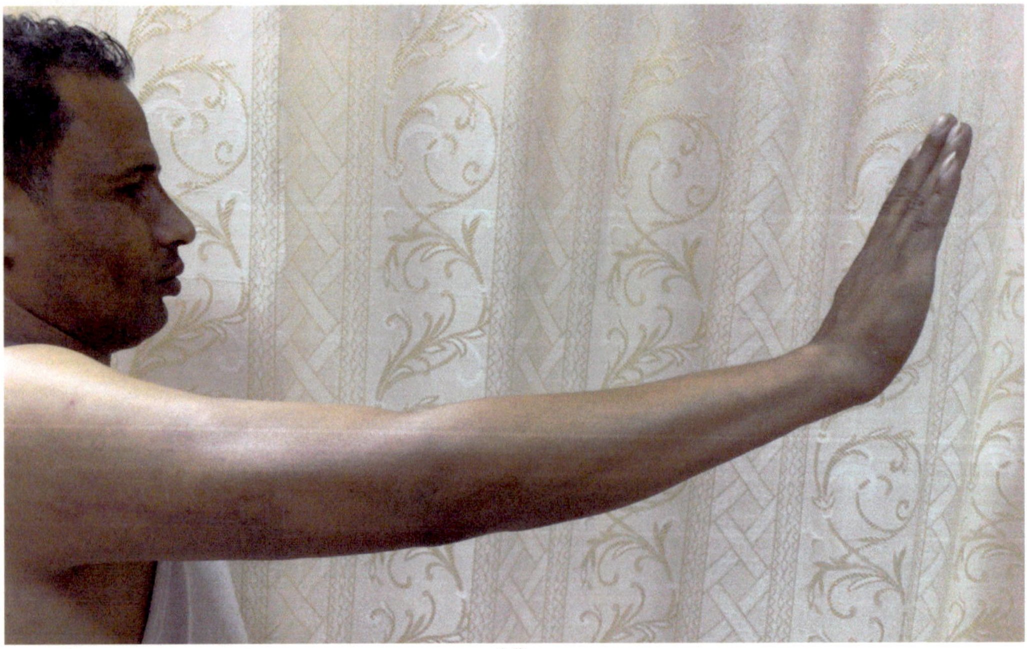

(d)

Fig. 4. Male patient 40 years old sustained motor car accident presented by fracture humerus with radial nerve injury, (a) early exploration revealed complete transaction of the radial nerve. (b) Micro-epi-neurorrhaphy after fixation of the humerus by plate and screws. (c) 9 months of follow up with complete wrist extension. (d) 9 months of follow up with complete finger extension.

5. Median nerve

5.1 Anatomy

The median nerve arises from the medial and lateral cords of the brachial plexus. It contains the nerve root fibers from C6-T1. It provides the motor supply to the pronator teres, the flexor digitorum sublimus, the palmaris longus, the flexor carpi radialis, the thenar muscles, and the radial two lumbricals. Its anterior interosseous branch supplies the flexor pollicus longus, the pronator quadratus, and the flexor digitorum profundus to the index and middle fingers. Its sensory distribution includes the palmar surface of the thumb, index, middle, and radial half of the ring finger. It lies lateral to the axillary artery, but then crosses medial to it at the level of the coracobrachialis. At the elbow, the median nerve travels behind the bicipital aponeurosis but in front of the brachialis. It enters the forearm between the two heads of the pronator teres and is adherent to the undersurface of the flexor digitorum sublimus muscle until it becomes superficial, 5 cm proximal to the wrist. It then passes underneath the carpal transverse ligament, giving off the recurrent motor branch and sensory branches to the thumb and fingers.

5.2 Above elbow

Median nerve injury is uncommon above the elbow. We present 12 patients who have median nerve injury above the elbow. Three patients had broken glass injury, 4 cases had firearm injuries and 5 cases associated with fractures around elbow. Exploration was performed for 10 cases while two patients recovered spontaneously. Primary repair was performed for 8 cases while 2 cases were repaired within one week of the trauma. The mean follow up was 7 years. The time of recovery was ranged from 6-12 month postoperatively. We used both Medical Research Council Grading and Noaman scoring system for evaluation of wrist and finger flexors, intrinsic muscles supplied by the median nerve, hand grip, lateral key pinch, opposition, hand deformity, and sensation. All patients had wrist and finger flexors M5, good opposition, normal hand grip, lateral key pinch and S3.

5.3 Below elbow

The most common cause of median nerve injury at our locality is broken glass; the next cause is firearm injuries while motor car accident with crushed forearm is not uncommon. We treated 40 patients who had median nerve injuries below elbow from 1999 to 2010. Twenty six were male and 14 were famales. Twenty two patients presented by cut wound caused by broken glass associated with muscles and musculotendinous injuries. Primary repair was performed in all cases. Time elapsed between injury and exploration was ranged from 2 to 6 hours. Eight cases had firearm injury. Open fracture radius was involved in 4 cases while fracture proximal ulna and radius was involved in one case. Debridement, open reduction and internal fixation and median nerve epineurorrhaphy were performed for 5 cases while debridement and epineurorrhaphy were performed for 3 cases. Seven cases had median nerve injury below the elbow caused by motor car accident. There were forearm complex injuries, i.e injuries of bone, muscles tendons, nerves, vessels and skin. Debridement, bone stabilization, vascular repair, nerve repair, and tendon repair were performed consequently. Machine injury was the leading cause in the remaining 2 cases of median nerve injury with complex forearm injuries.

Wrist and finger flexors were M5 in 28 (70%) patients (Fig. 5), M4 in 10 (25%) and M3 in 2 patients. S3 was gained in 32 (80%), and S2+ in 8 patients. Hand grip was 90% in 32 (80%), and 75% in 8 (20%) patients.

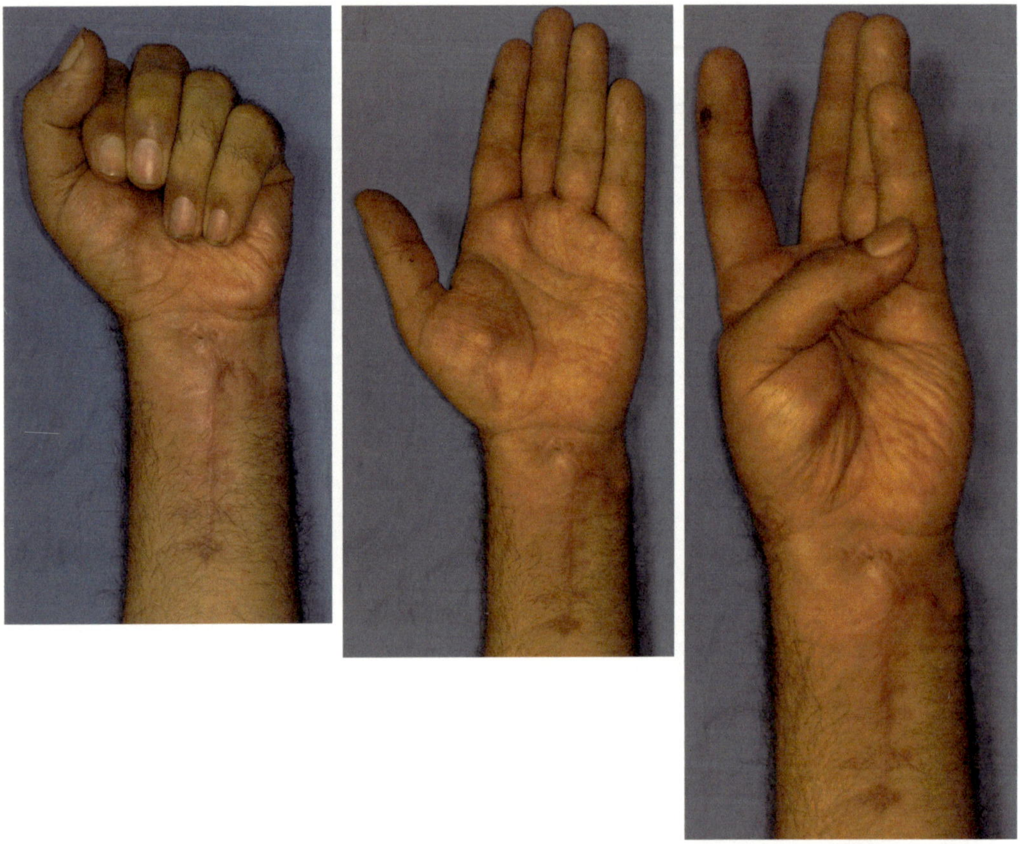

(a) (b) (c)

Fig. 5. Male patient 32 years old had cut wound at mid- forearm presented by median nerve injury. Primary exploration of the median nerve and repair were done. Post operative follow up after 24 month showed: (a) Complete finger flexion. (b) Complete finger extension. (c) Normal thumb opposition.

5.4 Median nerve injury at wrist

It is rarely to have isolated median nerve injury at the wrist. It is usually associated with injuries of one or more of the following structures; flexor tendons, radial artery, ulnar nerve, ulnar vessels and bone (distal radius and/or carpal bones). A retrospective review of 42 patients with spaghetti wrist lacerations operated on by the author between June 1997 and May 2005 was completed. A total of 31 males and 11 females, average age of 17.1 years (range, 2–40 years), sustained spaghetti wrist injuries. The most frequent mechanisms of injury were accidental glass lacerations (55%), knife wounds (24%), and electrical saw injuries (11%). An average of 9.16 structures was injured, including 6.95 tendons, 1.4 nerves, and 0.8 arteries. The most frequently injured structures were median nerve (83%), flexor digitorum superficialis 2-4 tendons (81%), flexor digitorum profundus 2-4 tendons (66%), ulnar nerve and ulnar artery (57%), and flexor pollicis longus (40%). Combined flexor carpi ulnaris, ulnar nerve, and ulnar artery (ulnar triad) injuries occurred in 31%, while combined median nerve, palmaris longus, and flexor carpi radialis injuries (radial triad) occurred in 43%. Simultaneous injuries of both median and ulnar nerves occurred in 40.5%. Simultaneous injuries of both ulnar and radial arteries occurred in 14%. Neither artery was injured in 30.9%. Follow-up has ranged from 1 to 8 years, with an average of 46 months. Only four patients have been completely lost to follow-up. Range of motion of all involved digits (tendon function) was excellent in 34 patients, good in 3 patients, and poor in only one patient. Opposition was excellent in 31 patients, good in 5 patients, and poor in 2 patients. Intrinsic muscle recovery was subjectively reported to be excellent in 29 patients, good in 7, and fair to poor in 2 patients. Minor deformity (partial clawing) was reported in 4 patients and one patient has major deformity (total clawing). Sensory recovery was reported, excellent in 32 patients, good in 5 patients, and fair in only one patient (Table 1) [28].

	Tendon function	Opposition	Intrinsics	Deformities	Sensation
Excellent	Individual tendon function was evident with 85% to full range of motion or finger flexion to 1.0 cm or less from the distal palmer crease	When the tip of the thumb moves freely over the three phalanges of the other four fingers	When the patient can do both finger abduction and adduction with -ve froment sign	Major if there is both clawing and ape hand	When the two point discrimination is less than 10 mm
Good	70-84% total normal range of motion or 2.0 cm from the distal palmer crease	When the tip of the thumb touches only the tip of the other four fingers	When the patient can do both finger abduction and adduction with +ve froment sign		When the two point discrimination is 10-20 mm
Fair	50-69% total normal range of motion	When the tip of the thumb cannot reach the tip of the other four fingers	When the patient can do either finger abduction or adduction with +ve froment sign	Minor if there is either clawing or ape hand	When the two point discrimination is more than 20 mm with light touch and pain prick sensation
Poor	Fixed contractures or adhesions		When the patient cannot do finger abduction or adduction with +ve froment sign		When there is trophic changes or skin ulceration

Table 1. Noaman's evaluation system for follow up results of spaghetti wrist

6. Ulnar nerve

The ulnar nerve arises from the medial cord of the brachial plexus. It contains the nerve root fibers from C8-T1. It provides the motor supply to the hypothenar muscles, the ulnar two lumbricals, the interosseous muscles, the adductor pollicis, the FCU, and the profundus to the ring and small fingers. Its sensory distribution includes the palmar surface of the small finger, the ulnar half of the ring finger, and the dorsoulnar carpus. It lies medial to the axillary artery and continues distally to the midarm, where it pierces the medial intermuscular septum. The nerve often is accompanied by the superior ulnar collateral artery. At the elbow, it lies between the medial epicondyle and the olecranon, where it is covered by Osborne's ligament. It enters the forearm between the two heads of the FCU covered by a fibrous aponeurosis (the cubital tunnel). It runs deep to the FCU until the distal forearm. At the wrist, it passes over the transverse carpal ligament, medial to the ulnar artery through Guyon's canal. The deep motor branch is given off at the pisiform and passes underneath a fibrous arch to lie on the palmar surface of the interossei. It crosses the palm deep to the flexor tendons, to terminate in the adductor pollicis and ulnar head of the flexor pollicis brevis.

6.1 Ulnar nerve injury above elbow

It is manifested by partial claw hand, loss of finger adduction and abduction, positive Froment test, loss of sensation over the medial one third of the palm and medial one and half fingers (Fig. 6). Retrospectively, we treated 22 cases of ulnar nerve injury above the elbow by microneurorrhaphy. Median, radial and musculocutaneous nerve injuries were also involved in 7 cases. Cut wound was responsible for 10 cases, firearm injuries in 4 cases, post reduction injury of supracondylar fracture humerus in 4 cases, machine injury in 3 cases, and motor car accident with open fracture humerus in one patient. The mean age was 23 years. Right side was injured in 14 patients. Primary repair was performed for all patients. The mean follow up was 46 months. We used British medical research council grading system for both motor and sensory evaluation and Noaman(28) evaluation system for intrinsic function . Wrist and finger flexors were M5 in 7 cases, M4 in 9 cases and M3 in 6 cases. Sensation was S3 in 10 patients, S2+ in 9 patients and S2 in 3 patients. Hand grip was 80% in 15 patients, 70% in 5 patients and 60% in 2 patients.

6.2 Below elbow

Retrospectively, we treated 27 cases of ulnar nerve injury below elbow by microneurorrhaphy. Median nerve was involved in 12 patients. Cut wound was responsible for 15 cases, firearm injuries in 6 cases, machine injury in 3 cases, and motor car accident with open fracture radius and ulna in three patients. The mean age was 23 years. Right side was injured in 11 patients. Primary repair was performed for all patients. The mean follow up was 42 months. We used British medical research council grading system for both motor and sensory evaluation and Noaman evaluation system for intrinsic function. Wrist and finger flexors were M5 in 15 cases, M4 in 8 cases and M3 in 4 cases. Sensation was S3 in 18 patients, S2+ in 7 patients and S2 in 2 patients. Hand grip was 80% in 16 patients, 70% in 9 patients and 60% in 2 patients.

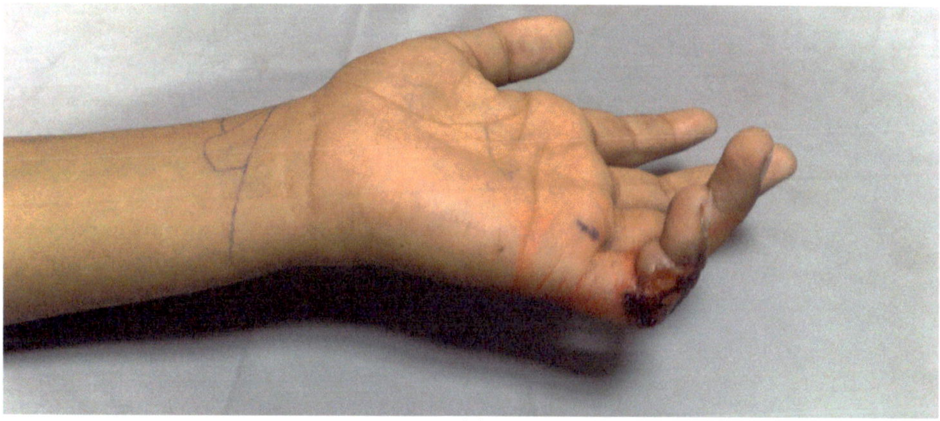

(a)

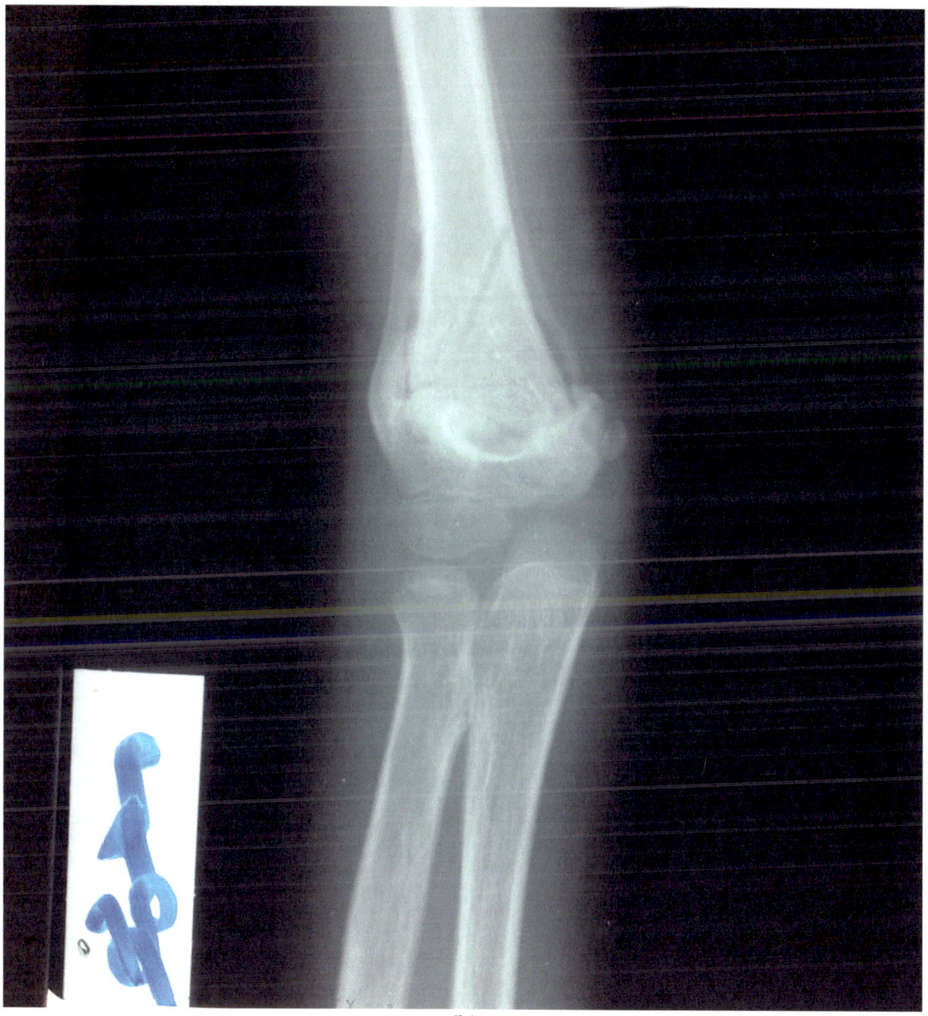

(b)

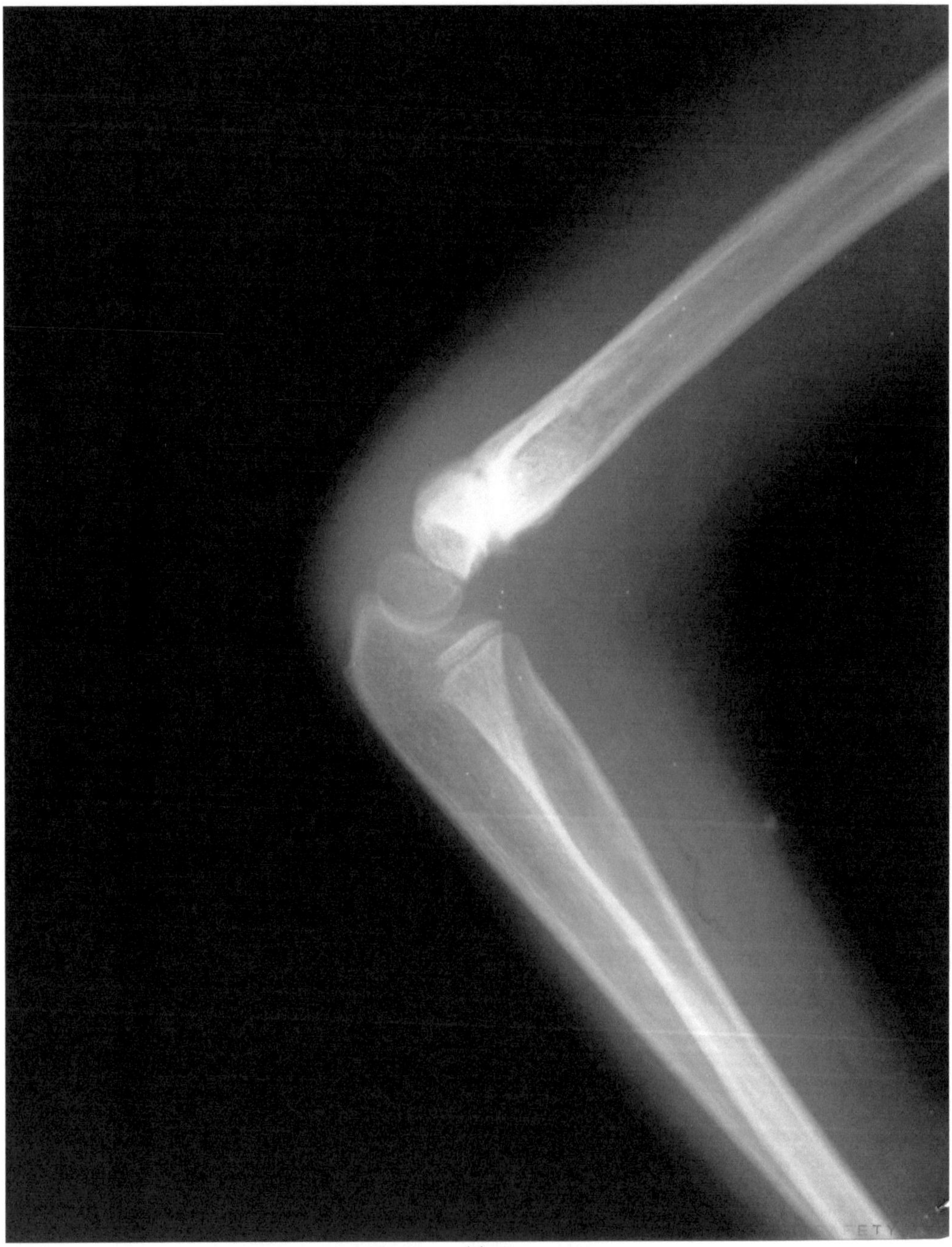

(c)

Fig. 6. Male patient 9 years old presented by ulnar nerve injury after percutaneous pinning of supracondylar fracture humerus, (a) Clinical manifestation of partial claw hand with trophic ulcer of the little finger. (B) And (C) antero-posterior and lateral views of the x-ray elbow with complete union of the supracondylar fracture humerus.

6.3 At the wrist

The ulnar nerve usually associated with other soft tissues (including tendons, vessels, and median nerve) at the wrist.

7. Sciatic nerve

Fortunately, the incidence of sciatic nerve injury is uncommon because its recovery (conservatively or after surgery) does not like the recovery of other peripheral nerves. This is most likely due to highly mixed nerve, thick nerve and very long nerve. The causes of sciatic nerve injury are variable. It is vulnerable for injury in cases of fracture acetabulum specially posterior column and posterior wall acetabulum fracture. Posterior hip dislocation, central hip fracture dislocation can be associated with sciatic nerve injury. These can be induced by motor car accident, fire arm injuries and falling from height. Iatrogenic sciatic nerve injury is the next common cause of sciatic nerve injury. It can be happened during posterior exposure of the hip e.g. (open reduction and internal fixation of fracture acetabulum, total hip replacement and even hemiarthroplasty). I noticed sciatic nerve injury after plate and screw fixation for fracture shaft femur. Sciatic nerve injury from intramuscular (gluteal) injection also is not uncommon.

The manifestations of sciatic nerve injury are variable. Usually the branches to the hamstring muscles (knee extensors) take off from the sciatic nerve before its vulnerable for injury. This is mean that the manifestations of sciatic nerve injury appear below the knee (flail ankle and loss of superficial and deep sensation over the leg and foot).

7.1 Tibial nerve injury

The tibial nerve is the larger of the two terminal branches of the sciatic nerve which separate about the middle of the back of the thigh. It supplies the muscles of the back of the leg and the sole of the foot, and the skin of the lower half of the back of the leg and the lateral side and sole of the foot. It is vulnerable to injury in cases with fracture lower femur and proximal tibia caused by high energy trauma e.g. motor car accident, falling from height, fire arm injury also caused tibial nerve injury without fracture. Cut wound in the popliteal fossa also can cause tibial nerve injury which is usually associated with popliteal artery injury.

The incidence of tibial nerve injury is not common. We treated 7 cases of tibial nerve injury from 1998 to 2010. Five cases were male and 2 cases were male. The average age was 13 years. The affected site was right side in 5 cases and left in 2 cases. The causative agent was fire arm injury in 3 cases, motor car accident in 2 cases and cut wound in 2 cases. Neurolysis was performed in 3 cases, repair in 3 cases and nerve graft in one case. The average follow up was 124 month. Plantar flexors of the ankle and toes were G5 in 2 cases of neurolysis, G4 in 3 cases, one of them had neurolysis and 2 had nerve repair, G3 in 2 cases (one treated by nerve repair and one treated by nerve graft). Sensation was gained in 7 cases.

7.2 Common peroneal nerve

This nerve is smaller than the tibial nerve. It supplies the muscles on the lateral and anterior surfaces of the leg and the dorsum of the foot and skin on the lateral side of the leg and the greater part of the dorsum of the foot.

It is usually vulnerable for injury because it is superficial and runs around the neck of the fibula. The causes of injury are the same like tibial nerve injury in addition to causes of entrapment neuropathy. It is common to be injured during squatting position so common in painters, farmers, and carpenters.

We treated 12 cases of common peroneal nerve injuries in the last 12 years. Six cases had entrapment neuropathy which did not recovered conservatively. Neurolysis was performed and full motor nad sensory recovery were gained 36 month postoperatively. Six cases treated by nerve repair, followed up to 54 month. Motor recovery was G5 in 2 cases, G4 in 3 cases and G3 in one case. Sensory recovery was satisfactory.

8. Methods to overcome nerve defect

There are several methods of closing gaps between nerve ends without appreciable damage to the nerve itself. The methods most often used are mobilization of the nerve ends and positioning of the extremity. Other methods include nerve transplantation, bone resection, bulb suture, nerve grafting, and nerve crossing (pedicle grafting).

1. Mobilization

It means lysis of the nerve through its course and to cut off small insignificant branches which tend to fix it through its pathway. It can be done to proximal and distal stump. It provides sufficient length in some cases. It needs wide nerve exposure.Most small gaps can be closed by mobilizing the nerve ends for a few centimeters proximal and distal to the point of injury. Mobilization of both nerve ends to some degree is required in all peripheral neurorrhaphies [(4)]. The exact amount of mobilization a peripheral nerve can tolerate before its regenerating potential is compromised is unknown; however, extensive dissection of a nerve from its surrounding tissues does disrupt the segmental blood supply, causing subsequent ischemia and increased intraneural scarring. Starkweather et al [(29)]. showed that mobilization is more detrimental to the distal nerve segment, as manifested by increased intraneural collagen production and collagen cross-linking. Seddon [(3)] suggested that extensive mobilization adversely affects recovery after median nerve repairs in the forearm. They found that if the gap was less than 2.5 cm, motor recovery was to the M3 level or better in 70%, whereas if the gap was 2.6 to 5 cm and required extensive mobilization, recovery was to the M3 level or better in only 50%. Large gaps require extensive dissection of the nerve from its adjacent tissues for a relatively tension-free epineurial repair. Before subjecting a peripheral nerve to extensive dissection, the surgeon should have some idea of the maximal nerve gap over which mobilization may become a futile endeavor. The nerve gap is determined at the time of surgery with the extremity in the anatomical position and after distal and proximal neuroma excision. Certain guidelines, although extremely variable, are found in the literature. Zachary [(30)] showed that the median and ulnar nerves can be mobilized 7 to 9 cm, and with anterior transposition an ulnar nerve gap of 13 cm can be overcome. Wilgis [(31)] cautioned against extensive mobilization to overcome gaps greater than 4 cm. Millesi [(32)] recommended that defects greater than 2.5 cm be treated by interfascicular nerve grafting rather than by extensive mobilization and positioning.

2. Positioning

Relaxing nerves by flexing various joints and occasionally by other maneuvers, such as abducting, adducting, rotating, and elevating the extremity, is as important as mobilization in closing large gaps in nerves. Through use of both methods, long gaps can be closed in nearly all of the peripheral nerves, and many unsatisfactory neurorrhaphies result from failure to make the most of their possibilities. When joints that are excessively flexed or awkwardly positioned are mobilized later, tension on the neurorrhaphy may be too great and may cause intraneural fibrosis that compromises axonal regeneration. Consequently, a joint should never be flexed forcibly to obtain end-to-end suture. It is a reasonable policy to flex the knee and elbow no more than 90 degrees. Also, flexion of the wrist more than 40 degrees is probably unwise. After the wound has healed sufficiently, the joint can be extended about 10 degrees per week until motion is regained. Flexing joints is most important in repairing gaps in the long nerves of the extremities. External rotation and abduction are helpful when repairing radial and axillary nerves, as in elevation of the shoulder girdle in brachial plexus injuries. Rarely, extension of a joint can be helpful, as in extension of the hip in sciatic injuries. Strong consideration should be given to nerve grafting in preference to drastic positioning of the extremity to produce a tension-free neurorrhaphy (4).

3. Nerve transposition

The anatomical course of some nerves can be changed to shorten the distance between severed ends. This is true especially of the ulnar nerve at the elbow. The median nerve also can be transposed anterior to the pronator teres if the lesion is distal to its branches to the long flexor muscles of the forearm, and the tibial nerve can be placed superficial to the soleus or gastrocnemius in the leg if the lesion is distal to its branches to the calf muscles. Most surgeons recommend transposition of the proximal end of the radial nerve anterior to the humerus and deep to the biceps to obtain needed length. Considerable length can be gained in most patients by the simpler maneuver of externally rotating the arm, provided that the mobilization has been carried into the axilla, and that the branches of the radial nerve to the triceps muscle have been dissected well up the nerve (4).

4. Bone shortening

In civilian injuries, bone resection almost never should be necessary to accomplish neurorrhaphy. Even in war wounds, it rarely was employed, and when it was used, it usually was because the joints of the extremity had become so stiff from immobilization caused by fracture or injudicious use of casts that limited flexion. Intact long bones and most bones in children rarely if ever should be shortened to aid in nerve repair. Bone resection is of particular value in the upper arm for closing large gaps in the ulnar, radial, or median nerves when the humerus already has been fractured. If early delayed suture is done in such patients before the fracture has healed, shortening the bone if necessary is not difficult. After the fracture has healed, however, osteotomy is more difficult. It rarely is worthwhile to shorten the femur in injuries of the sciatic nerve, unless this bone already has been fractured; shortening of the bone can be helpful. Both bones of the forearm or leg in the absence of a fracture should never be shortened (4).

5. Nerve graft

Interfascicular nerve grafting as described by Seddon (3) (and later by Millesi (32) is indicated when primary nerve repair cannot be done without excessive tension. In general, a nerve gap that is caused simply by elastic retraction usually can be overcome with local nerve mobilization, limited joint positioning, and primary repair. If the defect is caused in part by loss of nerve tissue, however, nerve grafting is our procedure of choice. When primary repair cannot be performed without undue tension, nerve grafting is required. Autografts remain the standard for nerve grafting material. Allografts have not shown recovery equivalent to that obtained with autogenous nerve and are still considered experimental. The three major types of autograft are cable, trunk, and vascularized nerve grafts. Cable grafts are multiple small-caliber nerve grafts aligned in parallel to span a gap between fascicular groups. Trunk grafts are mixed motor-sensory whole-nerve grafts (e.g., an ulnar nerve in the case of an irreparable brachial plexus injury). Trunk grafts have been associated with poor functional results, in large part due to the thickness of the graft and consequent diminished ability to revascularize after implantation. Vascularized nerve grafts have been used in the past, but with conflicting results. They may be considered if a long graft is needed in a poorly vascularized bed. Because donor-site morbidity is an issue, vascularized grafts have been most widely utilized in irreversible brachial plexus injuries. Autogenous sural nerve is the preferred source of graft. We do not use vascularized nerve grafts, trunk grafts, or allografts. The most common source of autograft is the sural nerve (Fig. 7), which is easily obtainable, the appropriate diameter for most cable grafting needs, and relatively dispensable. Other graft sources include the anterior branch of the medial antebrachial cutaneous nerve, the lateral femoral cutaneous nerve, and the superficial radial sensory nerve. The technique of nerve grafting involves sharply transecting the injured nerve ends to excise the zone of injury (Fig. 8). The nerve ends should display a good fascicular pattern. The defect is measured, and the appropriate length of graft is harvested to allow reconstruction without tension. If the injured nerve has a large diameter relative to the nerve graft, several cable grafts are placed in parallel to reconstruct the nerve. The grafts are matched to corresponding fascicles and sutured to the injured nerve with epineurial sutures, as in the primary neurorrhaphy technique (Fig. 9). Fibrin glue may be used to connect the cable grafts, thus decreasing the number of sutures and minimizing additional trauma to the nerve grafts. The surgeon can make fibrin glue intraoperatively by mixing thrombin and fibrinogen in equal parts, as originally described by Narakas [33]. Although nerve grafts have not generally been considered polarized, it is recommended that the graft be placed in a reversed orientation in the repair site. Reversal of the nerve graft decreases the chance of axonal dispersion through distal nerve branches. A well-vascularized bed is critical for nerve grafting. The graft should be approximately 10% to 20% longer than the gap to be filled, as the graft inevitably shortens with connective tissue fibrosis. From their clinical experience, Millesi et al [34] reported good results using an interfascicular nerve autografting technique to close gaps without undue tension. In the upper extremity especially, good results were achieved in repairing injuries to the digital, median, ulnar, and radial nerves. Of 38 patients with median nerve grafts, 82% achieved useful motor recovery (M3 or better), and all but 1 regained protective sensibility. Of 39 patients with ulnar nerve grafts, all achieved useful motor recovery (M2+ or better), and 28% regained 2-point discrimination. Of 13 patients with radial nerve grafts, 77% achieved an M4 or M5 level of function.

9. Allografts

Allografts have several potential clinical advantages: (1) grafts can be banked; (2) there is no need for sacrifice of a donor nerve; and (3) surgical procedures are quicker without the need to harvest a graft. However, allografts are not as effective as autografts, mainly due to the immunogenic host response. Ansselin and Pollard [35] studied rat allograft nerves and found an increase in helper T cells and cytotoxic/suppressor T cells, implying immunogenic rejection. The cellular component of allografts.and with it, their immunogenicity.can be destroyed by freeze-thawing. This leads to the production of cell debris, which in turn impairs neurite outgrowth. Dumont and Hentz [36] reported on a biologic detergent technique that removes the immunogenic cellular components without forming cell debris. Their experiments in rats have shown that allografts processed with this detergent had equivalent post repair results compared with autografts.

9.1 Role of the nerve graft

The nerve graft acts to provide a source of empty endoneurial tubes through which the regenerating axons can be directed. Any tissue that contains a basil lamina, such as freeze-dried muscle or tendon, can be substituted [37], but only the autogenous nerve graft also provides a source of viable Schwann cells. To be effective, the graft must acquire a blood supply. If the nerve graft survives, the Schwann cells also survive [38].

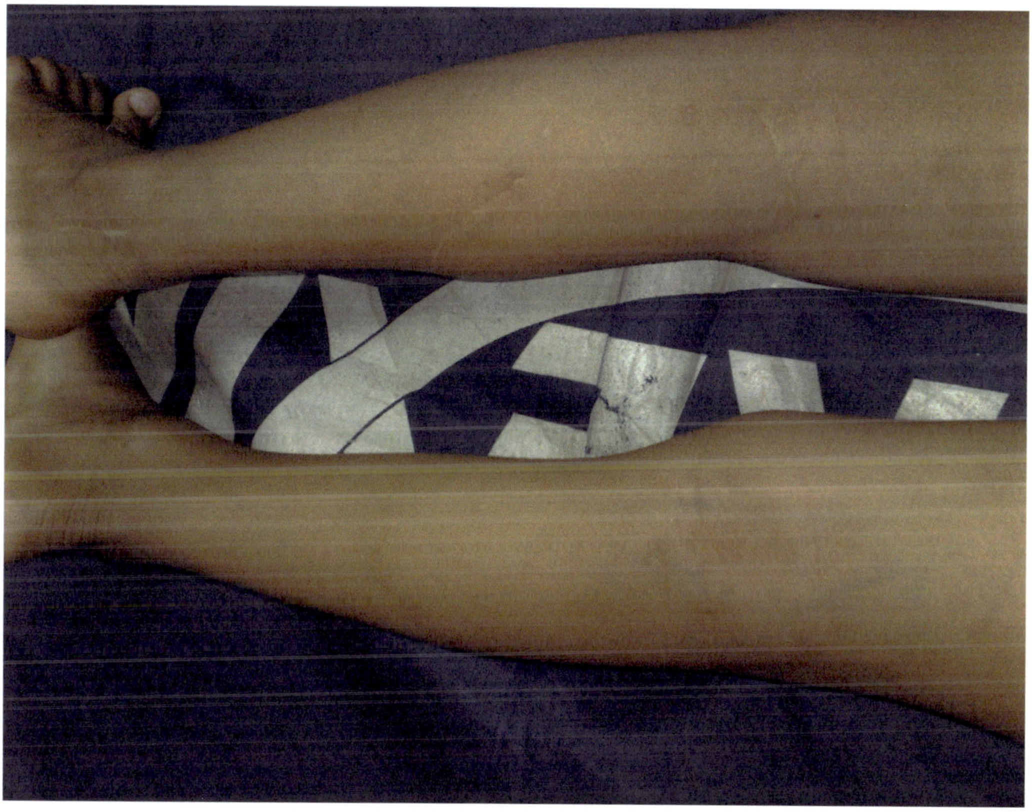

Fig. 7. Post operative photo showing a nice scar after sural nerve taken from both legs.

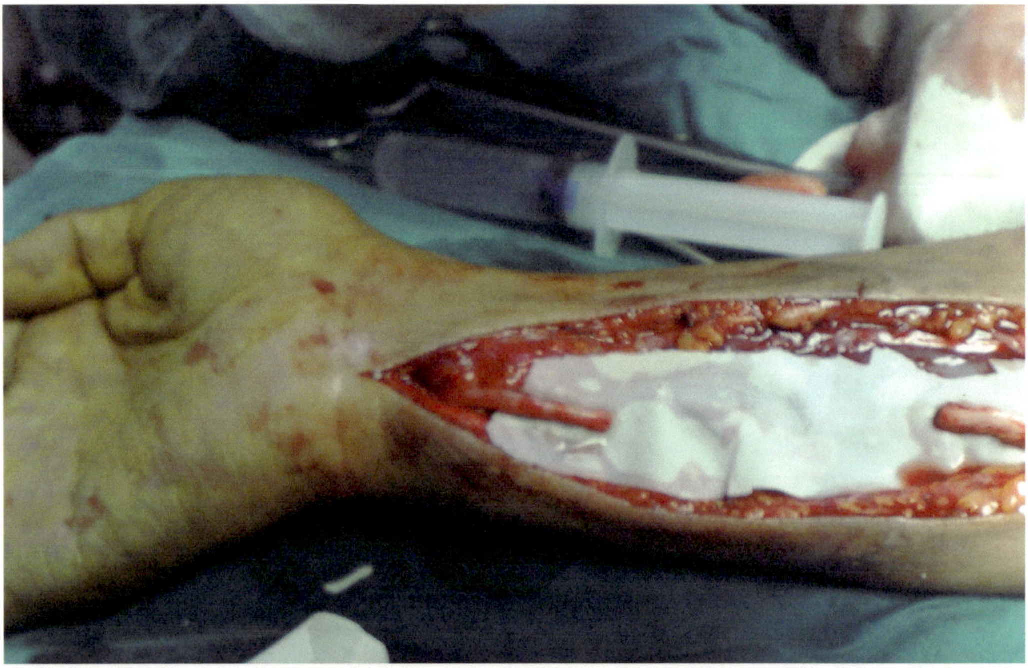

Fig. 8. Intra-operative photo showing a long median nerve defect at the forearm.

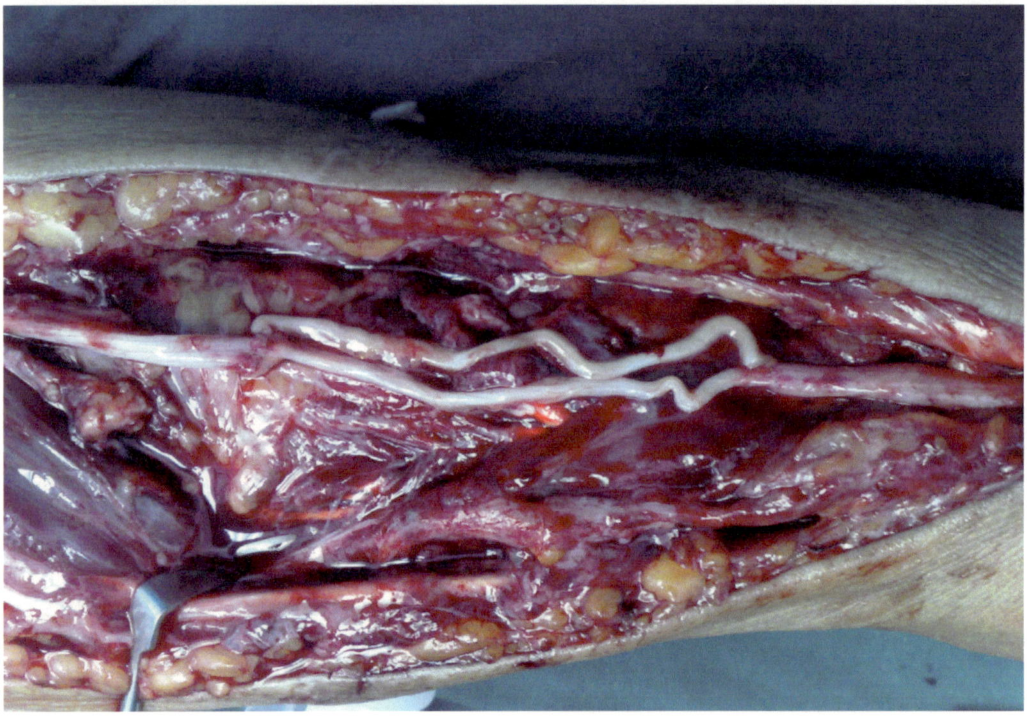

Fig. 9. Intraoperative photo showing 2 cable grafts bridging the median nerve defect with micro-epi-neurorrhaphy at both sides of the graft.

9.2 Graft incorporation

When separated from its blood supply, the graft undergoes wallerian degeneration. Schwann cells can survive 7 days, depending purely on diffusion (39). By 3 days after implantation, there is invasion of the nerve graft by endothelial buds from the surrounding tissue bed, with evidence of high nerve blood flows by 1 week (40,41). This segmental vascular sprouting from extraneural vessels is not limited by the length of the graft (42,43). The length of the graft is, within certain limits, of no significance to the end result, provided that there is a tension-free anastomosis.

The ingrowth of vessels from the ends of the graft (inosculation) does not seem to be of major importance, unless the recipient bed is poorly vascularized . The late phase of nerve graft incorporation shows migration of Schwann cells from the proximal nerve end into the graft and from the graft into both host nerve ends (44).

9.3 Graft diameter

Small-diameter grafts spontaneously revascularize, but large-diameter grafts do so incompletely (45). Thick grafts undergo central necrosis with subsequent endoneurial fibrosis. This fibrosis ultimately impedes the advancement of any ingrowing axon sprouts. Cable nerve grafts are similar to thick grafts. They consist of numerous nerve grafts that are sutured or glued together to match the caliber of the recipient nerve. Because a large percentage of the surface is in contact with another graft and not in contact with the recipient bed, the central portions may not revascularize. With large-diameter recipient nerves, it is preferable to use multiple smaller caliber grafts to bridge fascicular groups in the proximal and distal stumps to increase the surface area that is in contact with the recipient bed (45).

9.4 Nerve biomechanics

A normal nerve has longitudinal excursion, which subjects it to a certain amount of stress and strain in situ. Peripheral nerve is initially easily extensible. It rapidly becomes stiff with further elongation as a result of the stretching of the connective tissue within the nerve. Chronically injured nerves become even stiffer. Elasticity decreases by 50% in the delayed repair of nerves in which wallerian degeneration has occurred. Experimentally, blood flow is reduced by 50% when the nerve is stretched 8% beyond its in vivo length. Complete ischemia occurs at 15%. Suture pullout does not occur until a 17% increase in length; this suggests that ischemia and not disruption of the anastomosis is the limiting factor in acute nerve repair. This observation also is applicable to nerve grafting. Nerve is a viscoelastic tissue in that when low loading in tension is applied over time, the nerve elongates, without deterioration in nerve conduction velocities. Stress relaxation results in recovery of blood flow within 30 minutes at 8% elongation. Intriguing experimental work has been done with gradual nerve elongation to overcome nerve gaps using tissue expansion and external fixation, but this cannot be considered an accepted standard of treatment as yet.

A normal nerve can compensate for the change in length with limb flexion and extension because it is surrounded by gliding tissue that permits longitudinal movement. The change in length is distributed over the entire nerve so that the elongation of each nerve segment is small. A nerve graft becomes welded to its recipient bed by the adhesions through which it becomes vascularized. As a consequence, the nerve graft is exquisitely sensitive to tension because it has no longitudinal excursion. The harvested length of the graft must be long enough to span the nerve gap without tension while the adjacent joints are extended; this is also the position of temporary immobilization. If the limb or digit is immobilized with joint flexion, the graft becomes fixed in this position. When the limb is mobilized at 8 days, the proximal and distal stumps are subject to tension even though the graft initially was long enough. Early attempts at lengthening the graft lead to disruption of the anastomosis (46-53).

9.5 Grafting versus primary repair

A tension-free repair is the goal for any nerve anastomosis. When there is a clean transaction of the nerve and the gap is caused by elastic retraction, an acute primary repair is indicated.When treatment of a nerve laceration is delayed, fibrosis of the nerve ends prevents approximation, and nerve grafting is indicated even though there is no loss of nerve tissue. As a general rule, primary nerve repair yields superior results to nerve grafting, provided that there is no tension across the anastomotic site. Grafting can obtain similar results to primary repair under ideal conditions. If a nerve is repaired under tension, however, the results are superior with an interpositional graft. Axon sprouts are able to cross two tension-free anastomotic sites more easily than crossing one anastomosis that is under tension. Nerve grafting is indicated to bridge a defect when greater than 10% elongation of the nerve would be necessary to bridge the gap. This is a better indication for grafting than the nerve gap per se, although 4 cm is often used as the critical defect for grafting in the limb. Defects less than this may be overcome by nerve rerouting and transposition in some instances (54-58).

9.6 Considerations for donor nerve grafts

Many conditions must be met for a nerve to be considered as a potential graft. First, the relationship between the surface area and the diameter of the graft must be optimal to allow rapid revascularization. The donor site defect from sacrifice of any given nerve must be acceptable for the patient. The harvested nerve must be long enough to ensure a tension-free anastomosis with the adjacent joints in full extension. Finally, the cross-sectional area and number of fascicles should match those of the recipient nerve at the level of injury as closely as possible. For these reasons, most of the available grafts are cutaneous nerves. Most donor grafts are imperfect matches of the recipient nerve. The fascicular arrangement of the nerve graft is dissimilar to the nerve being repaired in size, number, and fascicular topography. The branching pattern of the grafts usually changes from an oligofascicular pattern proximally to a polyfascicular pattern distally, which typically corresponds to the branching pattern of the recipient nerve. There may be some loss of axon sprouts owing to growth down peripheral branches that leave the nerve graft. Some authors have recommended inserting the grafts in a retrograde manner for this reason, but others belief this is not warranted (31). The choice of nerve graft is dictated by the length of the nerve gap, the cross-sectional area of the recipient nerve, the available expendable donor nerves for that particular nerve injury, and the surgeon's preference.

9.7 Donor nerve grafts

As a general rule, it is good practice to divide the donor nerve in an intermuscular plane rather than in the subcutaneous tissue to diminish the risk of a painful neuroma. Some commonly used donor nerves are summarized here. Sunderland (1) emphasized that a cutaneous nerve for nerve grafting should be selected with great care. The sural nerve is the most commonly used, and in most situations it is recommended. From each leg, 40 cm of graft material can be obtained. McFarlane and Mayer (1976) (59), Wilgis and Maxwell (1979) (60), and Tenny and Lewis (1984) (61) used the lateral antebrachial cutaneous nerve for digital nerve grafts so that another limb would not be involved in the surgical procedure. Anatomical studies have shown no significant difference in fascicular area, area of the entire nerve bundle, and percentage of the nerve bundle occupied by the actual nerve fascicles. The lateral antebrachial cutaneous nerve is found most easily just lateral to the biceps tendon alongside the cephalic vein. Through a longitudinal incision, 20 cm of graft material can be obtained. The medial antebrachial cutaneous nerve, the terminal articular branch of the posterior interosseous nerve, and the dorsal sensory branch of the ulnar nerve also have been used for digital nerve grafting. The medial antebrachial cutaneous nerve is found adjacent to the basilic vein. The posterior interosseous nerve is located at the wrist just ulnar to the extensor pollicis longus tendon lying on the interosseous membrane. The superficial radial nerve is an excellent source of graft material when used in grafting a high radial nerve laceration because the neurological deficit that otherwise would be created already exists. It is not recommended as a routine source because its sensory contribution to the hand is significant, especially when the median nerve is deficient (4, 62).

9.8 Motor sensory differentiation

The use of intraoperative motor and sensory nerve differentiation can diminish the risk of fascicular mismatch when grafting a nerve. Available methods are the anatomic method, based on separate identification of groups of fascicles; the electrophysiologic method, using awakened stimulation and histochemical methods, which rely on staining for enzymes specific to motor or sensory nerves.

Electrical fascicle identification awaked stimulation requires the cooperation of the anesthesiologist and the patient. It is based on the observation that motor and sensory fascicles can be differentiated by direct stimulation. The median and ulnar nerves in the distal forearm are most amenable to this technique. It is especially useful when there is a nerve defect, owing to the dissimilar fascicular pattern between the proximal and distal nerve ends. The initial nerve dissection is performed under a regional block with tourniquet control. The wound is infiltrated with local anesthetic before release of the tourniquet. After 20 minutes, the patient is awakened. A lowamperage stimulator is applied to the major fascicles of the proximal nerve end in a systematic manner, starting at 0.2 to 0.5 mA. Sensory fascicles elicit pain and may be localized to a specific digit. Motor fascicles elicit no response at lower intensities and poorly localized pain at higher intensities. A cross-sectional sketch of the proximal stump is made. The sensory fascicles are tagged with 10–0 nylon, and the patient is placed under general anesthesia. The distal stump is stimulated in a similar fashion. The reverse picture is seen, with motor fascicles eliciting a muscle twitch and sensory fascicles being silent. A cross-sectional map is made again and used to match the proximal and distal motor and sensory fascicles (63-69).

9.9 Nerve lesions in continuity

Electrical stimulation is useful to determine if there are any intact fascicles in a neuroma in continuity. Bipolar hook electrodes are used with the stimulating and recording electrodes separated by at least 4 cm. The stimulus frequency is two to three times per second with pulse duration of less than 0.1 ms. The intensity is slowly increased to the range where a response is expected (3-15 V). The recorder sensitivity is increased to a maximum of 20 ľV/cm. The nerve is stimulated proximal to, across, and below the lesion. It is estimated that there must be at least 4000 myelinated axons for a recordable nerve action potential to conduct through a neuroma. A neurolysis is performed to single out any normal-appearing fascicles; this is confirmed electrically. Non conducting fascicles are excised and grafted (70).

- Grafting specific nerves
- Median nerve
- Injury at the elbow
- The Ulnar nerve

10. Factors affecting the results of nerve surgery

Few worthwhile reports have been published on the results of neurorrhaphy and the factors that influence them, first because few investigators have had access to a large enough group of patients to make evaluations statistically significant, and second because reports have only rarely been based on sound criteria of regeneration. Valuable reports have been compiled from studies of such injuries incurred in World War II and later conflicts. As a result of these studies, the influence of many factors on regeneration after nerve suture is now better understood. Rarely should a fracture interfere with nerve repair. In the usual situation, a nerve may be explored if the fracture requires open reduction. In many open injuries, the nature of the wound may be such that early repair of the nerve cannot be done satisfactorily. Every effort should be made by repeated débridement of necrotic material to promote rapid healing of any open wounds without sepsis. Nerves may be repaired successfully during a second débridement, followed by closure and healing. Associated vascular injury can adversely affect nerve regeneration because of tissue ischemia (4).

Several important factors that seem to influence nerve regeneration are (1) the age of the patient, (2) the gap between the nerve ends, (3) the delay between the time of injury and repair, (4) the level of injury, (5) the condition of the nerve ends, (6) type of nerve, (7) specific nerve involved, (8) associated vascular injury, and (9) the experience and techniques of the surgeon.

10.1 Age

Age undoubtedly influences the rate and degree of nerve regeneration. All other factors being equal, neurorrhaphies are more successful in children than in adults and are more likely to fail in elderly patients; why this is true has not been completely explained, but it may relate to the potential for central adaptation to the peripheral nerve injury. We do not know precisely what results can be expected in either of the extremes of age, for practically all significant studies have dealt with military personnel, whose average age was 18 to 30 years. Omer (71), in reviewing peripheral nerve injuries in upper extremities incurred in the Vietnam War, found the most successful results after neurorrhaphy in patients younger than 20 years. The work of Onne (72) suggests a close correlation between the age at the time of neurorrhaphy and the 2-point discrimination obtained after median and ulnar nerve repairs. Most of his patients between the ages of 20 and 40 years were found to have 2-point discrimination values in the range of 30 mm. During the teens, the values did not exceed 15 mm, and in patients 10 years old or younger, the values, with one exception, were less than 10 mm. Onne (72) observed, however, that after digital nerve repair the final 2-point discrimination was not as closely related to age. Kankaanpää and Bakalim (73), in studying sensory recovery after 137 peripheral neurorrhaphies in 96 patients, found that a higher percentage of patients younger than 20 years at the time of repair had 2-point discrimination of less than 6 mm than did patients older than 20.

10.2 Gap between nerve ends

The nature of the injury is the most important factor in determining the defect remaining between the nerve ends after any neuromas and gliomas are resected. When a sharp instrument, such as a razor or knife, severs a nerve, damage is slight proximally and distally, and although the nerve ends inevitably do retract, the gap usually can be overcome easily. Conversely, when a high-velocity missile severs a nerve, proximal and distal nerve damage is extensive. Ultimately, both ends must be widely resected to expose normal funiculi, producing a larger gap. The gap is increased further if part of the nerve is carried away by a missile, as in shrapnel injuries. Methods of closing troublesome gaps include (1) nerve mobilization, (2) nerve transposition, (3) joint flexion, (4) nerve grafts, and (5) bone shortening. The greater the defect, the more dissimilar the funicular pattern of the two ends because of the constantly changing arrangement of fibers within the nerve as it progresses distally. This is particularly important in the more proximal portion of peripheral nerves. Agreement is widespread that excessive tension on a neurorrhaphy harms nerve regeneration. Brooks advised nerve grafting if, after the nerve is mobilized, the gap cannot be closed by flexing the main joint of the limb 90 degrees. Sunderland cautioned against excessive tension on the line of suture after surgery to avoid excessive fibrosis. He advised a combination of transplantation, transposition, and mobilization of the nerve to close gaps. After experimental and clinical observations, Millesi (32) concluded that tension at the line of suture is the most important factor influencing the results of neurorrhaphy. He advised intrafascicular nerve grafting to close the large gaps. Nicholson and Seddon (3) and Sakellarides (75) observed that the upper limit of a gap beyond which results deteriorate is approximately 2.5 cm. The observations of Kirklin, Murphey, and Berkson (76) in 1949 that recovery is slightly better when the gap is relatively small remain valid.

10.3 Delay between time of Injury and repair

Delay of neurorrhaphy affects motor recovery more profoundly than sensory recovery. Scarff suggested that this is related to the survival time of denervated striated muscle.

Sunderland reported that satisfactory reinnervation of human muscle can occur after denervation of 12 months. The observations of patients with peripheral nerve injuries during World War II revealed that for every delay of 6 days between injury and repair, there is a variable loss of potential recovery that averages about 1% of maximal performance; after 3 months, this loss increases rapidly. In addition, return of function in distal muscles is poor when suture is late. The influence of delay on sensory return is unclear; in the Veterans Administration study, little influence could be found, and useful sensation returned in a few patients when suture was performed 2 years after injury. The critical limit of delay beyond which sensation does not return is unknown (4).

The British found early suture important in reducing the number of painful paresthesias and in regaining a useful degree of sensation. Kankaanpää and Bakalim (73) studied sensory return after 137 neurorrhaphies and found that, if done within 3 months after injury, the results usually were better after secondary repair than after primary repair; 21% of the 85 primary repairs and 38% of the 52 secondary repairs regained 2-point discrimination of 6 mm or less. The difference in return of sensation was most marked in digital nerve repairs. No difference in return between the primary and secondary repairs was noted in the nerve injuries at the wrist or in the forearm. The experimental work of Ducker et al (77) revealed a consistent timetable for intracellular metabolic events after nerve injury. They found that between 3 and 6 weeks the degenerative and reparative changes within the nerve cell body and the proximal and distal nerve trunks were well established. Kleinert et al (78) reported their clinical impression that a delayed primary repair done 7 to 18 days after injury is best for return of satisfactory function. In Omer's (71) study, 70% of successful repairs of lacerated nerves in the upper extremity had been done within 6 weeks after injury, and all successful repairs had been done within 3 months. Our practice is to perform neurorrhaphies in clean, sharp wounds immediately or during the first 3 to 7 days. In the presence of extensive soft-tissue contusion, laceration, crushing, or contamination in which the proximal and distal extent of the nerve injury is impossible to delineate, a delay of 3 to 6 weeks is preferred.

10.4 Level of injury

The more proximal the injuries, the more incomplete the overall return of motor and sensory function, especially in the more distal structures. Sunderland observed that conditions are more favorable for recovery in the more proximal muscles because (1) the neurons that innervate the distal portions of the limb are more severely affected by retrograde changes after proximal injury, (2) a greater proportion of the cross-sectional area of the nerve trunk is occupied by fibers to the proximal muscles, and (3) the potential for disorientation of regrowing axons and for axon loss during regeneration is greater for the distal muscles than for the muscles more proximally situated after a proximal injury. Boswick et al (79) in a review of 102 peripheral nerve injuries in 81 patients, found that of injuries below the elbow, 87% regained protective sensation, and 14% regained normal 2-point discrimination. Sakellarides (75) found that after closed peripheral nerve injuries above the elbow, return of function was delayed compared with such injuries below the elbow. Of patients treated surgically, 143 were followed for 12 months or more after neurorrhaphy. Recovery of good clinical function was found in 13 (27%) of 48 lesions above the elbow and in 37 (39%) of 95 lesions below the elbow. Except for parts of the brachial plexus, useful function at times returns regardless of the level of injury if the critical limit of delay has not passed.

10.5 Condition of nerve ends

Sunderland (1) stressed the importance of the condition of the nerve ends at the time of neurorrhaphy. He suggested that meticulous handling of the nerve ends, asepsis, care with nerve mobilization, preservation of neural blood supply, avoidance of tension, and provision of a suitable bed with minimal scar all exert favorable influences on nerve regeneration. Distal stump shrinkage has been found maximal at about 4 months, leaving the distal fascicular cross-sectional area diminished to 30% to 40% of normal size. Intraneural plexus formation and fascicular dispersal make accurate fascicular alignment and appropriate axonal regeneration more difficult. Edshage (80) showed that a neurorrhaphy with a satisfactory external appearance is no guarantee of optimal internal fascicular alignment. Fascicular malalignment was a common finding in his specimens taken from human nerve repairs. He used, in addition to a special miter box for nerve trimming, a variety of special knives and scissors designed to ensure satisfactory fascicular identification during neurorrhaphy. It is generally agreed that the nerve ends should be prepared in such a way that a satisfactory fascicular pattern is apparent in the proximal and distal stumps. No scar, foreign material, or necrotic tissue should be allowed to remain around the ends to interfere with axonal regeneration. Sometimes resection of the nerve ends so that satisfactory fasciculi are exposed leaves a gap that cannot be closed by end-to-end repair. As noted previously, clinical and experimental evidence indicates that excessive tension on the neurorrhaphy at the time of repair and when an acutely flexed limb is mobilized later causes excessive intraneural fibrosis. These findings and the promising results achieved after the interfascicular nerve grafting technique advocated by Millesi (32) and by Millesi, Meissl, and Berger (33) suggested that such a technique is preferable to repair of nerves under too much tension or with limbs in acutely flexed or awkward positions.

10.6 Type of nerve

The type of nerve injured (pure motor, pure sensory, sudomotor, or mixed) has same bearing on outcome. Repair of a pure motor or sensory nerve will lead to better results than mixed nerves, due to a decreased chance of fascicular mismatching (sensory axon growing into motor endoneurial tubes and vice versa). The specific prognosis for motor VS sensory recovery is more controversial.

10.7 Specific nerve involved

The specific peripheral nerve involved affects functional recovery. Radial nerve injuries are more likely to have functional motor return in the forearm than median or ulnar nerve lesions of similar level. As discussed before, if all other factors are comparable, a mixed motor-sensory nerve (e.g. ulnar) demonstrate inferior recovery compared to a primarily motor (e.g. radial) or sensory (e.g. digital) nerve.

11. References

[1] Sunderland S: *Nerve Injuries and Their Repair: A Critical Appraisal.* New York: Churchill Livingstone, 1991.

[2] Lee,S and Wolfe S. Peripheral Nerve Injury and Repair J Am Acad Orthop Surg 2000;8:243-252.

[3] Seddon HJ: Surgical Disorders of the Peripheral Nerves. Baltimore: Williams & Wilkins, 1972, pp 68-88.

[4] Canale & Beaty: Early management of nerve injuries. Campbell's Operative Orthopaedics, 11th ed.

[5] Noaman H, Khalifa A, ALam El-den M, Shiha A. Early surgical exploration of radial nerve injury associated with fracture shaft humerus. Microsurgery 2008;28:635–642.

[6] DeFranco MJ, Lawton JN. Radial nerve injuries associated with humeral fractures. J Hand Surg Am 2006;31:655–663.

[7] Shao YC, Harwood P, Grotz MRW, Limb D, Giannoudis PV. Radial nerve palsy associated with fractures of the shaft of the humerus: A systematic review. J Bone Joint Surg Br 2005;87:1647–1652.

[8] Crenshaw AH. Fracture of humeral shaft with radial nerve palsy. In: Crenshaw AH, editor. Campbell's Operative Orthopaedics, Vol. 2, 8th ed. St. Louis: Mosby Year Book; 1992. p 1016.

[9] Rockwood CA Jr, Green DP, Bucholz RW, Heckman JD. Rockwood and Green's Fracture in Adults, 4th ed. Philadelphia: Lippincott- Raven Publishers; 1996. pp 1043–1045.

[10] Holstein A, Lewis GM. Fractures of the humerus with radial nerve paralysis. J Bone Joint Surg Am 1963;45:1382–1388.

[11] Packer JW, Foster RR, Garcia A, Grantham SA. The humeral fracture with radial nerve palsy: Is exploration warranted? Clin Orthop 1972;88:34–38.

[12] Foster RJ, Swiontkowski MF, Bach AW, Sack JT. Radial nerve palsy caused by open humeral shaft fractures. J Hand Surg Am 1993;18: 121–124.

[13] Dabezies EJ, Banta CJ II, Murphy CP, d'Ambrosia RD. Plate fixation of the humeral shaft for acute fractures, with and without radial nerve injuries. J Orthop Trauma 1992;6:10–13.

[14] Larsen LB, Barfred T. Radial nerve palsy after simple fracture of the humerus. Scand J Plast Reconstr Surg Hand Surg 2000;34:363–366.

[15] Samardzic M, Grujicic D, Milinkovic ZB. Radial nerve lesions associated with fractures of the humeral shaft. Injury 1990;21:220–222.

[16] Shah JJ, Bhatti NA. Radial nerve paralysis associated with fractures of the humerus: A review of 62 cases. Clin Orthop 1983;172:171–176.

[17] Pollock FH, Drake D, Bovill EG, Day L, Trafton PG. Treatment of radial neuropathy associated with fractures of the humerus. J Bone Joint Surg Am 1981;63:239–243.

[18] Kettelkamp DB, Alexander H. Clinical review of radial nerve injury. J Trauma 1967;7:424–432.

[19] Shaw JL, Sakellarides H. Radial-nerve paralysis associated with fractures of the humerus: A review of forty-five cases. J Bone Joint Surg Am 1967;49:899–902.

[20] Amillo S, Barrios RH, Martinez-Peric R, Losada JI. Surgical treatment of the radial nerve lesions associated with fractures of the humerus. J Orthop Trauma 1993;7:211–215.

[21] Sonneveld GJ, Patka P, van Mourik JC, Broere G. Treatment of fractures of the shaft of the humerus accompanied by paralysis of the radial nerve. Injury 1987;18:404–40.

[22] Mackinnon SE: New directions in peripheral nerve surgery. *Ann Plast Surg* 1989;22:257-273.

[23] Hentz VR, Rosen JM, Xiao SJ, McGill KC, Abraham G: The nerve gap dilemma: A comparison of nerves repaired end to end under tension with nerve grafts in a primate model. *J Hand Surg [Am]* 1993;18:417-425.

[24] Lundborg G, Rosén B, Dahlin L, Danielsen N, Holmberg J: Tubular versus conventional repair of median and ulnar nerves in the human forearm: Early results from a prospective, randomized, clinical study. *J Hand Surg [Am]* 1997;22:99-106.

[25] Giddins GEB, Wade PJF, Amis AA: Primary nerve repair: Strength of repair with different gauges of nylon suture material. *J Hand Surg [Br]* 1989; 14:301-302.

[26] Gu XS, Yan ZQ, Yan WX, Chen CF: Rapid immunostaining of live nerve for identification of sensory and motor fasciculi. *Chin Med J* 1992;105:949-952.

[27] Sanger JR, Riley DA, Matloub HS,Yousif NJ, Bain JL, Moore GH: Effects of axotomy on the cholinesterase and carbonic anhydrase activities of axons in the proximal and distal stumps of rabbit sciatic nerves: A temporal study. *Plast Reconstr Surg* 1991;87:726-740.

[28] Noaman H. Management and functional outcomes of combined injuries of flexor tendons, nerves and vessels at the wrist. Microsurgery 2007;27:536-543.

[29] Starkweather RJ, Neviaser RJ, Adams JP, et al: The effect of devascularization on the regeneration of lacerated peripheral nerves: an experimental study. *J Hand Surg* 1978; 3:163.

[30] Zachary RB: *Results of nerve suture*. In: Seddon HJ, ed. *Peripheral nerve injuries*, London: Her Majesty's Stationery Office; 1954.

[31] Wilgis EFS: Techniques for diagnosis of peripheral nerve loss. *Clin Orthop Relat Res* 1982; 163:8.

[32] Millesi H: Techniques for nerve grafting. *Hand Clin* 2000; 16:73.

[33] Narakas A: The use of fibrin glue in repair of peripheral nerves. *Orthop Clin North Am* 1988;19:187-199.

[34] Millesi H, Meissl G, Berger A. Further experience with interfascicular grafting of the median, ulnar, and radial nerves. *J Bone Joint Surg* 1976; 58A:209.

[35] Ansselin AD, Pollard JD: Immunopathological factors in peripheral nerve allograft rejection: Quantification of lymphocyte invasion and major histocompatibility complex expression. *J Neurol Sci* 1990;96:75-88.

[36] Dumont CE, Hentz VR: Enhancement of axon growth by detergent-extracted nerve grafts. *Transplantation* 1997;63: 1210-1215.

[37] Nishiura Y, Brandt J, Nilsson A, et al. Addition of cultured Schwann cells to tendon autografts and freeze-thawed muscle grafts improves peripheral nerve regeneration. Tissue Eng 2004;10:157.

[38] Aguayo AJ, Kasarjian J, Skamene E, et al. Myelination of mouse axons by Schwann cells transplanted from normal and abnormal human nerves. Nature 1977;268:753.

[39] Fansa H, Schneider W, Keilhoff G. Revascularization of tissue-engineered nerve grafts and invasion of macrophages. Tissue Eng 2001;7:519.

[40] Daly PJ, Wood MB. Endoneural and epineural blood flow evaluation with free vascularized and conventional nerve grafts in the canine. J Reconstr Microsurg 1985;2:45.

[41] Lind R, Wood MB. Comparison of the pattern of early revascularization of conventional versus vascularized nerve grafts in the canine. J Reconstr Microsurg 1986;2:229.

[42] Penkert G, Bini W, Samii M. Revascularization of nerve grafts: an experimental study. J Reconstr Microsurg 1988; 4:319.

[43] Prpa B, Huddleston PM, An KN, et al. Revascularization of nerve grafts: a qualitative and quantitative study of the soft-tissue bed contributions to blood flow in canine nerve grafts. J Hand Surg 2002;27A:1041.

[44] Trumble TE, Parvin D. Physiology of peripheral nerve graft incorporation. J Hand Surg 1994;19A:420.

[45] Best TJ, Mackinnon SE, Evans PJ, et al. Peripheral nerve revascularization: histomorphometric study of small- and large-caliber grafts. J Reconstr Microsurg 1999;15:183.

[46] Slutsky D. A practical approach to nerve grafting in the upper extremity. Atlas Hand Clin 10 (2005) 73–92.

[47] Kwan MK, Savio L- YW. Biomechanical properties of peripheral nerve. In: Gelberman R, editor. Operative nerve repair and reconstruction, vol. I. Philadelphia: JB Lippincott; 1991. p. 47.

[48] Beel JA, Groswald DE, Luttges MW. Alterations in the mechanical properties of peripheral nerve following crush injury. J Biomech 1984;17:185.

[49] Trumble TE, McCallister WV. Repair of peripheral nerve defects in the upper extremity. Hand Clin 2000;16:37.

[50] Lundborg G, Rydevik B. Effects of stretching the tibial nerve of the rabbit: a preliminary study of the intraneural circulation and the barrier function of the perineurium. J Bone Joint Surg Br 1973;55:390.

[51] Clark WL, Trumble TE, Swiontkowski MF, et al. Nerve tension and blood flow in a rat model of immediate and delayed repairs. J Hand Surg 1992;17A:677.

[52] Matsuzaki H, Shibata M, Jiang B, et al. Distal nerve elongation vs nerve grafting in repairing segmental nerve defects in rabbits. Microsurgery 2004;24:207.

[53] Ruch DS, Deal DN, Ma J, et al. Management of peripheral nerve defects: external fixator-assisted primary neurorrhaphy. J Bone Joint Surg Am 2004;86:1405.

[54] Terzis J, Faibisoff B, Williams B. The nerve gap: suture under tension vs. graft. Plast Reconstr Surg 1975;56:166.

[55] Millesi H. The current state of peripheral nerve surgery in the upper limb. Ann Chir Main 1984;3:18.

[56] Kalomiri DE, Soucacos PN, Beris AE. Nerve grafting in peripheral nerve microsurgery of the upper extremity. Microsurgery 1994;15:506.
[57] Millesi H. Healing of nerves. Clin Plast Surg 1977;4:459.
[58] Stevens WG, Hall JD, Young VL, et al. When should nerve gaps be grafted? An experimental study in rats Plast Reconstr Surg 1985;75:707.
[59] McFarlane RM, Mayer JR: Digital nerve grafts with the lateral antebrachial cutaneous nerve. *J Hand Surg* 1976; 1A:169.
[60] Wilgis EFS, Maxwell GP: Distal digital nerve grafts: clinical and anatomical studies. *J Hand Surg* 1979; 4A:439.
[61] Tenny JR, Lewis RC: Digital nerve-grafting for traumatic defects: use of the lateral antebrachial cutaneous nerve. *J Bone Joint Surg* 1984; 66A:1375.
[62] Nunley J. Donor nerves for grafting. In: Gelberman R, editor. Operative nerve repair and reconstruction, vol. I. Philadelphia: JB Lippincott; 1991. p. 545.
[63] Chow JA, Van Beek AL, Meyer DL, et al. Surgical significance of the motor fascicular group of the ulnar nerve in the forearm. J Hand Surg 1985;10A:867.
[64] Jabaley ME, Wallace WH, Heckler FR. Internal topography of major nerves of the forearm and hand: a current view. J Hand Surg 1980;5A:1.
[65] Watchmaker GP, Lee G, Mackinnon SE. Intraneural topography of the ulnar nerve in the cubital tunnel facilitates anterior transposition. J Hand Surg 1994;19A:915.
[66] Williams HB, Jabaley ME. The importance of internal anatomy of the peripheral nerves to nerve repair in the forearm and hand. Hand Clin 1986;2:689.
[67] Gaul JS Jr. Electrical fascicle identification as an adjunct to nerve repair. Hand Clin 1986;2:709.
[68] Deutinger M, Girsch W, Burggasser G, et al. Peripheral nerve repair in the hand with and without motor sensory differentiation. J Hand Surg 1993;18A.426.
[69] Hakstian RW. Funicular orientation by direct stimulation: an aid to peripheral nerve repair. J Bone Joint Surg Am 1968;50:1178.
[70] Happel LT, Kline DG. Nerve lesions in continuity. In: Gelberman R, editor. Operative nerve repair and reconstruction, vol. I. Philadelphia: JB Lippincott; 1991. p. 601.
[71] Omer Jr GE: Reconstructive procedures for extremities with peripheral nerve defects. *Clin Orthop Relat Res* 1982; 163:80.
[72] Onne L: Recovery of sensibility and sudomotor activity in the hand after nerve suture. *Acta Chir Scand Suppl* 1962; 300:1.
[73] Kankaanpää U, Bakalim G: Peripheral nerve injuries of the upper extremity. Sensory return of 137 neurorrhaphies. *Acta Orthop Scand* 1976; 47:41.
[74] Brooks D: The place of nerve-grafting in orthopaedic surgery. *J Bone Joint Surg* 1955; 37A:299.
[75] Sakellarides H: A follow up study of 172 peripheral nerve injuries in the upper extremity in civilians. *J Bone Joint Surg* 1962; 44A:140.
[76] Kirklin JW, Murphey F, Berkson J: Suture of peripheral nerves. *Surg Gynecol Obstet* 1949; 88:719.
[77] Ducker TB, Kempe LG, Hayes GJ: The metabolic background for peripheral nerve surgery. *J Neurosurg* 1969; 30:270

[78] Kleinert HE, Cook NM, Wayne L, et al: Post-traumatic sympathetic dystrophy. *Orthop Clin North Am* 1973; 4:917.

[79] Boswick Jr JA, Schneewind J, Stromberg Jr W: Evaluation of peripheral nerve repairs below elbow. *Arch Surg* 1965; 90:50.

[80] Edshage S: Peripheral nerve suture: a technique for improved intraneural topography: evaluation of some suture materials. *Acta Chir Scand Suppl* 1964; 331:1.

8

Peripheral Nerve Surgery: Indications, Surgical Strategy and Results

Jörg Bahm[1,2] and Frédéric Schuind[2]
[1]*Euregio Reconstructive Microsurgery Unit, Franziskushospital Aachen,*
[2]*Department of Orthopaedics and Traumatology, ULB University Hospital Erasme, Brussels,*
[1]*Germany*
[2]*Belgium*

1. Introduction

So far, peripheral nerve surgery is not a recognized surgical speciality or competence and is currently performed by dedicated colleagues trained either in neurosurgery, plastic and/or hand surgery, or general surgery all over the world. Like the vascular surgeon who needs sound understanding of blood flow dynamics when planning and performing a macro- or microvascular anastomosis, the peripheral nerve surgeon must be aware of the increasing knowledge on *nerve regeneration*, a complex and multifactorial biological repair process with a defined time course and known actors, promoters and inhibitors.

Surgery of peripheral nerves is always *microsurgery*, therefore addressing the microscopic anatomy of the nerves (42), the need for magnification loops or a microscope and specific instruments, and the necessary skill to handle the structures carefully when performing neurolysis, nerve sutures and grafts with a high technical standard, an important factor to provide a good functional outcome.

Basic knowledge in peripheral nerve surgery has already been established for over twenty years. The reader should be familiar with basics like the microanatomy of a peripheral nerve (12), the technique of end to end and end to side anastomosis, and the indications and techniques of neurolysis, as described by Millesi (35). Furthermore, sound understanding of neurophysiologic examination techniques (46) (including various nerve conduction studies like conduction velocity, distal latency, sensory and motor evoked potentials, and special stimulation techniques like transcranial magnetic stimulation) and neuropathologic nerve staining techniques (42) are also mandatory. Refined imaging techniques (ultrasound, MRI) and new image processing technologies like tension- weighted tractography should be looked at, as they may increase our preoperative knowledge and thus may change reconstructive strategies in the near future.

Why then another article on that topic? The aim of this chapter is a *personal view* summarizing clinical skills and regular surgical experience in peripheral nerve surgery and especially brachial plexus operations of the last 15 years. For the novice, both the anatomy of neural networks like the brachial or lumbosacral plexus and the surgical strategy might look complex and fastidious. Our aim is to insist on specific landmarks, clinical decision points, and important technical details - all of which should help to improve the functional outcome for our patients.

2. Nerve regeneration (12,17,43,54)

After a severe nerve injury and/or transsection, Wallerian degeneration occurs at the distal nerve stump as a clearing process to prepare for reinnervation (arrival of the growth cones). This degenerative process removes axonal debris and myelin and is initiated by the Schwann cells, and complemented by activated macrophages. Schwann cells proliferate and arrange into clusters (bands of Büngner) which will orientate the newly arriving growth cones. In addition, the remaining connective tissue basal membrane forms endoneural tubes. On the proximal edge, the neuronal cell body undergoes chromatolysis with peripheral migration of the nucleus and changes in the endoplasmic reticulum characteristic of the production of molecules for growth and repair. Growth cones emerge from the proximal edge into the nerve segment distal to the lesion and migrate down to the target, thereby progressively reconstructing the nerve structure and function.

Neurotrophic factors like Nerve Growth Factor (NGF), Ciliary Neurotrophic Factor (CNTF) and Insulin-like Growth Factors (IGFs) and neurite-promoting factors including laminin, fibronectin, neural cell adhesion molecules (N-CAM) and N-cadherin are nerve growth promoting factors. They act locally or within the neural cell conducted there by retrograde axoplasmic transport.

3. Patient examination and decision making

Peripheral nerve trauma occurs in the upper or lower limb, as an isolated or combined injury.

The birth process might be complicated by shoulder dystocia in a macrosomic child, and lead to an upper or total obstetric brachial plexus palsy (3). Children may undergo soft tissue laceration by broken glass and suffer from undiscovered peripheral nerve section, or present progressive paralysis of muscle groups after a fall (like weakness of shoulder abductors due to an unrecognized axillary nerve lesion within the quadrangular space, deep in the axilla). Young adults are at risk to become polytraumatized victims of motorcycle accidents including severe injury to the brachial plexus. Pelvic fractures affect the lumbosacral plexus (12, 23). At all ages, bone or soft tissue tumours growing inside the extremities may create nerve lesions, by compression or structural invasion, with progressive destruction of the nerve morphology and function.

Especially brachial plexus lesions in adults and children require a particular consideration, taking also into account in neonates the disturbances in growth (table 1).

Any major peripheral nerve injury needs a quick assessment including a complete patient examination and a complete motor and sensory evaluation.

Of course, the difficult clinical condition of a polytraumatized patient, including alterations of consciousness and/or hemodynamic instability, must be considered. Some initial neurologic deficiencies also resolve spontaneously within the first days after the trauma. Recently, Wiberg (53) stressed that a substantial brachial plexus lesion in an adult is a diagnostic emergency, as the most proximal root lesions induce neuronal cell apoptosis in the anterior medullar horn and thus preclude later motor nerve regeneration.

Adult	Child
High velocity injury (motorcycle)	Traction forces (shoulder dystocia)
Avulsions and ruptures	(partial) ruptures, rare avulsions
Polytrauma	Isolated, rare bone trauma
Slow & incomplete nerve regeneration	Fast regeneration, cortical plasticity
„Fixed“ anatomy	*Growing, adaptative anatomy*
Adult limb	*Growing limb, proportional muscle masses*
Organized lifeplan	Progressive task development
Highly compliant	Non compliant

Table 1. Comparison of brachial plexus lesions in adult and children

This paradigm is in clear contradiction with the actual daily practice in most Traumatology departments, where the polytraumatized patient is stabilized, multi-operated, then eventually sent for rehabilitation and left with a flail arm, often even without imagery and clear strategy about exposure and repair of the brachial plexus or nerve trunk injuries. We propose the following guidelines for any (hypothetic or proven) severe peripheral nerve injury:

3.1 Complete clinical (neurological) examination

As early as possible, and then after two weeks (identification of neurapraxia), six weeks and three months.

3.1.1 Signs of severity

Any *rapid muscle waste* is a sign of a severe nerve dysfunction or nerve root avulsion. *Deafferentation neuropathic pain* also signs avulsion of sensitive rootlets. *Horner's sign* associated to complete brachial plexus palsy signs an avulsion of the Th1 root and is even alone a reason for surgical exploration.

3.1.2 Pain

Where children suffering an obstetric brachial plexus palsy don't experience pain, adult patients are mostly concerned by severe, untreatable, excruciating neuropathic pain attacks, sometimes making discussion about a sound reconstructive strategy impossible unless the pain is managed correctly.

3.1.3 General patient condition

When preparing one or more reconstructive procedures for severe nerve injury, especially when including exposure of the brachial or lumbosacral plexus with the need for harvesting donor nerves, patients will undergo longlasting and iterative procedures. This strategy should be adapted to the general health situation, the extent of the polytrauma and related surgeries, and the social background.

3.1.4 Neurophysiology

There is still controversy about a regular use of nerve conduction studies and CMAP (EMG) recordings, as global findings do very rarely help for surgical decisions. After a severe isolated nerve injury, signs of early recovery might be an argument to delay surgery and to repeat the measurements after four to six weeks. In severe plexus root injuries, the signs distinguishing pre- and postganglionic injuries might be of help when planning a reconstructive strategy. Presence of muscle fibrillations is a strong indicator that a given muscle is still re-innervatable and that thus neurotisation is still of worth. SSEP and MEP are of limited value to judge nerve root quality; we therefore prefer a combination of imagery and intraoperative macro- and microscopic findings.

3.1.5 Imagery

In suspected nerve root avulsions (breech presentations in babies, high velocity motorway injuries), we ask for a MyeloCT or an MRI. Frequently, patients arrive at the first consultation with already performed imagery of variable quality. Ultrasound examination, eventually combined with intraoperative assessment, is a new and promising strategy to assess lesions-in-continuity. Diffusion MRI technique measuring water diffusion along preferential guiding structures ("tractography" of peripheral nerves) (16) may show functional connections and the progression of reinnervation along defined axes (nerve trunks).

4. Counselling

The patient needs a good understanding of the extent of the nerve trauma, global nerve function, the aim of the reconstructive surgery and the anticipated maximal and minimal results. Sometimes, primary or secondary procedures compete for a same clinical issue. An example is a proximal radial nerve injury (associated to a humeral shaft fracture) where we have to decide between a cable graft, selective nerve transfers or a classic tendon transfer procedure. There is no golden standard so far and the pro´s and con´s will have to be outlined more clearly. The final decision has to be taken as a consent between the patient and the surgical staff, including a summary of postoperative and rehabilitation requirements.

In adults, important socio- professional requirements must be clarified. Waiting for the recovery of a nerve graft may take six or nine months at minimum, severely increasing the work's leaves, where a tendon transfer might be functional six to eight weeks after surgery.

5. Team organisation

Any "emergent" or early indication should be operated on according to that rationale, which could cause important organisation challenges and eventual postposure of other patients with regular, not time-dependant surgeries. The Operation Room crew should be aware of the potential time schedule (a brachial plexus exposure and reconstruction in an adult patient may take easily eight to eleven hours). Sometimes a two-team approach is helpful (eg when harvesting donor nerves at the lower leg or when performing a free functional muscle transfer). After a longlasting procedure, we prefer to observe the patient the first night under cardiovascular monitoring at the intensive care unit.

5.1 Primary nerve surgery: Exposure and techniques

Every nerve should be exposed according to its topography (22), allowing clear identification of the lesion itself and the unaffected proximal and distal ends.

As these surgeries may require a long operation time, prevention of pressure sores using special cushions and monitoring of the body temperature including the use of heating envelopes may be mandatory.

Our preferred exposure of the brachial plexus in adults and children is a straight supraclavicular approach, dividing the platysma lateral to the sternocleidomastoideus muscle with reclination of the adipolymphatic pad to discover the interscalenic triangle with the nerve trunks and the subclavian artery (3,6,8). In rare conditions, we have to isolate the clavicle, separating the insertions of the pectoralis major muscle and hooking up the bone on a silicone loop to explore the retro- and infraclavicular spaces. An osteotomy of the clavicle is rarely mandatory. An additional delto-pectoral approach might be helpful in extended injuries in the adult patient.

For elective nerve transfers, other more direct approaches might be useful (22), including a dorsal approach to the suprascapular and spinal accessory nerve for a classic extraplexic XI onto SSC neurotisation (7).

After the exposure of the traumatized nerve segment(s) and clear identification of healthy proximal (if feasible) and distal edges, a careful *neurolysis* is performed under magnification according to Millesi´s classification of nerve fibrosis (table 2) (35). Type C fibrosis and non-conducting neuromas are resected. Direct electrical stimulation on both proximal and distal areas with decreasing current intensity (from 5 to 1 mA by 1mA steps, and from 1 down by 0.1 steps) is helpful to make the decision, when there is a lack of electrical conductivity and insufficient distal motor response. After resection of the injured segment, the remaining stumps are prepared for grafting and donor nerves are harvested, while waiting for the neuropathologic examination results.

Type A: epifascicular epineurium	epineurotomy
Type B: interfascicular epineurium	epi- or interfascicular epineuriectomy
Type C: perineurium and endoneurium	nerve grafting

Table 2. Sites of nerve fibrosis and surgical treatment according to Millesi (35)

Considering the extent of resection of a neuroma, there is still controversy on how far the back-cut should be. On the distal edge, fascicular pattern should be visible on magnification and, for the beginner, a pathological quality assessment is useful. At the proximal level, where the remaining nerve stump or plexus root is a precious part of the potential reinnervation source, the morphologic appearance and indirect information about the reinnervation potential are of very high importance and correlate directly to the functional prognosis. We rely on a reduced amount of perineural and endoneural fibrosis, a homogenous fascicular architecture and a sufficient density of newly built myelin sheaths, which constitute indirect signs of reinnervation by the growth cone advancements (42). Peripheral microfascicles should not be too numerous, as they are representative of the neuroma and its disorganized fascicular pattern. Eventually, a more proximal back-cut is performed, although we have to assume that if the remnant of a plexus root is near the foramen, the grafting becomes technically difficult and the lesion might extend into the foramen, represent a very proximal rupture responsible for more neuronal apoptosis or an in situ root avulsion. We don't trust this type of root quality; and the stump becomes a second line donor, eg for the middle trunk.

Some neurosurgeons used to perform (hemi)laminectomies perform a dorsal neck approach to evaluate the root quality and confirm the diagnosis of root avulsions suspected on MRI images, and even perform rootlet reimplantations (13,14).

5.2 Neuropathologic examination of proximal and distal nerve stumps: Technique of harvest and microscopic examination

All specimens to be sent are cut with a fresh surgical knife, marked either proximally or distally using a vital blue pen, and sent on a moist swab.

The neuropathologist performs an immediate (fast) examination and a more remote appreciation. We receive a phone call discussing the fast result after some 50 minutes and a written report 10 to 14 days later, including an analysis of all staining techniques.

The fast examination is performed on frozen sections (Cryostat), after Hematoxylin Eosin (HE) and trichrome Gomorri staining. Morphometry is performed on these specimens to evaluate the size of the fascicles, the thickness of myeline sheaths, and their proportion in a nerve section area. The delayed examination of Epon imbedded tissue cut into semi-thin slices after toluidine blue staining is aimed to confirm the structural observations made within the first examination and concludes the written report.

While waiting for the neuropathologic appreciation of the stump quality, *grafts* are harvested from the lower legs (one or two sural nerves), the cervical subcutaneous tissue or the ipsilateral forearm (superficial branch of the radial nerve). All grafts are conditioned in a wet swab and brought into the defect without tension, in an antidromic direction, to avoid lost collateral sprouting during the reinnervation. Simple nerve gaps are bridged by an interfascicular cable graft, made of numerous graft segments to fill the gap. If there is information about the clockwise orientation of fascicles within the proximal and distal segment, this information is integrated to avoid any mismatch. The longer the gap, the more "hazardous" is the topographic reinnervation due to the intraneural plexiform arrangement of the different fascicles, a well known microanatomical characteristic more present in the proximal nerve segments than in the distal parts, close to the target.

number of roots	*children*	*adult*
one	LT, lat UT, XI-MC	UT, IC-R, XI-SSC
two	LT+MT, UT	UT, MT
three or more	Anatomic reconstruction	

UT upper trunk, MT middle trunk, LT lower trunk (lat=lateral part) XI spinal accessory nerve, MC musculocutaneous nerve, R radial nerve, IC intercostal nerves

Table 3. Priorities of reinnervation in brachial plexus repair

A brachial plexus repair is normally made out of a combination of intraplexic ("anatomic") and extraplexic repair (3,8,12):

Intraplexic repair is performed by cable grafts, without tension, including very precise positioning and fibrin glue fixation, between the remaining roots of good morphological quality and the preferential distal nerve targets (priorities are given in table 3).

5.3 Extraplexic adjuncts

Are either added in the same procedure (when they can be performed within reasonable time and access limits, like the transfer of the distal branch of the spinal accessory nerve onto the suprascapular nerve) or in a second procedure (eg multiple intercostal nerve transfers for elbow flexion or extension). An overview of routine extraplexic nerve transfers is given in table 4, summarizing the currently used nerve transfer procedures (34,37).

5.4 Nerve coaptation technique

End-to-end coaptation of nerve ends requires very precise tissue arrangement and absence of tension. When fascicular groups may be arranged according to the cross sectional pattern, more direct and complete regeneration is expected. The microsurgical technique using epi-perineural stitches is actually believed to be the gold standard; but fibrin glue used as a *peripheral* stump fixation substance (creating a stable peripheral sheath around both stumps which should be perfectly coapted) has proven its high quality.We use fibrin glue for every nerve coaptation, either in addition to the sutures, to create a smooth and protective environnement to the anastomosis, either as the only fixation, especially in children and for interposition grafts when there is no tension at all on the stumps. In nerve transfers, sometimes tiny fascicles have to be coaptated to selective motor or sensory fibers and this connexion is crucial for the good functional outcome: then we use 10 or 11 /0 sutures and very high magnification under the microscope. On the other hand, when repairing very proximal root ruptures after brachial plexus injury, the proximal stump might be so close to the foramen that sutures are impossible and than fibrin glue alone will allow to fix the coaptation.The only drawback with fibrin glue is that once the site is glued, there is no further visual control possible. We never would use fibrin glue as an *interposition* substance between nerve stumps, as this would impair the nerve regeneration through the local fibrosis.Unfortunately, there is so far evident lack of experimental data comparing the use of stitches and fibrin glue under ideal (no tension) conditions.

5.5 Nerve imbedding

Nerve grafts are made of newly denervated fresh nerve segments which need concomittant revascularization to insure good reinnervation. Therefore, a healthy, not scarred and well vascularized surrounding tissue is mandatory. In a longer cable graft, fascicles might be separated to favour the revascularization. Longer interposition nerve grafts, like those for a free functional muscle transfer, should be placed in an unconstrained, well vascularized environment like an unoperated subcutaneous layer, as we already have observed severe graft constriction and increasing fibrosis when the graft was positioned between muscles, eg between delto-pectoral muscle layers.

Immobilisation of the head-neck segment is mandatory for three weeks postoperatively.

5.6 Nerve transfers

This concept includes a growing group of specific fascicle transfer techniques (26,37,39,48,50) where a donor nerve (harvest of redundant fascicles sorted out by an intraoperative selective low intensity electrostimulation) is transferred to a specific motor or sensitive target. A selective end-to-side anastomosis with an epineural window is the final achievement of this selective transfer concept (36).

Table 4 gives an overview of the actually known nerve transfers in the reconstruction of upper limb nerve defects.

In specific indications, motor nerve ends may be directly implanted into target muscles (24).

Donor nerve	Target nerve	Author
XI	SSC (spinati)	Malessy 2004 (32), Bahm 2005 (7), Pondaag 2005 (41)
XI	MC (biceps)	Narakas (37)
IC	MC (biceps)	Malessy 1998 (30)
IC	AX (deltoid)	Malungpaishrope 2007 (33)
U	MC (biceps or brachialis)	Oberlin 2002 (38), Teboul 2004 (49), Liverneaux 2006 (27)
U	R (triceps)	Gilbert 2011 (18)
M	MC (biceps or brachialis)	Oberlin 2008 (39)
M	R (PIN)	Mackinnon 2007 (29), Bertelli 2010 (11)
R	AX (deltoid)	Leechavengvongs 2003 (25), Colbert and McKinnon 2006 (15), Bertelli 2007 (10)
MC (brachialis)	M (finger flexion)	Palazzi 2006 (40)
ThD	ThL (serratus ant.)	Uerpairojkit 2009 (52)
Ph	MC	Gu 1989 (20), Siqueira 2009 (45)
Ph	SSC	Sinis 2009 (44)
cC7	multiple	Gu 1987 (19,21), Songcharoen 2001 (47), Terzis 2009 (51)

Table 4. Currently performed nerve transfers

6. Principles of secondary surgery

Most indications of secondary corrections arise once the reinnervation process after the primary nerve reconstruction comes to an end, dependant on the distance between the proximal nerve stump / fascicle donor and the motor target, i.e. generally after one to three years (5). When the functional result of a primary nerve surgery is expected to be poor (e.g. grafting of a proximal radial nerve lesion), a secondary procedure with tendon transfers may be indicated early; and the eventual gain from reinnervation will improve the result of tendon transfers.

Only some rare clinical conditions in children with soft tissue contractures and joint subluxations need sometimes an early decision, without considering the nerve recovery, but focusing on potential joint and bone growth disturbances (9). Secondary surgery may be directed at:

- tendon and/ or muscle transfer(s) to increase or balance key muscle functions in the affected extremity,
- correct soft tissue contractures at the shoulder or elbow level,
- newly orientate a limb segment by (de)rotational osteotomy,
- recreate a mandatory limb function by functioning free muscle transfer,
- increase protective sensibility in special skin areas by distal nerve transfers (eg using the intercostobrachialis nerve to supply the lateral part of the median nerve);
- perform corrections at the hand level, e.g. correction of clawing, difference of flexion power between long fingers, increasing thumb mobility (e.g. opposition).

In the growing child, muscle transfers are best performed before school age, when the limb weight is still not prohibitive for the transferred muscle to achieve good active ROM against gravity (minimum M3 recovery).

Specific technical points concern:

- the tendon suture(s) (preferred interweaving Pulvertaft technique),
- the tendon re-attachment to the bone (direct suture into the periosteum or using a bone anchor).

After six weeks of immobilisation, specific rehabilitation is prescribed for a minimum of 6-12 months and, later on, strengthening exercices are mandatory.

7. Results

A good result is characterized by a useful return of function in sensory and/or motor skills. Indications for primary and secondary surgery focus on this expectation: any reconstructive surgery in this field is acceptable only when a real functional goal can be met.

Results remain very individual, present several facets and depend on many factors. Therefore, evidence based medecine criteria don't apply easily to this individualized surgery.

Ongoing reinnervation might be clinically detected by a progressing Hofmann-Tinel sign along the nerve axis. In a near future, repetitive diffusion tensor imaging (16) should be able to visualize the progressing line of growth cones by the intense metabolic activity.

Recovery of motion is measured by the increase of the active range of motion (aROM) in the powered joint; and force by the BRMC grading system (M1 to M5). It is accepted today that only a motor power above M3 (movement against gravity) is of functional worth. Recent developments in video-assisted motion analysis of the upper limb (4) allow parallel recordings of the motion pattern, active ROM and EMG, and also forces and torques applied to the analyzed joints. These multifactorial records are useful once conducted under repeatable and objective measurement conditions (e.g. using a robot arm for a standardized movement sequence) both before an operation and within the postoperative rehabilitation period. Nevertheless, muscle strength and fatigue-resistance, important characteristics when looking at activities of daily life, are rarely studied so far.

Measurements of recovery of sensation and the value of sensitive rehabilitation are a wide field of research and beyond the scope of this review (12,28).

From the patient's view, recoveries of activities useful in his private and professional life are important. Questionnaires about performance of activities in daily living and pain intensity altogether with functional scores may address some of these particular issues, but any general conclusion drawn from these might be hazardous, as so many - controlled and also unknown - factors interfere with the outcome.

One also has to consider that the possible ergonomic and financial compensations existing in Western culture countries, making some extended surgeries less accepted here, as patients with very severe nerve injury (a young adult suffering a total brachial plexus palsy with four or five root avulsions) may prefer a rehabilitation program associated with social help and reintegration much better than repetitive and longlasting surgeries with sometimes doubtful outcomes.

The litterature is made of presentations of techniques and often small retrospective clinical series restricted to one technique or a specific injury pattern or target. Some contributions would make believe that there are more or less good nerves, as far as regeneration or recovery is concerned. In fact, we have to remember the microanatomy: anastomosis or grafting of a mixed nerve, containing motor and sensory fibers, always will be hazardous concerning fiber redistribution and functional outcome; the same applies to end-to-side connections between mixed nerves. The main negative predictive factors are the severity of injury, the amount of intraneural fibrosis, the delay for surgery and the distance to the target. These factors all interfere with the surgical technical attempts to restore motor or sensory function.

8. Scientific purposes and future directions

Especially at the upper limb level, movements are executed by groups of muscles working together as a team. Furthermore, agonist and antagonist activities should harmonize for a goal-directed motion. Therefore, we should perhaps look more at muscle groups, like the analytic work in physiotherapy and ongoing research in motion analysis starts to show.

Sensation is a very complex topic and should not been treated as a second-choice subject in reconstructive nerve surgery and rehabilitation (12,14,28).

The interface between the human body, its muscles and myoelectric prostheses has gained new interest through multi-channel, highly specialized "bionic prostheses", aiming at restoration of multiple degree of freedom movements (2). The sensory glove (28) represents one field of research of rehabilitation of a sensory loss introducing other CNS functions like audition to complement the sensorial lack within the recovery process.

Another field concerns the experimental and clinical work around nerve root reimplantation (13,14) achieving motion (although parasitized by cocontractions) and restoration of simple reflex arcs.

Bioartificial nerve grafts and also allografts could increase our capacity to bridge numerous and large nerve defects in the adult (e.g. long defect of a sciatic nerve), but are at present worthless in numerous indications and especially in children.

The pain management in adult patients with severe nerve injury may be very challenging. Sometimes, this priority is higher than the functional reconstruction, as the patient not only is totally incapacitated by the pain in his daily living, but also has to consider the numerous side effects of a longlasting treatment with multiple drugs. Finally, cortical plasticity after reconstructive neurosurgery is a promising field to understand how we learn to use nerve transfers and adapt to newly recreated functions (1,31).

9. Acknowledgement

We want to express our gratitude to Baxter Germany represented by S. Ehrle MD who supported the manuscript edition financially and thus concretized the publication.

10. References

[1] Anastakis DJ, Malessy MJ, Chen R, Davis KD, Mikulis D: Cortical plasticity following nerve transfer in the upper extremity. Hand Clinics 2008 24 425-444

[2] Aszmann OC, Dietl H, Frey M: Selective nerve transfers to improve the control of myoelectrical arm prostheses. Handchir Mikrochir Plast Chir 2008 40 60-65

[3] Bahm J : Obstetric brachial plexus palsy – clinics, pathophysiology and surgical treatment. Handchir Mikrochir Plast Chir 2003 35 83-97

[4] Bahm J, Meinecke L, Brandenbusch V, Rau G, Disselhorst-Klug C : High spatial resolution electromyography and video-assisted movement analysis in children with obstetric brachial plexus palsy. Hand Clinics 2003 19 393-399

[5] Bahm J : Secondary procedures in obstetric brachial plexus lesions. Handchir Mikrochir Plast Chir 2004 36 37-46

[6] Bahm J, Becker M, Disselhorst-Klug C, Williams C, Meinecke L, Müller H, Sellhaus B, Schröder JM, Rau G : Surgical Strategy in Obstetric Brachial Plexus Palsy - the Aachen Experience. Seminars in Plastic Surgery 2004 18 285-299

[7] Bahm J, Noaman H, Becker M : The dorsal approach to the suprascapular nerve in neuromuscular reanimation for obstetric brachial plexus lesions. Plast Reconstr Surg 2005 115 240-244

[8] Bahm J, Ocampo-Pavez C, Noaman H : Microsurgical technique in obstetric brachial plexus repair : a personal experience in 200 cases over 10 years. J Brachial Plexus Peripheral Nerve Injury 2007 2 1-7

[9] Bahm J, Wein B, Alhares G, Dogan C, Radermacher K, Schuind F : Assessment and treatment of glenohumeral joint deformities in children suffering from obstetric brachial plexus palsy. J Ped Orthop 2007 16B 243-251

[10] Bertelli JA, Santos MA, Kechele PR, Ghizoni MF, Duarte H: Triceps motor nerve branches as a donor or receiver in nerve transfers. Neurosurgery 2007 61:333-338

[11] Bertelli JA, Ghizoni MF: Transfer of supinator motor branches to the posterior interosseous nerve in C7-T1 brachial plexus palsy. J Neurosurg 2010 113 129-132

[12] Birch R, Bonney G, Wynn Parry CB: Surgical Disorders of the Peripheral Nerves. Churchill Livingstone Edinburgh 1998

[13] Carlstedt T: Central Nerve Plexus Injury. Imperial College Press London 2007

[14] Carlstedt T: Spinal Cord Surgery Restores Motor and Sensory Function in Patients with Brachial Plexus Avulsion Injury. Invited lecture at the FESSH congress Oslo May 2011

[15] Colbert SH, Mackinnon S: Posterior approach for double nerve transfer for restoration of shoulder function in upper brachial plexus palsy. Hand 2006 1 71-77

[16] Filler A: Magnetic Resonance Neurography and Diffusion Tensor Imaging: Origins, History, and Clinical Impact of the First 50 000 Cases With An Assessment of Efficacy and Utility in A Prospective 5000-Patient Study Group. Neurosurgery 2009 65 A29-A43

[17] Frostick SP, Yin Q: Schwann cells, neurotrophic factors, and peripheral nerve regeneration.Microsurgery 1998 18: 397-405

[18] Gilbert A: personal communication at the Narakas meeting Lisboa 2011

[19] Gu YD, Wu MM, Zhen YL et al: Microsurgical treatment for root avulsion of the brachial plexus. Chin Med J 1987 100 519-522

[20] Gu YD, Wu MM, Zhen YL et al: Phrenic nerve transfer for treatment of brachial plexus root avulsion. Report at Brachial Plexus Symposium Lausanne 1989

[21] Gu YD, Zhang GM, Chen DS et al: Cervical nerve root transfer from healthy side for treatment of brachial plexus root avulsion. Report at Brachial Plexus Symposium Lausanne 1989

[22] Kline DG, Hudson AR, Kim DH: Atlas of peripheral nerve surgery Saunders Philadelphia 2001

[23] Lang EM, Borges J, Carlstedt T: Surgical treatment of lumbosacral plexus injuries. Neurosurg 2004 1:64-71

[24] Lassner F, Becker M, Fansa H, Mawrin C; Pallua N: [Reconstruction of defects at the neuromuscular junction]. Handchir Mikrochir Plast Chir 2003 35: 127-131

[25] Leechavengvongs S, Witoonchart K, Uerpairojkit C, Thuvasethakul P: Nerve transfer to deltoid muscle using the nerve to the long head of the triceps. Part II A report of 7 cases. J Hand Surg Am 2003 28 633-638

[26] Leechavengvongs S, Witoonchart K, Uerpairojkit C; Thuvasethakul P; Malungpaishrope K: Combined nerve transfers for C5 and C6 brachial plexus avulsion injury. J Hand Surg Am 2006 31 183-189

[27] Liverneaux PA, Diaz LC, Beaulieu JY, Durand S, Oberlin C: Preliminary results of double nerve transfer to restore elbow flexion in upper type brachial plexus palsies. Plast Reconstr Surg 2006 117 915-919

[28] Lundborg G: Nerve Injury and Repair (2nd edition) Churchill Livingstone New York 2005

[29] Mackinnon SE, Roque B, Tung TH: Median to radial nerve transfer for treatment of radial nerve palsy. Case report. J Neurosurg 2007 107666-671

[30] Malessy MJ, Thomeer RT: Evaluation of intercostals to musculocutaneous nerve transfer in reconstructive brachial plexus surgery. J Neurosurg 1998 88 266-271

[31] Malessy MJ, Thomeer RT, van Dijk JG: Changing central nervous system control following intercostals nerve transfer. J Neurosurg 1998 89 568-574

[32] Malessy MJ, de Ruiter GC, de Boer KS, Thomeer RT: Evaluation of suprascapular nerve neurotisation after nerve graft or transfer in the treatment of brachial plexus traction lesions. J Neurosurg 2004 101 377-389

[33] Malungpaishrope K, Leechavengvongs S, Uerpairojkit C, Witoonchart K, Jitprapaikulsarn S, Chongthammakun S: Nerve transfer to deltoid muscle using the intercostal nerves through the posterior approach: an anatomic study and two case reports. J Hand Surg Am 2007 32 218-224

[34] Merrell GA, Barrie KA, Katz DL, Wolfe SW: Results of nerve transfer techniques for restoration of shoulder and elbow function in the context of a meta-analysis of the English literature. J Hand Surg Am 2001 26 303-314

[35] Millesi H: Neurolysis. In Boome RS (ed): The Brachial Plexus. The Hand and Upper Extremity (volume 14) Churchill Livingstone New York 1997

[36] Millesi H, Schmidhammer R: Nerve fiber transfer by end-to-side coaptation. Hand Clin 2008 24 461-483

[37] Narakas AO: Neurotization in the treatment of brachial plexus injuries. In: Gelberman RH (ed): Operative nerve repair and reconstruction. JB Lippincott Company Philadephia 1991 (1329-1358)

[38] Oberlin C, Ameur NE, Teboul F, Beaulieu JY, Vacher C: Restoration of elbow flexion in brachial plexus injury by transfer of ulnar nerve fascicles to the nerve to the biceps muscle. Tech Hand Up Extrem Surg 2002 6 86-90

[39] Oberlin C, Durand S, Belheyar Z, Shafi M, David E, Asfazadourian H: Nerve transfers in brachial plexus palsies. Chir Main 2008 25 S1297-1302

[40] Palazzi S, Palazzi JL, Caceres JP: Neurotization with the brachialis muscle motor nerve. Microsurg 2006 26 330-333

[41] Pondaag W, de Boer R, van Wijlen-Hempel MS, Hofstede-Buitenhuis SM, Malessy MJ: External rotation as a result of suprascapular nerve neurotization in obstetric brachial plexus lesions. Neurosurgery 2005 57 530-537

[42] Schröder JM: Pathology of Peripheral Nerves Springer Berlin 2001

[43] Schuind F, Phan QD, Cermak K, El Kazzi W, Bahm J: Stimulation biologique de la régénération axonale. Cours européen de pathologie chirurgicale du membre supérieur et de la main Paris january 2011

[44] Sinis N, Boettcher M, Werdin F, Kraus A, Schaller HE: Restoration of shoulder abduction function by direct muscular neurotization with the phrenic nerve fascicles and nerve grafts: a case report. Microsurgery 2009 29 552-555

[45] Siqueira MG, Martins RS: Phrenic nerve transfer in the restoration of elbow flexion in brachial plexus avulsion injuries: how effective and safe is it? Neurosurgery 2009 65 A125-131

[46] Smith SJM: The role of neurophysiological investigation in traumatic brachial plexus injuries in adults and children. J. Hand Surgery 1996 21B 145-148

[47] Songcharoen P, Wongtrakul S; Mahaisavariya B; Spinner RJ: :Hemi-contralateral C7 transfer to median nerve in the treatment of root avulsion brachial plexus injury. J Hand Surg Am 2001 26 1058-1064

[48] Songcharoen P, Wongtrakul S, Spinner RJ: Brachial plexus injuries in the adult. nerve transfers: the Siriraj Hospital experience. Hand Clin 2005 21 83-89

[49] Teboul F, Kakkar R, Ameur N, Beaulieu JY; Oberlin C: Transfer of fascicles from the ulnar nerve to the nerve to the biceps in the treatment of upper brachial plexus palsy. J Bone Joint Surg Am 2004 86 1485-1490

[50] Terzis JK, Kostas I, Soucacos PN: Restoration of shoulder function with nerve transfers in traumatic brachial plexus palsy patients. Microsurg 2006 26 316-324

[51] Terzis JK, Kokkalis ZT: Selective contralateral c7 transfer in posttraumatic brachial plexus injuries: a report of 56 cases. Plast Reconstr Surg 2009 123 927-938

[52] Uerpairojkit C, Leechavengvongs S, Witoonchart K, Malungpaishorpe K, Raksakulkiat R: Nerve transfer to serratus anterior muscle using the thoracodorsal nerve for winged scapula in C5 and C6 brachial plexus root avulsions. J Hand Surg Am 2009 34 74-78

[53] Wiberg M, Vedung S, Stalberg E: Neuronal loss after transsection of the facial nerve: a morphological and neurophysiological study in monkeys. Scand J Plast Reconstr Surg Hand Surg 2001 35 135-140

[54] wikipedia: Overview of events in peripheral regeneration (http://en.wikipedia.org/wiki/Peripheral_nerve_injury)

[55] wikipedia: Muscular fibrillation (http://en.wikipedia.org/wiki/Fibrillation)

9

Neural - Glial Interaction in Neuropathic Pain

Homa Manaheji
Department of Physiology and Neuroscience Research Center of Shahid Beheshti University of Medical Sciences, Tehran, Iran

1. Introduction

Lesioning of the nervous system can produce a form of pathological pain called "neuropathic pain" that is characterized by sensory deficit, burning sensation, hyperalgesia and allodynia (Cui et al., 2000). The mechanisms underlying neuropathic pain have been studied extensively. Abundant evidence has indicated that aside from the neural component, the non-neural cells of the CNS, such as glial cells, have important roles in the pathogenesis of pain (Coyle, 1998). To a certain extent, glial activation is triggered secondary to injury. Glial cells play an important role in the initiation, development and maintenance of persistent neuropathic pain. Both microglia and astrocytes are activated in the spinal cord after nerve injury, and pain is amplified when glia become activated (Mika, 2008). It has been hypothesized that neuropathic pain and morphine tolerance share some common pathological mechanisms (Mayer et al., 1999). Many studies have indicated that neuropathic pain leads to reduced morphine efficacy and the rapid development of morphine tolerance. The glia become activated in response to the repeated administration of morphine, which leads to the release of proinflammatory mediators and may oppose opioid analgesia by altering neuronal excitability (Campbell et al., 2006). It is not clear how opioids activate microglia in the spinal cord, but previous work by Hutchinson's team suggested the possible involvement of toll-like receptor 4 (TLR4) (Tanga et al., 2005). In this study, we tried to understand the role of microglia in morphine tolerance and also examine some possible methods for improving the efficacy of morphine to control neuropathic pain.

2. Basic mechanisms of neuropathic pain

Pain is a sensory system that, under normal conditions, is protective and adaptive. It serves as a warning signal for the body (tissue inflammation and damage) and induces behavioral changes that facilitate wound healing and recuperation and help to prevent further tissue damage (Bridges et al., 2001). Lesioning of the nervous system can produce a form of pathological pain called "neuropathic pain". Neuropathic pain is a debilitating condition that affects millions of individuals worldwide (Colburn et al., 1999; Zimmermann, 2001). It is characterized by sensory deficit, burning sensation, hyperalgesia and allodynia (Coyle, 1998). Changes in signal processing in the nervous system may contribute to or may become the sole cause for hyperalgesia and allodynia (DeLeo & Yezierski, 2001). A lesion in the peripheral nervous system may induce pain, but simply severing dorsal roots seems to have little chance of causing lasting pain (Li et al., 2000).

Combining inflammatory substances with nerve injury enhances pain behavior (Clatworthy et al., 1995), and there is a strong correlation between the presence of mechanical allodynia in different nerve injury models (Cui et al., 2000; Mirzaei et al., 2010). A neuroma forms when the nerve is injured. The spontaneous activity and ectopic sensitivity to mechanical, thermal, and chemical stimuli that originate from the traumatic neuroma have been well documented (Devor, 2006). It has been demonstrated that there is a large increase in the level of spontaneous firing in the afferent neurons linked to the injury site. Abnormal pain after peripheral nerve injury is dependent on the activation of spontaneous and persistent abnormal discharge from ectopic foci at the site of injury (Wall & Gutnik, 1974) and the dorsal root ganglia (DRG) (C. N. Liu et al., 2000). This spontaneous discharge has been termed ectopic discharge and has also been demonstrated in humans suffering from neuropathic pain (Nordin et al., 1984). Pain is exacerbated in part because of a reorganization of spinal cord circuitry in the setting of persistent injury (Basbaum, 1999). This leads to the prolonged hyperexcitability of spinal cord neurons, which alters transmission of the pain message. Enhanced sensitivity to pain may persist long (months and years) after the primary tissue damage has healed (Dworkin et al., 2003; DeLeo & Yezierski, 2001). Chemical and neural changes occur, at the site of tissue injury, at the nerve endings of pain fibers, along their axons, at first -order synapses, and both pre-and post synaptically in the dorsal horn of the spinal cord or in supra-spinal pain-processing areas. This processing, from the normal condition to a pain - facilitatory state, in the dorsal horn of the spinal cord is collectively known as central sensitization (G. Woolf & Salter, 2000). Pain can transform from a symptom to a disease when injury or inflammation is prolonged (Hucho & Levine, 2007; C. J. Woolf & Mannion, 1999). The alteration of central sensory processing by sensitization of the spinal cord seems to be the key step for many sensory abnormalities in the context of neuropathic pain (Gracely et al., 1993; Roberts, 1986). There has been a great deal of research into the mechanisms of chronic pain, with a strong focus on the development of central sensitization. Changes in dorsal horn neuronal excitability can be achieved by increasing the excitatory input or by decreasing the inhibitory tone. This concept of disinhibition has been of considerable interest as a key mediator of the transmission of augmented sensory input to higher CNS regions in neuropathic pain states. The majority of currently used neuropathic pain models display similar alterations in hind-limb cutaneous sensory thresholds following partial injury of a peripheral (usually sciatic) nerve. In particular, the demonstration of hyperalgesia to noxious thermal stimuli and allodynia to cold and mechanical stimuli are used as outcome measures (Bridges et al., 2001; Bennett, 2005). The three most commonly used models are the chronic constriction injury (CCI) of the sciatic nerve (Bennett & Xie, 1988), the partial sciatic nerve ligation model (PNL) (Seltzer et a1., 1990) and the spinal nerve ligation model (SNL) (Kim et al., 1999). We investigated the characteristics of a CCI neuropathic model from behavioral, molecular and electrophysiological perspectives. In our laboratory, the CCI model produced robust behavioral changes in terms of pain sensation. Findings reveal that the CCI procedure produces long-lasting cold and mechano-allodynia as well as hypersensitivity to noxious stimulation (Hamidi et al., 2006). Microscopic studies of the injured nerves have revealed pathological changes distal to the injured site (see Fig. 1). There is massive degeneration of myelinated axons and less marked damage to unmyelinated axons (Basbaum et al., 1991; Manaheji et al., 2005). It is believed that allodynia is a central phenomenon mediated by large myelinated fibers (Yamamoto & Yaksh, 1992). In the injured nerve, the evoked compound action potentials (CAPs) including conduction velocity (CV), amplitude and rising time have become standard tools for the evaluation of peripheral nerve disorders and the investigation of the function of the sciatic nerve. Recent research has shown that reduced CV can be caused by demyelination in the zone of the lesion (Basbaum et al., 1991). In our study, we found that the injury leads to a decrease in the CV and amplitude as well as an increase in the rising time of the CAPs (see Fig. 2). These changes are more pronounced in the recordings obtained distally to the ligated site. It seems that the sciatic nerve injuries yield changes in behavioral responses that are in accordance with the electrophysiological events that occur only in the distal part of the ligation site (Hamidi et al., 2006). Peripheral nerve injury is associated with inflammatory responses at the site of tissue damage. CNS injury is accompanied by the release of proinflammatory cytokines (Verri et al., 2006). Proinflammatory cytokines, especially tumor necrosis factor-α (TNF- α), interleukin (IL)-1 and IL-6, induce long-term alteration of synaptic transmission in the CNS and play a critical role in the development and maintenance of neuropathic pain (DeLeo & Yezierski, 2001).

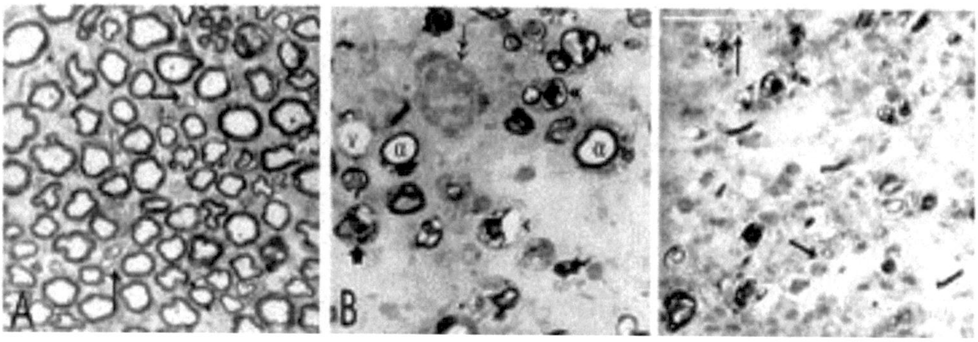

Fig. 1. Photomicrographs of toluidine blue stained semi-thin cross sections from normal sciatic (control or A). CCI 2 or B = two weeks after CCI. CCI 8 or C = eight weeks after CCI Small myelinated fibers (arrows) are shown in A&C, ruffled basal lamina (double head arrow) in B, Schwann cells or phagocytic cells containing myelin debris (thin arrows) in B, damaged axons (thick arrows)in B. Atrophic axons (double arrow heads) and Schwann cells (arrow head)and blood vessel(V) in B.

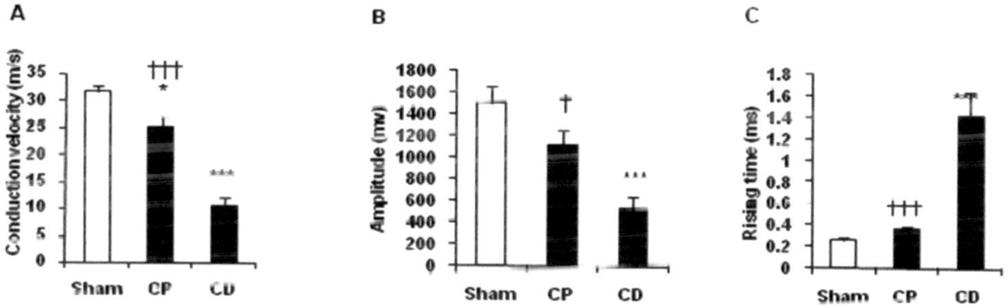

Fig. 2. Histograms of conduction velocity (CV) of the compound action potential (CAP) recorded from the sciatic nerve proximally. Location of stimulation was proximal (CP) or distal (CD) to the level of the constriction. A: The CV decreased in both operated CCI rats compared to the sham animals. B: amplitude of CAPs decreased in both CD and CP groups when compared to the sham animals. C: comparison of the rising time of CAPs represents a significant increased between the CD and CP and the sham animals. Asterisks indicate significant differences between CP and CD with sham. Crosses indicate significant difference between CD and CP.

3. Opioid tolerance in neuropathic pain

The perception of pain is modulated by pain-inhibitory and pain-facilitatory systems. The activation of several areas in the dorsal horn of the spinal cord results in the secretion of modulatory compounds that produce pain suppression (analgesia) or pain facilitation (hyperalgesia). Pain facilitation is mediated by many substances, including cholecystokinin (CCK), prostaglandins, dynorphin, substance P, and sympathetic amines (Mayer et al., 1999; Verri et al., 2006), and can be blocked by NMDA-receptor antagonists (Ben-Eliyahu et al., 1992; Parsons, 2001). Researchers are working to characterize the changes that occur in the nervous system during the development of neuropathic pain in animal models. An understanding of how neuropathic pain develops is necessary to guide the development of new pain therapies. Unfortunately, neuropathic pain is generally resistant to currently available treatments, so treatment options for neuropathic patients are limited, as opioids and other available pharmacological treatments are not able to adequately control associated spontaneous pain (Colburn et al., 1999). Non-steroidal anti-inflammatory drugs, antidepressants and local anesthetic agents are generally ineffective or have substantial drawbacks due to side effects. Generally, these treatments do not protect neurons from stress or death. Recent evidence suggests that NMDA receptor antagonists may have a role in attenuating the features of neuropathic pain. Glutamate concentration increases in the ipsilateral dorsal horn after CCI (Kawamata & Omote, 1996). It has been established that hyperalgesia can be prevented in the CCI model by continual pre- and post-injury i.p. administration of the NMDA receptor antagonist MK-801 (Davar et al., 1991). The endogenous opioid system plays a pivotal role in pain suppression. The administration of exogenous opioid drugs can also activate this system (Shavit et al., 2007). Notably, opioid compounds (e.g., morphine) have been used for centuries to combat many extremely painful conditions. Opioids are among the most effective analgesics for many types of pain (Rashid et al., 2004). However, opioids are reported to have suboptimal therapeutic efficacy against neuropathic pain (Bleeker et al., 2001; Cherny et al., 1994). There have been reports that chronic morphine treatment leading to 'morphine tolerance' may indeed induce the death of neurons (Hameed et al., 2010; Mao et al., 2002). The ineffectiveness of morphine in the context of neuropathic pain may be due to the reduced number of presynaptic opioid receptors due to the degeneration of primary afferent neurons, which is in turn caused by nerve damage. In our study, we treated rats with morphine and MK-801 both separately and together prior to CCI injury. This anti-nociceptive treatment prevents the establishment of altered central processing, which amplifies post-CCI pain. Therefore the application of morphine or MK-801 exerts a minimal effect on allodynia and hyperalgesia phenomena. However, the co-administration of morphine and MK-801 effectively modulates some aspects of neuropathic pain related to behavioral disorders in allodynia induced by extreme cold (Hamidi et al., 2006; Nichols et al., 1997). It has been hypothesized that neuropathic pain shares cellular and molecular mechanisms of neural plasticity with opioid tolerance. Additional evidence for this hypothesis came from a study by (Ossipov et al. 1995), which observed the same result with experimental animal models of neuropathic pain. A reduction in the number of μ-opioid receptors may be an important factor in diminishing the efficacy of morphine and μ-opioid receptor agonists (Przewlocki & Przewlocka, 2001). Partial sciatic nerve injury caused a drastic decrease in μ-opioid receptor expression in the injured DRG neurons (Rashid et al., 2004). Most previous studies examined the reasons behind the decreased effectiveness of spinal morphine in neuropathic pain, which includes reduced μ-opioid receptor (mOR) expression in the spinal dorsal horn (Porreca et al., 1998). It is well known that mOR expression is greatly decreased in the dorsal root ganglion neurons after peripheral nerve injury (Zang et al., 1998). In contrast, the functional activity of the central and peripheral opioid systems is enhanced by inflammation (Bilevicute-Ljungar et al., 2006). It has been shown that during inflammation, the effect of μ-opioid receptor agonists increases by approximately 10-fold (Cook & Nickerson, 2005). In a study from our laboratory, the effect of persistent arthritis inflammation on spinal μ-opioid receptor expression and variation in hyperalgesia was examined. The results indicated a significant increase in spinal μ-opioid receptor mRNA expression, which was demonstrated by semiquantitative RT-PCR in the first week after arthritis induction. There were also significant ipsilateral changes in thermal hyperalgesia after arthritis. However, in a 21-day study, both μ-opioid receptor mRNA expression and thermal hyperalgesia gradually decreased and achieved levels that were close to normal. It seems that μ-opioid receptor fluctuation may be involved in changes in hyperalgesia during the 21 days after arthritis (see Fig. 3).

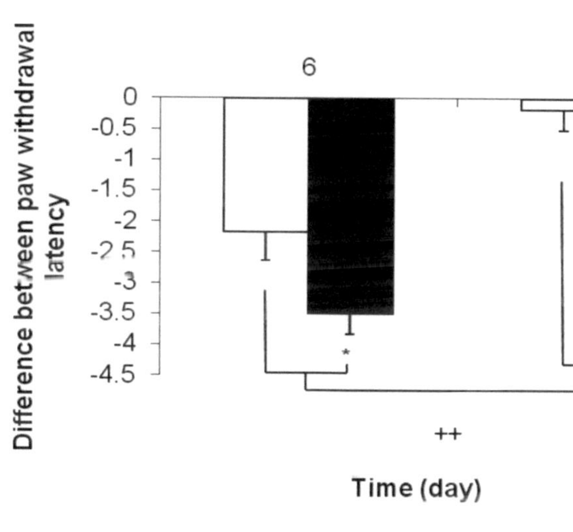

Fig. 3. Comparison of variation in thermal hyperalgesia after naloxone injection on day 6 and 21 days after induction of adjuvant arthritis (AA). (□), AA; (■), AA + naloxone. Data are the mean ±SEM (n= 6-7/ group). $P < 0.001$. *** $P < 0.01$, ** $P < 0.05$, *

Our results demonstrate that opioid receptor mRNA expression and variation in hyperalgesia are time dependent (Zaringhalam et al., 2008). Cytokines may play an important role in this mechanism by up-regulating mOR expression in the CNS. It is believed that excess IL-6 plays a pathogenic role in inflammation. In another set of experiments in our lab, we considered the role of IL-6 in arthritis. IL-6 is a multifunctional cytokine with pro- and anti-inflammatory properties. IL-6 mediates both acute and chronic phases of inflammatory responses and is therefore involved in both the early and late stages of inflammation (Moller & Villiger, 2006). Our study demonstrated that serum IL-6 and spinal mOR expression increased with concurrent decreases in hyperalgesia during the chronic phase of arthritis. This finding supports the hyperalgesic role of IL-6 during chronic inflammation. Our previous studies demonstrated that IL-6 administration resulted in analgesia, which was blocked by naloxone. This analgesia for sustained inflammatory pain was attributed to a local release of endogenous opioid peptide by immune cells after IL-6 challenge (Tekieh et al., 2011). These results demonstrated an anti-inflammatory effect of serum IL-6 during the chronic phase of arthritis (see Fig. 4). It has been suggested that IL-6 may serve as a regulator of inflammatory pain and may be essential in the immune-opioid pathway (De Jongh et al., 2003). Systemic administration of anti-IL-6 antibody reduced spinal mOR expression and subsequently increased hyperalgesia. IL-6 is an important cytokine for transitioning between acute and chronic inflammation and is involved in different stages of arthritis (Nishimoto & Kishimot, 2006). In another study we revealed an increase in the serum level of IL-6 in CCI animals which was blocked by minocyline and produced antinocicepion (Zanjani et al., 2006). These results suggest that the stages of inflammation in arthritis and the pain behaviors in CCI must be considered to achieve effective anti-hyperalgesic and anti-inflammatory intervention via anti-IL-6 antibody and analgesic effect of minocycline treatment respectively.

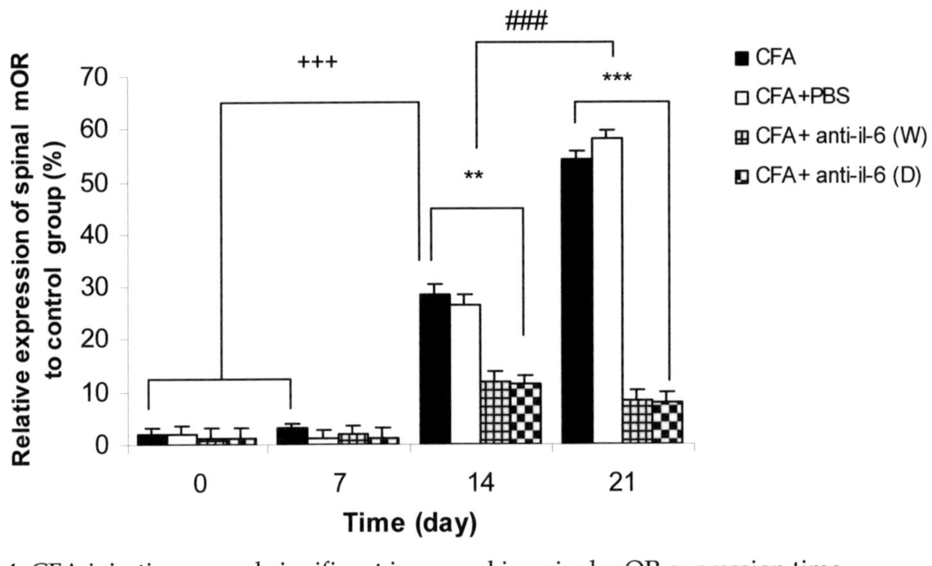

Fig. 4. CFA injection caused significant increased in spinal mOR expression time dependently. Anti- IL-6 antibody administration significantly reduced spinal mOR expression during different stages of AA. Ratio of spinal mOR protein band intensity in AA group significantly decreased at 14th and 21th days after anti-IL-6 antibody treatment compared to AA control group. Data are presented as mean ±SEM (n=6/ group). +++ $P < 0.001$ comparison of ratio of spinal mOR protein band intensity between different days of AA. ** $P < 0.01$, *** $P < 0.001$ comparison of spinal mOR protein band intensity between AA and AA + anti-IL-6 antibody treated rats. ### $P < 0.001$ indicated spinal mOR protein band intensity difference in AA and AA + anti-IL-6 antibody treated rats between 14th and 21th days.

4. Glial and opioid tolerance

As with peripheral mechanisms, much evidence supports the view that the initiation but not the maintenance of neuropathic pain behaviors is associated with immune mechanisms (Xu et al., 2006). Central glial activation is a player in this complicated nociceptive signaling cascade. It has become evident that spinal cord glial cells play a major role in pain facilitation (Campbell & Meyer, 2006; Watkins & Maier, 2002). It is proposed that neuropathic pain leads to reduced morphine efficacy and to the development of morphine tolerance. The results of many studies support the idea that the modulation of glial and neuroimmune activation may be a potential therapeutic mechanism to enhance morphine-induced analgesia (Mika, 2008). The analgesic potency of both systemic and intrathecal morphine is greatly reduced in animal models of neuropathic pain (Idanpaan et al., 1997). Recent evidence suggests that nerve damage evokes a cascade of immune responses and that glia play a crucial role in the maintenance of neuronal homeostasis in the central nervous system (Nakajima & Kohsaka, 2001; Stoll & Jander, 1999). In recognizing that glial cells play a role in chronic pain, one of the most important findings was that P2X receptors resided on glial cells, not on neurons (Sutherland, 2004). P2X receptors, or pain-signaling molecules, have long been associated with pain, but they were perceived to be associated with nerve cells. As a result of this discovery, researchers began inspecting the mechanisms of glial activation more closely (DeLeo, 2006). The mechanisms for this activation might be multifactorial. The glia become activated in response to the repeated administration of morphine, which leads to the release of proinflammatory mediators and may oppose opioid analgesia by altering the level of neuronal excitability. It has been increasingly recognized that spinal cord glial cells such as microglia and astrocytes play a critical role in the induction and maintenance of neuropathic pain by releasing powerful neuromodulators such as proinflammatory cytokines and chemokines. Recent evidence identifies chemokines as new players in pain control (Gao & Ji, 2010). Targeting glial activation is a clinically promising method for the treatment of neuropathic pain (Mika, 2008). Glial cells represent 70% of the cells in the central nervous system (CNS), and microglia represent 5–10% of glial cells under normal conditions. Microglia cells have a small soma bearing thin and branched processes under normal conditions. They are the first non-neural cells to respond to a CNS perturbation such as nerve injury or chronic opioid administration (Raghavendra et al., 2002; Tanga et al., 2004). They play a crucial role in the maintenance of neuronal homeostasis in the central nervous system. It seems that microglia might be responsible for the initiation of neuropathic pain states (Marchand et al., 2005), and their production of immune factors is believed to play an important role in nociceptive transmission (Colburn, 1999; Watkins, et al., 2001). Nerve injury distal to the dorsal root ganglia leads to microglial activation. However, activation after dorsal rhizotomy is much reduced, in keeping with the observation that dorsal rhizotomy leads to less impressive hyperalgesia as compared to spinal nerve lesions involving the identical root (Willis et al., 2006). After activation, microglia cells change morphology from a resting, ramified shape into an active, amoeboid shape (Stoll & Jander, 1999). Activated microglia have dual regulatory functions in the maintenance and facilitation of tissue homeostasis in the CNS. They remove dead cells or dangerous debris by releasing toxic factors and phagocytosis, but they also repair injured cells by releasing neurotrophic factors (Quattrini et al., 1996). The exact mechanism of microglia cell activation may involve the release of algesic factors such as ATP, glutamate and nitric oxide from injured or hyperactive neurons (Inoue, 2006; Watkins & Maier, 2005). Microglial activation can alter the activity of opioid systems, and neuropathic pain is characterized by resistance to morphine. The major proinflammatory cytokines (IL-1, IL-6 and TNF-α) oppose acute opioid analgesia. Their effects may interact because suppressing the action of any single cytokine unmasks continuing analgesia (Hutchinson et al., 2008). The spinal cellular source of the proinflammatory signal was also of interest. Studies of normal spinal cord document the basal expression of proinflammatory cytokines in glia and to some extent in neurons, suggesting that under acute conditions, both glial and neural stores may be available to oppose opioid analgesia. The potentiation of acute morphine analgesia by minocycline suggests that microglia may prove to be a significant source of mediators that oppose opioid analgesia (Fu et al., 2006). Nevertheless, later reports that studied hyperalgesia in the spinal cord revealed that cytokines were indeed being secreted in a chronic pain state (Wieseler-Frank et al., 2005). These proinflammatory cytokines, specifically tumor necrosis factor (KB-TNF-α), interleukin-1 (IL-1), and interleukin-6 (IL-6), are proteins that are vital in immune-to-brain communication (Sweitzer et al., 2002; Watkins & Maier, 2005; Watkins & Milligan, 2001). It has been found that propentofylline, pentoxifylline, fluorocitrate, ibudilast and minocycline decrease microglial and astroglial activation and inhibit proinflammatory cytokines, thereby suppressing the development of neuropathic pain (Mika, 2008; Raghavendra et al., 2004). Interathecal delivery of the antibiotic minocycline, an inhibitor of microglial activation, attenuates neuropathic pain (Raghavendra et al., 2003). Some glial inhibitors, which are safe and clinically well tolerated, are potentially useful agents for the treatment of neuropathic pain and for the prevention of tolerance to morphine analgesia. Evidence exists for a role of the ATP receptors P2X4 and/or P2X7, both of which are expressed on microglia. The chemokine fractalkine may also be involved, as blockade of its receptor, CX3CR1, attenuates hyperalgesia in neuropathic pain models (Milligan et al., 2005).

Pentoxifylline is a non-specific cytokine inhibitor and an inhibitor of phosphodiesterase that can inhibit the synthesis of TNF-a, IL-1β and IL-6. Some studies have demonstrated that pentoxifylline influences the development of neuropathic pain behavior in rats and mice (J. Liu et al., 2007; Mika et al., 2007). The local injection of pentoxifylline reduced inflammatory pain by decreasing TNF-a (Dorazil-Dudzik et al., 2004). When injected in a preemptive analgesia schema, it reduces postoperative pain in patients (Dobrogowski et al., 2005).The anti-nociceptive effects of pentoxifylline are correlated with a reduced production of TNF-a, IL-1β, and IL-6 through the inhibition of nuclear factor-KB as well as the stimulation of IL-10 expression in the spinal cord and brain (Vale et al., 2004). However, the therapeutic effects of pentoxifylline on developed neuropathic pain remain to be determined by future studies.

Minocycline, a semi-synthetic second-generation tetracycline with adequate penetration into the brain and cerebrospinal fluid (Colovic & Caccia, 2003), has emerged as a potent inhibitor of microglial activation and proliferation, without any known direct action on astrocytes or neurons (Tikka et al., 2001). The effects of minocycline are mediated by microglial cells and are distinct from the antimicrobial actions of this drug (He et al., 2001). The administration of minocycline either systemically or intrathecally attenuated hyperalgesia in rat models of neuropathy. The effect is associated with an inhibition of spinal microglial activation and the attenuated expression of proinflammatory cytokines (Ledeboer et al., 2005; Mika et al., 2007). It is emphasized that minocycline attenuated the development of behavioral hypersensitivity in the rat model of neuropathic pain when the inhibitor was injected preemptively (Raghavendra et al., 2003). However, the analgesic effects of minocycline in a rat model of neuropathic pain result from attenuated expression of IL-1β, IL-6, TNF-a, IL-1β-converting enzyme, TNF-α-converting enzyme, an IL-1β receptor antagonist and IL-10 in the lumbar dorsal spinal cord.

Activation of microglial cells occurs in the dorsal horn, and this activation may play a vital role in initiating central sensitization. The role of this activation in ongoing neuropathic pain is less clear. The sensation of pain begins with a simple thesis: nociceptors encode information about noxious stimuli and propagate these messages to the CNS; then, pain is felt. In the case of neuropathic pain, however, we see that a complex biology is at play (Campbell et al., 2006). Recent studies indicate that preemptive treatment with glial inhibitors seems to be more effective than their administration after glial cells have already been activated (Raghavendra et al., 2003). We observed similar results with minocycline. Preemptive treatment with minocycline in our study attenuated hyperalgesia and allodynia in CCI. We observed that minocycline, which was reported to have a neuroprotective effect in some neurodegenerative diseases, reversed hyperalgesia and allodynia due to sciatic nerve ligation and inhibited interleukin-6 production (see Fig. 5).

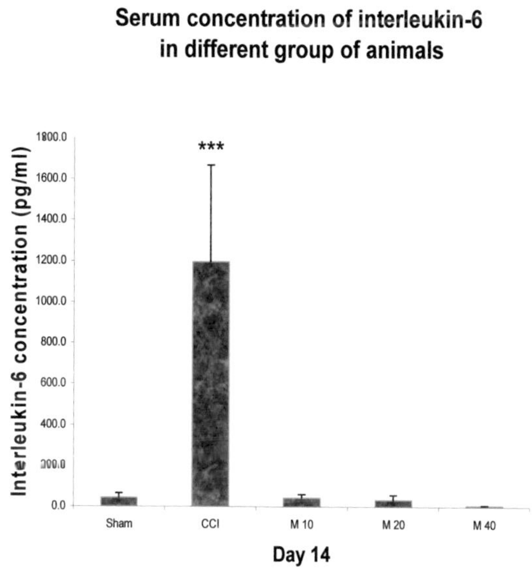

Fig. 5. Serum concentration of interleukin-6 in CCI saline-treated, sham-operated and CCI minocycline – treated rats on day 14 post- ligation. Data are presented as mean ±SEM of 6 rats in each group. *** $P < 0.001$ indicate a statistically significant difference when compared to CCI saline - treated rats. M10 = minocycline 10 mg/kg, M20 = minocycline 20 mg/kg, M40 = minocycline 40 mg/kg

It seems that minocycline could have an anti-inflammatory and analgesic effect in some chronic pain states (Zanjani et al., 2006). As chronic morphine activates spinal cord glia, glial activation causes morphine tolerance, and both neuropathic pain and morphine tolerance share the same mechanism (Mayer et al., 1999), we sought to understand the role of microglia in the morphine tolerance observed following the administration of glial inhibitors (pentoxifylline and minocycline) *after* glial cells have already been activated. We administered Pentoxifylline and Minocyclines i.p. after chronic opioid treatment in a CCI model. Interestingly, the results demonstrated the attenuation of hyperalgesia and allodynia. This suggests a glial contribution in changing nociceptive processing, which could be blocked by glial inhibitor agents and enhance the analgesic effect of morphine. Some studies have suggested that glial-derived fractalkine is an endogenous regulator of morphine analgesia. It is involved in increasing pain sensitivity, which occurs after chronic opioid treatment (Verge et al., 2004). Several other possible mechanisms involving activated glia have been suggested, such as morphine-induced p^{38} MAPK activation in microglia, changes in the glial regulation of glutamatergic NMDA receptors and the release of excitatory amino acids, prostaglandins and dynorphin (Svensson et al., 2006). Recent works have indicated that microglia are responsible for opioid tolerance and dependence (Guo & Schluesener, 2007). It is not clear how opioids activate microglia in the spinal cord, but previous work by Hutchinson's team suggested the possible involvement of toll-like receptor 4 (TLR4). The results indicate a role for the pattern recognition receptor TLR4 in microglial activation, which provides a link between central sensitization and innate immune responses. Levels of spinal mRNA for TLR4 are increased after L5 SNL (Tanga et al, 2005). TLR4 is involved in neuropathic pain and the dysregulation of opioid actions (Hutchinson et al, 2008). Notably, morphine upregulates TLR4 expression in microglia (Hutchinson et al., 2007). The neuropathic pain arising from CCI is created in part via activation of TLR4, which contributes to microglial activation. These data suggest that TLR4 may prove to be a target worth exploring to improve clinical pain control (Hutchinson et al., 2008).

5. Conclusion

These findings suggest that the analgesic efficacy of opioid is reduced by glial activation, and the release of proinflammatory cytokines may have implications for the treatment of pain. Blocking agents may improve the effectiveness of morphine. Blocking glial activation and the subsequent release of proinflammatory cytokines may minimize the development of opiate tolerance, providing more effective treatment for chronic pain, which is particularly advantageous for the treatment of neuropathic pain.

6. Acknowledgement

This work was supported by grants from the neuroscience research center of Shahid Beheshti University of Medical Sciences.The author would like to thank their outstanding support.

7. References

Basbaum, A. I. (1999). Spinal Mechanisms of Acute and Persistent Pain. *Regional Anesthesia and Pain Medicine*, Vol. 24, No. 1, pp. 59–67. ISSN, 10987339

Basbaum, A. I., Gautron, M., Jazat, F., Mayes, M. & Guilbaud, G. (1991). The Spectrum of Fiber Loss in a Model of Neuropathic Pain in Rat: An Electron Microscopic Study. *Pain*, Vol. 47, No. 3, pp. 359–367. ISSN, 03043959

Ben-Eliyahu, S., Marek, P., Vacccarino, A. L., Mogil, J. S., Sternberg, W. F. & Liebeskind J. C. (1992). The NMDA Receptor Antagonist MK-801 Prevents Long-Lasting Non-Associative Morphine Tolerance in the Rat. *Brain Research*, Vol. 575, No.2 , pp. 304–308. ISSN, 00068993

Bennett, G. J. (2005). Experimental Neuropathic Pain in Animals: Models and Mechanisms, In: *Pain: An Update Review*, D.J. Justins (Ed). pp. 97–105, IASP Press, ISBN, 9780931092633 , Seattle, WA.

Bennett, G. J. & Xie, Y. K. (1988). A Peripheral Mononeuropathy in Rat That Produces Disorders of Pain Sensation Like Those Seen in Man. *Pain*, Vol. 33, No. 1, pp. 87–107. ISSN, 03043959

Bileviciute-Ljungar, I., Saxne, T. & Spetea, M. (2006). Anti- Inflammatory Effects of Contralateral Administration of the Kappa-Opioid Agonist U-50 488H in Rats with Unilaterally Induced Adjuvant Arthritis. *Rheumatology*, Vol. 45, No. 3, pp. 295–302. ISSN, 0315162x

Bleeker, C. P., Bremer, R. C., Dongelmans, D.A., van Dongen, R.T. & Crul, B. J. (2001). Inefficacy of High-Dose Transdermal Fentanyl in a Patient with Neuropathic Pain: A Case Report. *European Journal of Pain*, Vol. 5, No. 3, pp. 325–329. ISSN, 10903801

Bridges, D., Thompson, S. W. N. & Rice, A. S. C. (2001). Mechanisms of Neuropathic Pain. *British Journal of Anesthesia*, Vol. 87, No. 1, pp. 12–26. ISSN, 00070912

Campbell, J. N., Basbaum, A. I., Dray, A., Dubner, R., Dworkin, R. H. & Sang, C. N. (Eds.). (2006). *Emerging Strategies for the Treatment of Neuropathic Pain*, IASP press, ISBN, 9780931092619, Seatle , WA.

Campbell, J. N. & Meyer, R. A. (2006). Mechanisms of Neuropathic Pain. *Neuron*, Vol. 52, No. 1 , pp. 77–92. ISSN, 08966273

Cherny, N. I., Thaler, H. T., Friedlander-Klar, H., Lapin, J. Foley, K. M. , Houde, R., & P0rtenoy, R. K. (1994). Opioid Responsiveness of Cancer Pain Syndromes Caused by Neuropathic or Nociceptive Mechanisms: A Combined Analysis of Controlled Single Dose Studies. *Neurology*, Vol. 44, No. 5 , pp. 857–861. ISSN,00283878

Clatworthy, A. L., Illich, P.A., Castro, G. A. & Walters, E. T. (1995). Role of Peri-Axonal Inflammation in the Development of Thermal Hyperalgesia and Guarding Behavior in a Rat Model of Neuropathic Pain. *Neuroscience Letters*, Vol. 184, No. 1 , pp. 5–8. ISSN, 03043940

Colburn, R. W., Rickman, A. J. & DeLeo, J. A. (1999). The Effect of Site and Type of Nerve Injury on Spinal Glial Activation and Neuropathic Pain Behavior. *Experimental Neurology*, Vol. 157, No. 2 , pp. 289–304. ISSN, 00144886

Colovic, M. & Caccia, S. (2003). Liquid Chromatographic Determination of Minocycline in Brain-to-Plasma Distribution Studies in the Rat. *Journal of Chromatography B*, Vol. 791, No. 1-2 , pp. 337–343. ISSN, 15700232

Cook, C. D. & Nickerson, M. D. (2005). Nociceptive Sensitivity and Opioid Antinociception and Antihyperalgesia in Freund's Adjuvant-Induced Arthritic Male and Female Rats. *Journal of Pharmacology and Experimental Therapeutics*, Vol. 313, No. 1 , pp. 449–459. ISSN, 00223565

Coyle, D. E. (1998). Partial Peripheral Nerve Injury Leads to Activation of Astroglia and Microglia Which Parallels the Development of Allodynic Behavior. *Glia*, Vol. 23, No. 1 , pp. 75–83. ISSN, 10981136

Cui, J-G., Holmin, S., Mathiesen, T., Meyerson, B.& Linderoth, B. (2000). Possible Role of Inflammatory Mediators in Tactile Hypersensitivity in Rat Models of Mononeuropathy. *Pain*, Vol. 88, No. 3 , pp. 239–248. ISSN, 03043959

Davar, G., Hama, A., Deykin, A., Vos, B. & Maciewicz, R. (1991). MK 801 Blocks the Development of Thermal Hyperalgesia in a Rat Model of Experimental Painful Neuropathy. *Brain Research*, Vol. 553, No. 2 , pp. 327–330. ISSN, 00068993

De Jongh, R. F., Vssers, K. C., Booij, L. H., De Jongh, K. L., Vincken, P. & Meert, T. F. (2003). Interleukin -6 and Perioperative Thermoregulation and HPA-Axis Activation. *Cytokine*, Vol. 21, No. 5 , pp. 248–256. ISSN, 10434666

DeLeo, J. A. (2006). Basic Science of Pain. *The Journal of Bone and Joint Surgery, American Volume*, Vol. 88, No.2 , pp. 58–62. ISSN, 00219356

DeLeo, J. A. & Yezierski, R. P. (2001).The role of Neuroinflammation and Neuroimmune Activation in Persistent Pain. *Pain*, Vol. 90, No. 1-2 , pp. 1–6. ISSN, 03043959

Devor, M. (2006). Response of nerves to injury in relation to neuropathic pain. In: *Wall and Melzack's Textbook of Pain*, S. B. McMahon & M. Koltzenburg, (Eds.). pp. 905–927, Elsevier, ISBN, 9780443072871 , London, UK.

Dobrogowski, J., Wrzosek, A. & Wordliczek, J. (2005). Radiofrequency Denervation with or without Addition of Pentoxifylline or Methylprednisolone for Chronic Lumbar Zygapophysial Joint Pain. *Pharmacological Reports*, Vol. 57, No. 4 , pp. 475–480. ISSN, 17341140

Dorazil-Dudzik, M., Mika, J., Schafer, M. K., Li, Y., Obara, I., Wordliczek, J. & Przewocka, B. (2004). The Effects of Local Pentoxifylline and Propentofylline Treatment on Formalin Induced Pain and Tumor Necrosis Factor Messenger RNA Levels in the Inflamed Tissue of the Rat Paw. *Anesthesia & Analgesia*, Vol. 98, No. 6 , pp. 1566–1573. ISSN, 00032999

Dworkin, R. H., Backonja, M., Rowbotham, M. C., Allen, R. R., Argoff, C. R., Bennet, G. J. (2003). Advances in Neuropathic Pain: Diagnosis, Mechanisms, and Treatment Recommendations. *Archives of Neurology*, Vol. 60, No. 11 , pp. 1524–1534. ISSN, 00039942

Fu, D., Guo, Q., Ai, Y., Cai, H., Yan, J. & Dai, R. (2006). Glial Activation and Segmental Up Regulation of Interleukin 1β (IL- 1β) in the Rat Spinal Cord after Surgical Incision. *Neurochemical Research*, Vol. 31, No. 3 , pp. 333–340. ISSN, 15736903

Gao, Y. J. & Ji, R. R. (2010). Chemokines, Neuronal-Glial Interactions, and Central Processing of Neuropathic Pain. *Pharmacology & Therapeutics*, Vol. 126, No. 1, pp. 56–68. ISSN, 01637258

Gracely, R. H., Lynch, S. A. & Bennet, G. J. (1993). Painful Neuropathy: Altered Central Processing Maintained Dynamically by Peripheral Input. *Pain*, Vol. 51, No. 2 , pp. 175–194. ISSN, 03043959

Guo, L. H. & Schluesener, H. J. (2007). The Innate Immunity of the Central Nervous System in Chronic Pain: The Role of Toll-Like Receptors. *Cellular and Molecular Life Sciences*, Vol. 64, No. 9 , pp. 1128–1136. ISSN, 1421682x

Hameed, H., Hameed, M. & Christo, P. J. (2010). The Effect of Morphine on Glial Cells as a Potential Therapeutic Target for Pharmacological Development of Analgesic Drugs. *Current Pain and Headache Reports*, Vol. 14, No.2 , pp. 96–104. ISSN, 15343433

Hamidi, G. A., Manaheji, H., Janahmadi, M., Noorbaksh, S. M. & Salami, M. (2006). Co-Administration of MK-801 and Morphine Attenuate Neuropathic Pain in Rat. *Physiology & Behavior*, Vol. 88, No.4-5 , pp. 628–635. ISSN, 00319384

He, Y., Appel, S. & Le, W. (2001). Minocycline Inhibits Microglial Activation and Protects Nigral Cells after 6-Hydroxydopamine Injection into Mouse Striatum. *Brain Research*, Vol. 909, No.1-2 , pp. 187–193). ISSN, 00068993

Hucho, T. & Levine, J. D. (2007). Signalling Pathways in Sensitization: Toward Nociceptor Cell Biology. *Neuron*, Vol. 55, No.3 , pp. 365–376. ISSN, 08966273

Hutchinson, M. R., Bland, S. T., Johnson, K. W., Rice, K. C., Maier, S. F. & Watkins, L. R. (2007). Opioid-Induced Glia Activation: Mechanisms of Activation and Implications for Opioid Analgesia, Dependence and Reward. *The Scientific World Journal*, Vol. 7, No. , pp. 98–111. ISSN, 1537744x

Hutchinson, M. R., Coats, B. D., Lewis, S. S., Zhang, Y., Sprunger, D. B., Rezvani, N., Baker, E. M., Jekich, B. M., Wieseler, J. L., Somogyi, A. A., Martin, D., Poole, S. , Judd, C. M., Maier, S. F. & Watkins, L. R. (2008). Proinflammatory Cytokines Oppose Opioid-Induced Acute and Chronic Analgesia. *Brain, Behavior, and Immunity*, Vol. 22, No. 8 , pp. 1178–1189. ISSN, 08891591

Idanpaan Heikkila, J. J., Guilbaud, G. & Kayser, V. (1997). Prevention of Tolerance to the Antinociceptive Effects of Systemic Morphine by a Selective Cholecystokinin-B Receptor Antagonist in a Rat Model of Peripheral Neuropathy. *Journal of Pharmacology and Experimental Therapeutics*, Vol. 282, No. 3 , pp. 1366–1372. ISSN, 00223565

Inoue, K. (2006). The Function of Microglia through Purinergic Receptors: Neuropathic Pain and Cytokine Release. *Pharmacology & Therapeuitcs*, Vol. 109, No.1-2 , pp. 210–226. ISSN, 01637258

Kawamata, M. & Omote, K. (1996). Involvement of Increased Excitatory Amino Acids and Intracellular Ca2+ Concentration in the Spinal Dorsal Horn in an Animal Model of Neuropathic Pain. *Pain*, Vol. 68, No. 1 , pp. 85–96. ISSN, 03043959

Kim, Y. I. & Chung, J. M. (1992). An experimental model for peripheral neuropathy produce by segmental spinal nerve ligation in the rat. *Pain*, Vol.50, No. 3 pp. 355-363. ISSN, 03043959

Ledeboer, A., Sloane, E. M., Milligan, E. D., Frank, M. G., Mahony, J. H., Maier, S. F. & Watkins, L. R. (2005). Minocycline Attenuates Mechanical Allodynia and Proinflammatory Cytokine Expression in Rat Models of Pain Facilitation. *Pain*, Vol. 115, No.1-2 , pp. 71 83. ISSN, 03043959

Li, Y., Dorsi, M. J., Meyer, R. A. & Belzberg, A. J. (2000). Mechanical Hyperalgesia after an L5 Spinal Nerve Lesion in the Rat Is not Dependent on Input from Injured Nerve Fibers. *Pain*, Vol. 85, No. 3 , pp. 493–502. ISSN, 03043959

Liu, J., Feng, X., Yu, M., Xie, W., Zhao, X., Li, W., Guan, R. & Xu, J. (2007). Pentoxifylline Attenuates the Development of Hyperalgesia in a Rat Model of Neuropathic Pain. *Neuroscience Letters*, Vol. 412, No. 3 , pp. 268–272. ISSN, 03043940

Liu, C. N., Wall, P. D., Ben-Dor, E., Michaelis, M., Amir, R., Devor, M., (2000). Tactile Allodynia in the Absence of C-fiber Activation: Altered Firing Properties of DRG Neurons Following Spinal Nerve Injury. *Pain*, Vol. 85, No. 3 , pp. 503–521 ISSN, 03043959

Manaheji, H., Nasirinezhad, F. & Behzadi, G. (2005). Effect of Intrathecal Transplantation of Adrenal Medullary Tissue on the Sciatic Nerve Regeneration Following Chronic Constriction Injury in the Rat. *Yakhteh*, Vol. 7, No. 2, pp. 68–73. ISSN, 15614921

Mao, J., Sung, B., Ji, R. R. & Lim, G. (2002). Neural Apoptosis Associated with Morphine Tolerance: Evidence for an Opioid-Induced Neurotoxic Mechanism. *Journal of Neuroscience*, Vol. 22, No.17 , pp. 7650–7661. ISSN, 02706474

Marchand, F., Perretti, M. & McMahon, S. B. (2005). Role of the Immune System in Chronic Pain. *Nature Reviews. Neuroscience*, Vol. 6, No. , pp. 521 532. ISSN, 14710048

Mayer, D. J., Mao, J., Holt, J. & Price, D. D. (1999). Cellular Mechanisms of Neuropathic Pain, Morphine Tolerance and Their Interactions. *Proceedings of the National Academy of Sciences USA*, Vol. 96, No. 14 , pp. 7731–7736. ISSN, 00278424

Mika, J. (2008). Modulation of Microglia Can Attenuate Neuropathic Pain Symptoms and Enhance Morphine Effectiveness. *Pharmacological Reports*, Vol. 60, No. 3 , pp. 297–307. ISSN, 17341140

Mika, J., Osikowicz, M., Makuch, W. & Przewocka, B. (2007). Minocycline and Pentoxifylline Attenuate Allodynia and Hyperalgesia and Potentiate the Effects of Morphine in Rat and Mouse Models of Neuropathic Pain. *European Journal of Pharmacology*, Vol. 560, No. , pp. 142–149. ISSN, 00142999

Milligan, E., Zapata, V., Schoeniger, D., Chacur, M., Green, P., Poole, S., Martin, D., Maier, S. F. & Watkins, L. R. (2005). An Initial Investigation of Spinal Mechanisms Underlying

Pain Enhancement Induced by Fractalkine, a Neuronally Released Chemokine. *European Journal of Neuroscience*, Vol. 22, No.11 , pp. 2775–2782. ISSN, 14609568

Mirzaei, V., Manaheji, H., Maghsoudi, N., Zaringhalam, J. (2010). Comparison of Changes in mRNA Expression of Spinal Glutamate Transporters Following Induction of Two Neuropathic Pain Modeles. Spinal Cord, Vol. 48, No. 11 , PP. 791-797. ISSN, 13624393

Moller, B. & Villiger, P. M. (2006). Inhibition of IL-1, IL-6 and TNF-Alpha in Immune-Mediated Inflammatory Diseases. *Seminars in Immunopathology*, Vol. 27, No.4 , pp. 391–408. . ISSN, 18632297

Nakajima, K. & Kohsaka, S. (2001). Microglia: Activation and Their Significance in the Central Nervous System. *Journal of Biochemistry*, Vol. 130, No. 2 , pp. 169–175. ISSN, 60219258

Nichols, M. L., Lopez, Y., Ossipov, M. H., Bian, D. & Porreca, F. (1997). Enhancement of the Antiallodynic and Antinociceptive Efficacy of Spinal Morphine by Antisera to Dynorphine A (1-13) or MK-801 in a Nerve-Ligation Model of Peripheral Neuropathy. *Pain*, Vol. 69, No. 3 , pp. 317–322. ISSN, 03043959

Nishimoto, N. & Kishimot, T. (2006). Interleukin 6: From Bench to Bedside. *Nature Clinical Practice. Rheumatology*, Vol. 2, No. 12 , pp. 619–626. ISSN, 0315162x

Nordin, M., Nystrom, B., Wallin, U. & Hagbarth, K. E. (1984). Ectopic Sensory Discharge and Paresthesiae in Patients with Disorders of Peripheral Nerves, Dorsal Roots and Dorsal Columns. *Pain*, Vol. 20, No. , pp. 231–245. ISSN, 03043959

Ossipov, M. H., Lopez, Y., Nicholos, M. L., Bian, D. & Porreca, F. (1995). Inhibition by Spinal Morphine of the Tail-Flick Attenuated in Rats with Nerve Ligation Injury. *Neuroscience Letters*, Vol. 199, No.12 , pp. 83–86. ISSN, 03043959

Parsons, C. G. (2001). NMDA Receptors as Targets for Drug Action in Neuropathic Pain. *European Journal of Pharmacology*, Vol.429, No. , pp. 71–78. ISSN, 00142999

Porreca, F., Tang, Q. B., Bian, D., Riedl, M., Elde, R. & Lai, J. (1998). Spinal Opioid Mu Receptor Expression in Lumbar Spinal Cord of Rats Following Nerve Injury. *Brain Research*, Vol. 795, No. 1-2 , pp. 197–203. ISSN, 00068993

Przewlocki, R. & Przewlocka, B. (2001). Opioids in Chronic Pain. *European Journal of Pharmacology*, Vol. 429, No.1-3 , pp. 79–91. ISSN, 00142999

Quattrini, A., Previtali, S., Feltri, M. L., Canal, N., Nemni, R. & Wrabetz, L. (1996). 4 Integrin and Other Schwann Cell Markers in Axonal Neuropathy. *Glia*, Vol. 17, No. , pp. 294–306. ISSN, 10981136

Raghavendra, V., Rutkowski, M. D. & DeLeo, J. A. (2002). The Role of Spinal Neuroimmune Activation in Morphine Tolerance- Hyperalgesia in Neuropathic and Sham-Operated Rats. *Journal of Neuroscience*, Vol. 22, No. 22, pp. 9980–9989. ISSN, 02706474

Raghavendra, V., Tanga, F. Y. & DeLeo, J. A. (2004). Attenuation of Morphine Tolerance, Withdrawal-Induced Hyperalgesia, and Associated Spinal Inflammatory Immune Responses by Propentofylline in Rats. *Neuropsychopharmacology*, Vol. 29, No. 2 , pp. 327-334. ISSN, 0893133x

Raghavendra, V., Tanga, F., Rutkowski, M. D. & DeLeo, J. A. (2003). Anti-Hyperalgesic and Morphine-Sparing Actions of Propentofylline Following Peripheral Nerve Injury In Rats: Mechanistic Implications of Spinal Glia and Proinflammatory Cytokines. *Pain*, Vol. 104, No.3 , pp. 655–664. ISSN, 03043959

Rashid, Md. H., Inoue, M., Toda, K. & Ueda, H. (2004). Loss of Peripheral Morphine Analgesia Contributes to the Reduced Effectiveness of Systemic Morphine in

Neuropathic Pain. *Journal of Pharmacology and Experimental Therapeutics*, Vol. 309, No. 1 , pp. 380–387 ISSN, 00223565.

Roberts, W. J. (1986). A Hypothesis on the Physiological Basis for Causalgia and Related Pains. *Pain*, Vol. 24, No. 3 , pp. 297–311. ISSN, 03043959

Shavit, Y., Wolf, G., Johnston, I. N., Westbrook, R. F., Watkins, L. R. & Yirmia, R. (2007). Proinflammatory Cytokines Modulate Neuropathic Pain, Opioid Analgesia, and Opioid Tolerance. In: *Immune and Glial Regulation of Pain*, J. A. DeLeo, L. S. Sorkin, & L. R. Watkins (Eds.), pp. 361–382, IASP Press, ISBN 9780931092671 , Seattle, WA.

Seltzer, Z., Dubner, R. & Shir, Y. (1990). A Novel Behavioral Model of Neuropathic Pain Disorders Produced in Rats by Partial Sciatic Nerve Injury. *Pain*, Vol. 43, No. 2 , pp. 205–218. ISSN, 03043959

Stoll, G. & Jander, S. (1999). The role of Microglia and Macrophages in the Pathophysiology of the CNS. *Progress in Neurobiology*, Vol. 58, No. 3 , pp. 233–247.

Sutherland, S. (2004). Glia Emerge as Pain Therapy Targets. *Drug Discovery Today*, Vol. 9, No. 14, p. 588. ISSN, 03010082

Svensson, C. I., Schafers, M., Jones, T. L., Yaksh, T. L. & Sorkin, L. S. (2006). Covariance Among Age, Spinal P38 MAP Kinase Activation and Allodynia. *Journal of Pain*, Vol. 7, No. 5 , pp. 337–345. ISSN, 15265900

Sweitzer, S. M., Hicky, W. F., Rutkowski, M. D., Pahl, J. L. & DeLeo, J. A. (2002). Focal Peripheral Nerve Injury Induces Leukocyte Trafficking into the Central Nervous System: Potential Relationship to Neuropathic Pain. *Pain*, Vol. 100, No.1-2 , pp. 163–170. ISSN, 03043959

Tanga, F. Y., Nutile-McMenemy, N. & DeLeo, J. A. (2005).The CNS Role of Toll-Like Receptor 4 in Innate Neuroimmunity and Painful Neuropathy. *Proceedings of the National Academy of Sciences USA*, Vol. 102, No. 16 , pp. 5856–5861. ISSN, 00278424

Tanga, F.Y., Raghavand, V. & DeLeo, J. A. (2004). Quantitative Real-Time RT-PCR Assessment of Spinal Microglial and Astrocytic Activation Markers in a Rat Model of Neuropathic Pain. *Neurochemistry International*, Vol. 45, No. 2-3 , pp. 397–407. ISSN, 01970186

Tekieh, E., Zaringhalam, J., Manaheji, H., Maghsoodi, N., Alani B. & Zardooz, H. (2011). Increased Serum IL-6 level Time-Dependently Regulates Hyperalgesia and Spinal Mu Opioid Receptor Expression During CFA-Induced Arthritis. *EXCLI Journal*, Vol. 10, No. , pp. 23–33. ISSN, 16112156

Tikka, T., Fiebich, B. L., Goldsteins, G., Keinanen, R. & Koistinaho J (2001). Minocycline, a Tetracycline Derivative, Is Neuroprotective Against Excitotoxicity by Inhibiting Activation and Proliferation of Microglia. *Journal of Neuroscience*, Vol. 21, No.8 , pp. 2580–2588. ISSN, 02706474

Vale, M. L., Benevides, V. M., Sachs, D., Brito, G. A., da Rocha, F. A., Poole, S., Ferreira, S. H., Cunha, F. Q. & Ribeiro, R.A. (2004). Antihyperalgesic Effect of Pentoxifylline on Experimental Inflammatory Pain. *British Journal of Pharmacology*, Vol. 143, No. 7 , pp. 833–844. ISSN, 14765381

Verge, G. M., Milligan, E. D., Maier, S. F., Watkins,L.R., Naeve, G. S. & Foster, A.C.(2004). Fractalkine (CXCL1) and Fractalkine Receptor (CX3CR1) Distribution in Spinal Cord and Dorsal Root Ganglia Under Basal and Neuropathic Pain Conditions. *European Journal of Neuroscience*, Vol. 20, No. 5 , pp. 1150–1160. ISSN, 0953816x

Verri Jr., W. A., Cunha, T. M., Parada, C. A., Poole, S., Cunha, F. Q. & Ferreira, S. H. (2006). Hypernociceptive Role of Cytokines and Chemokines: Target for Analgesic Drug

Development? *Pharmacology & Therapeutics*, Vol. 112, No. 1 , pp. 116–138. ISSN, o1637258

Wall, P. D. & Gutnick, M. (1974). Ongoing Activity in Peripheral Nerves: The Physiology and Pharmacology of Impulses Originating from a Neuroma. *Experimental Neurology*, Vol. 43, No. 3 , pp. 580–593. ISSN, 00144886

Watkins, L.R., Hutchinson, M.R., Johnson, I.N. & Maier, S. F. (2005). Glia: Novel Counter-Regulators of Opioid Analgesia. *Trends in Neurosciences*, Vol. 28, No. 12 , pp. 661–669. ISSN, 01662236

Watkins, L. R. & Maier, S. F. (2002). Beyond Neurons: Evidence that Immune and Glial Cells Contribute to Pathological Pain States. *Physiological Reviews*, Vol. 82, No. 4 , pp. 981–1011. ISSN, 00319333

Watkins, L. R. & Maier, S. F. (2005). Immune Regulation of Central Nervous System Functions: From Sickness Responses to Pathological Pain. *Journal of Internal Medicine*, Vol. 257, No. , pp. 139–155. ISSN, 13652796

Watkins, L.R., Milligan, E. D. & Maier S. F. (2001). Spinal Cord Glia: New Players in Pain. *Pain*, Vol. 93, No.3 , pp. 201–205. ISSN, 03043959

Wieseler-Frank, J., Maier, S. & Watkins, L. (2005). Immune-to-Brain Communication Dynamically Modulates Pain: Physiological and Pathological Consequences. *Brain Behavior and Immunity*, Vol. 19, No. 2, pp. 104–111. ISSN, 08891591

Willis Jr., W. D., Hammond, D. L., Dubner, R., Merzenich, M., Eisenach, J. C., Salter, M. W., Lyengar, S. & Shippenberg, T. (2006). Central Nervous System Targets: Rapporteur Report. In: *Emerging Strategies for the Treatment of Neuropathic Pain*, J. N. Campbell, A. I. Basbaum, A. Dray, R. Dubner, R. H. Dworkin & C. N. Sang, (Eds.), pp. 105–122, IASP Press, ISBN, 9780931092619 , Seattle, WA.

Woolf, C. J. & Mannion, R. J. (1999). Neuropathic Pain: Etiology, Symptoms, Mechanisms, and Management. *Lancet*, Vol. 353, No. , pp. 1959–1964. ISSN, 01406736

Woolf, G. & Salter, M. W. (2000). Neuronal Plasticity: Increasing the Gain in Pain. *Science*, Vol. 288, No.5472 , pp. 1765–1768. ISSN, 00368075

Xu, J. T., Xin, W. J., Zang, Y., Wu, C. Y. & Liu, X. G. (2006). The Role of Tumor Necrosis Factor-Alpha in the Neuropathic Pain Induced by Lumbar 5 Ventral Root Transaction in Rat. *Pain*, Vol. 123, No.3 , pp. 306–321. ISSN, 03043959

Yamamoto, T. & Yaksh, T. L. (1992). Studies on the Spinal Interaction of Morphine and the NMDA Antagonist MK-801 on the Hyperesthesia Observed in a Rat Model of Sciatic Mononeuropathy. *Neuroscience Letters*, Vol. 135, No.1 , pp. 67–70. ISSN, 03043940

Zang, X., Bao L., Shi, T. J., Ju, G., Elde, R. & Hokfelt, T. (1998). Down-Regulation of Mu-Opioid Receptors in Rat and Monkey Dorsal Root Ganglion Neurons and Spinal Cord after Peripheral Axotomy. *Neuroscience*, Vol. 82, No. 1 , pp. 223–240. ISSN, 03064522

Zanjani, T. M., Sabetkasaei, M., Mosaffa, N., Manaheji, H., Labibi, F. & Farokhi, B. (2006). Suppression of Interleukin-6 by Minocycline in a Rat Model of Neuropathic Pain. *European Journal of Pharmacology*, Vol. 538, No. 1-3 , pp. 66–72. ISSN, 00142999

Zaringhalam, J., Manaheji, H., Maghsoodi, N., Farokhi, B. & Mirzaie, V. (2008). Spinal μ-Opioid Receptor Expression and Hyperalgesia with Dexamethasone in Chronic Adjuvant-Induced Arthritis in Rats. *Clinical and Experimental Pharmacology and Physiology*, Vol. 35, No. 11 , pp. 1309–1315. ISSN, 03051870

Zimmermann, M. (2001). Pathobiology of Neuropathic Pain. *European Journal of Pharmacology*, Vol. 429, No. 1-3 , pp. 23–37. ISSN, 00142999

10

An Approach to Identify Nerve Injury-Evoked Changes that Contribute to the Development or Protect Against the Development of Sustained Neuropathic Pain

Esperanza Recio-Pinto[1,2], Monica Norcini[1] and Thomas J.J. Blanck[1,3]
[1]Department of Anesthesiology,
[2]Department of Pharmacology,
[3]Department of Neuroscience and Physiology,
[1,2,3]New York University Langone Medical Center
USA

1. Introduction

Chronic neuropathic pain is a huge public health problem that compromises the quality of life of millions of individuals. There are many causes for chronic neuropathic pain, one of them being peripheral nerve injury occurring during surgery or trauma. Even when considering only those cases resulting from surgery about 2-10% of patients undergoing various surgeries (amputation, breast surgery, thoracotomy, inguinal hernia, coronary artery bypass surgery, caesarean section) develop chronic severe (disabling) pain (Kehlet et al., 2006). In the USA alone, there are approximately 80 million surgeries performed each year (Apfelbaum et al., 2003); if only 5% of those patients went on to develop severe chronic pain, ~4 million people would be added to the list of chronic pain patients each year. Of the patients attending chronic pain clinics, 20% have implicated surgery as one of the causes of their chronic pain and, in about half of these, it was the sole cause (Macrae, 2001). The intensity of acute postoperative pain is a good predictor of long-term pain; however, adequate control of acute postoperative pain does not always lead to a decrease in the incidence of developing long term pain (Perkins and Kehlet, 2000). To reduce the level of tissue injury during surgery, surgical procedures have been modified including those used for joint repair (Kehlet et al., 2006); mastectomy and breast reconstruction (Galun et al.; 2010; Vadivelu et al., 2008) and herniorraphy (Nathan and Pappas, 2003; Pokorny et al., 2008); however, a significant percentage of patients still develop chronic pain. Hence, there is a need to develop treatments that can be used before and during the early phases following nerve injury (as a result of surgery or trauma) to prevent the development of chronic pain. The development of chronic pain following surgery correlates with the presence of peripheral nerve injury (Macrae, 2001). Studies using various peripheral nerve injury models have shown that these models share some, but not all, of the injury-induced molecular changes that may be contributing to chronic neuropathic pain (Berger et al., 2011; Xu and Yaksh, 2011). Moreover, whether changes in a given molecule contribute to neuropathic pain also appears to depend in their anatomical location (neuroma at the site of the peripheral nerve injury, dorsal root ganglia somata, spinal cord etc). Hence there is a need to not only identify the molecules but their relevant location with respect to their contribution to neuropathic pain. Those studies have also shown that not all of the underlying causes for neuropathic pain are shared between the various peripheral nerve injury models, for example in the "sciatic nerve ligation" model blocking the excitability of the nerve prior to its ligation (injury) and for a period following the injury (~week) eliminates the development of sustained neuropathic pain (mechanical allodynia)(Kim and Nabekura, 2011). On the other hand in the "sural spared nerve injury model", in which the common peroneal and the tibial branches of the sciatic nerve are cut, blocking the nerve impulses before and during one week after the nerve injury does not eliminate the development of sustained neuropathic pain (Suter et al., 2003). The latter picture more closely resembles the clinical outcome of many surgical patients that endure peripheral nerve injuries (Perkins and Kehlet, 2000). Since dorsal root ganglia sensory neurons are the first sensory neurons that are affected following a peripheral nerve injury; then another approach for treatment could be to modulate (rather than block) their activity. Pharmacological modulation should be directed to either prevent or compensate for the injury-evoked functional alterations that contribute to the initiation and probably maintenance (at least at early stages) of chronic pain and in this way prevent/limit central sensitization and in turn the level of sustained neuropathic pain.

Studies directed towards detecting injury-evoked changes that correlate with the presence of neuropathic pain have identified changes in the expression of a large number of molecules that appear to contribute to neuropathic pain states (Berger et al., 2011; Xu and Yaksh, 2011). This information has provided many insights for possible treatments; sadly, for the most part effective sustained neuropathic pain treatment still remains evasive. Hence studies identifying not only the changes that contribute to neuropathic pain but also those that limit the magnitude of neuropathic pain following a nerve injury should provide additional information that could improve treatment. In this chapter we will touch on two points: first why the dorsal root ganglia is an attractive pharmacological target to prevent as well as reverse neuropathic pain states (at least at the early stages) resulting from peripheral nerve injury. Second, we will describe an approach (using two modalities of an already established animal model, the spared nerve injury (Decosterd and Woolf, 2000)) to distinguish peripheral nerve injury-induced changes within the dorsal root ganglia (or at any level of the sensory pathway) that contribute to the development of chronic neuropathic pain from those that represent a protective response and hence limit the development and the level of chronic neuropathic pain.

2. The dorsal root ganglia provides an interesting pharmacological target for treating neuropathic pain resulting from peripheral nerve injury

2.1 Dorsal root ganglia morphology

The arrangement of the dendrites, cell body and axon in dorsal root ganglia sensory neurons is different from that of most neurons. In early embryonic stages these neurons are bipolar (Matsuda et al., 1996) (Figure 1). During late embryonic development the proximal regions of the two processes coalesce into a T-shaped process and these neurons progressively become pseudounipolar such that by birth most of them are pseudounipolar (Matsuda et al., 1996). The pseudounipolar conformation appears to ensure as well as allow for modulation of the impulses being transmitted from the periphery to the central terminals of dorsal root ganglia sensory neurons (Amir and Devor, 2003a; Amir and Devor, 2003b; Devor, 1999). Within the dorsal root ganglia there are no synaptic contacts between neurons however, the somata have microvilli that appear to contribute to the observed interactions between the neuronal somata and between neuronal somata and their surrounding satellite glia cells (Pannese, 2002; Takeda et al., 2009). Moreover, the lack of a nerve-blood barrier also exposes the somata within the dorsal root ganglia to plasma molecules that can modulate their function (Abram et al., 2006; Hirakawa et al., 2004). Each soma is completely surrounded by a layer of satellite glia cells (Figure 1); and together the soma and satellite glia cells form a single anatomical and functional unit (Hanani, 2005; Pannese, 1981). These individual units can have one to three neuronal somata, and occasionally some of the somata within a unit are not surrounded by satellite glia cells (Pannese et al., 1991). The units are in turn separated by areas of connective tissue (Pannese et al., 1991). Following nerve injury satellite glial cells, as their glia counterparts in the CNS, undergo functional changes (release of cytokines and neurotrophins, changes in neurotransmitter-scavenging capacity) and hence they may also contribute to the initiation and maintenance of chronic pain (Gosselin et al., 2010; McMahon and Malcangio, 2009; Milligan and Watkins, 2009; Romero-Sandoval et al., 2008; Scholz and Woolf, 2007; Takeda et al., 2009; Watkins et al., 2001; Watkins and Maier, 2002).

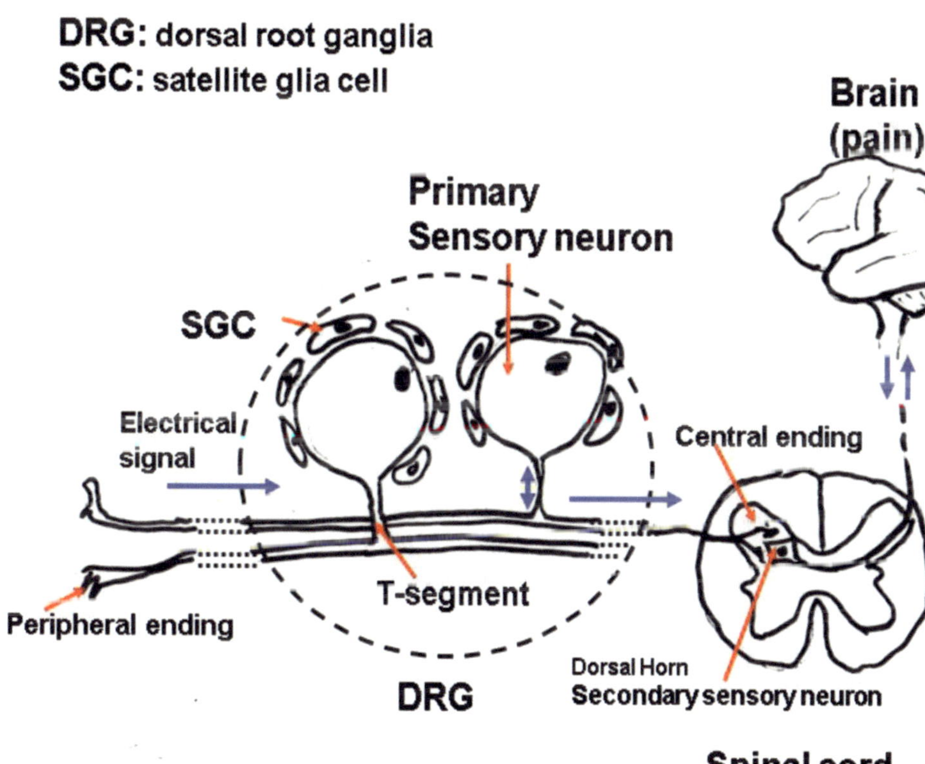

Fig. 1.

2.2 Dorsal root ganglia as a pharmacological target to avoid the development of chronic pain following peripheral nerve injury

The dorsal root ganglia is a good pharmacological target for preventing the initiation and limiting the level of chronic neuropathic pain following peripheral nerve injury because: First, the dorsal root ganglia sensory neurons are the first neurons in the sensory pathway that are affected following a peripheral nerve injury. It is known that within the dorsal root ganglia there is crosstalk between the sensory neurons and signals from the injured sensory neurons can modulate the activity of the uninjured neurons within the same ganglia (Ali et al., 1999; Wu et al., 2002). Even during peripheral nerve injuries that do not directly affect the dorsal root ganglia sensory neurons; for example when the injury solely involves motor axons (e.g. during ventral L5 transection) (He et al., 2010; Li et al., 2002); the dorsal root ganglia sensory neurons still undergo functional changes that have been found to correlate with the development of neuropathic pain (He et al., 2010; Wu et al., 2002; Xu et al., 2006). Some of the peripheral nerve injury-induced functional changes in the dorsal root ganglia sensory neurons are believed to be important for the initiation and sustained alteration of the activity of the spinal cord neurons and in turn of the brain neurons (central sensitization) that underly chronic neuropathic pain (Harris et al., 1996; Jang et al., 2007; Lee et al., 2003; Liu and Salter, 2010; Obata et al., 2003; Ringkamp and Meyer, 2005). Second, although the dorsal root ganglia is surrounded by a thick connective tissue capsule, the dorsal root ganglia is not protected by a "blood-nerve barrier", as it is the rest of the peripheral nervous system (Abram et al., 2006; Hirakawa et al., 2004). Hence the somata of dorsal root ganglia sensory neurons as well as their surrounding satellite glia cells can be specifically targeted (with respect to the rest of the nervous system including the central nervous system that is also protected by the "blood-brain barrier") with pharmacological agents. Third, the excitability of dorsal root ganglia somata and their T segments (both located within the dorsal root ganglia) facilitate and regulate the transmission of the electrical signal from the periphery to the central dorsal root ganglia sensory terminals (Amir and Devor, 2003a; Amir and Devor, 2003b; Devor, 1999); hence one could also pharmacologically and locally alter the electrical activity of the somata and their T segments in order to compensate for the injury-evoked changes in sensory activity (from periphery to central endings) that contribute to the initiation and establishment of chronic pain.

2.3 Peripheral nerve injury alters the dorsal root ganglia environment and function

Following peripheral nerve injury, the properties for generating afferent impulses (action potentials) are modified and such modifications are believed to contribute to the initiation of central sensitization which includes several components including activation of the NMDAr and increased AMPA subunit expression (at the spinal cord) (Harris et al., 1996; Liu and Salter, 2010). Peripheral nerve injury-evoked changes in impulse generation include the appearance of ectopic afferent impulses and the modification of the stimuli-evoked impulses. Following sciatic nerve injury (constriction or cutting), ectopic discharges (firing of action potentials) from the injured site (Tal and Eliav, 1996; Wall and Gutnick, 1974a; Wall and Gutnick, 1974b; Wall and Devor, 1983) and the dorsal root ganglia (Amir et al., 2002; Liu et al., 2000a; Liu et al., 1999; Liu et al., 2000b) correlate with the development of neuropathic pain. The frequency of ectopic discharges shows a transient increase within the first 24 hrs following spinal nerve ligation (Sun et al., 2005). Based on this it was concluded that ectopic discharges may only contribute to the initiation of mechanical allodynia (Sun et al., 2005). In that same study, however, the pattern of the discharges was altered throughout the observation period (14 days) (from tonic and bursting to irregular). This suggests that not only the presence but also the pattern of ectopic discharges could be important to the development and/or maintenance of neuropathic pain. In addition to "ectopic" discharges, changes in the "stimuli-evoked" discharges have also been found to be altered following spinal nerve ligation (Sun et al., 2005). Therefore, both ectopic discharges and alterations of stimuli-evoked discharges appear to contribute to the initiation and maintenance of neuropathic pain.

Studies characterizing the expression of various ion channel proteins that underlie the electrical excitability of dorsal root ganglia neurons show that many of them undergo changes following a peripheral nerve injury, including various sodium channels (Dib-Hajj et al., 2010), potassium channels (Abdulla and Smith, 2001; Chien et al., 2007; Kim et al., 2002) and calcium channels (Abdulla and Smith, 2001;).

Since excitability of sensory neurons involve activation of voltage-dependent sodium channels, many studies have been directed to understand whether their changes (if any) following injury contribute to neuropathic pain. Those studies have been recently reviewed (Amir et al., 2006; Dib-Hajj et al., 2010; Liu and Wood, 2011). Here we will just describe some of the results mostly to indicate the complexity of the problem. There are nine isoforms of voltage-dependent sodium channels and some of the isoforms are expressed by dorsal root ganglia sensory neurons but not by muscle tissue, which make them potential pharmacological targets (Amir et al., 2006). What it has been found is that their role in neuropathic pain following peripheral nerve injury is a complex one (Dib-Hajj et al., 2010; Liu and Wood, 2011). The Nav1.3 is increased in dorsal root ganglia somata following various peripheral nerve injuries, however a decrease of their expression (with antisense) has been reported to either decrease (Hains et al., 2003; Hains et al., 2004) or have no effect in the development of chronic pain (Lindia et al., 2005). Nav1.8 and Nav1.7 accumulate within injured axons in painful human neuromas (Kretschmer et al. 2002, Bird et al. 2007, Black et al. 2008). Nav1.8 is upregulated in the uninjured L4 and L5 dorsal root ganglia after L5 ventral root transection (Chen et al., 2011; He et al., 2010). Moreover, the increased membrane expression of Nav1.8 leads to spontaneous repetitive discharge. However, the increase in Nav1.8 (Amir et al., 2006; Nassar et al., 2005), and of Nav1.7 (Nassar et al., 2004; Nassar et al., 2005) appears to underlie purely inflammatory pain but not neuropathic pain. Finally, Nav1.8 (as well as Nav1.9), is downregulated in axotomized neurons (Dib-Hajjet al. 1998b, Sleeper et al. 2000, Decosterd et al. 2002) and within the injured human dorsal root ganglia neurons (Coward et al. 2000, 2001) Similarly to sodium channels, there are also reported changes in potassium channels (Chien et al., 2007; Kim et al., 2002;) and calcium channels (Abdulla and Smith, 2001; Luo et al., 2001; Newton et al., 2001) that have been postulated to contribute to the excitability changes of sensory neurons and to contribute to neuropathic pain. Hence, although injury-induced changes in excitability of dorsal root ganglia neurons is believed to contribute to the development of chronic pain; the players involved as well as their role are less clear and they may not be the same in different types of injury.

Another approach has been to identify soluble factors that are altered following injury and are responsible for evoking the excitability changes of dorsal root ganglia neurons. Following nerve injury there is an invasion of immune cells into the nervous system that is promoted largely by the Wallerian degeneration of the injured nerve as well as by damage of the tissue surrounding the nerve (Chung et al., 2007; Dubovy et al., 2007; Hu and McLachlan, 2002). The immune cells alter the neuronal environment in part by changing the level of various cytokines/chemokines produced by the immune cells and by the neurons and glial cells in response to those released by the immune cells (Austin and Moalem-Taylor; Brazda et al., 2009; Dubovy et al., 2006; Dubovy et al., 2010a; Dubovy et al., 2010b). Since some of the immune mediators have been shown to contribute to neuropathic pain by altering the excitability of both primary and secondary sensory neurons one approach that has been investigated to treat/prevent chronic pain is to pharmacologically alter their production. This approach however, has been limited because some of these factors also have been found to be involved in axonal regeneration or neuroprotection (e.g. IL-6) (Murphy et al., 1999; Osamura et al., 2005; Wang et al., 2007; Wang et al., 2009) or in muscle regeneration (e.g. CCL2)(Lu et al., 2011; Van Steenwinckel et al., 2011; Wang et al., 2010). The contribution of immune mediators to neuropathic pain appears to involve alterations of excitability of primary and secondary sensory neurons; therefore, a more targeted approach such as decreasing their level (and/or production by) at the dorsal root ganglia, and in this way blocking their effects on excitability of primary sensory dorsal root ganglia neurons, could improve their use for treating neuropathic pain.

In addition to changes in cytokines/chemokines, there are many other genes/proteins that have been found to be upregulated or downregulated in the dorsal root ganglia sensory neurons following nerve injury but in many cases their contribution to chronic pain is also complex (Birder and Perl, 1999; Krekoski et al., 1996; Lee et al., 2002; Schafers et al., 2003; Seijffers et al., 2006; Xiao et al., 2002; Zhou et al., 1999). For example, following sciatic nerve injury there is an increase in the BDNF expression in large dorsal root ganglia sensory neurons and in satellite glia cells, while its expression is decreased in small dorsal root ganglia sensory neurons (Zhou et al., 1999), moreover the magnitude of the change in BDNF expression in dorsal root ganglia neurons depends on the site of the peripheral nerve injury (proximal vs distal) (Obata et al., 2006). These studies suggested that increases in BDNF expression in the large dorsal root ganglia sensory neurons contribute to neuropathic pain following peripheral nerve injury (Obata et al., 2006; Zhou et al., 1999). However, blocking production of BDNF by dorsal root ganglia sensory neurons, showed that BDNF in dorsal root ganglia sensory neurons, while it contributed to inflammatory pain (induced by injections of either Carrageean, NGF or Formalin), it did not contribute to the development of neuropathic pain (following L5 spinal nerve ligation) (Zhao et al., 2006). Moreover, intrathecal application of BDNF has been shown to have both pronociceptive (Yajima et al., 2002; Yajima et al., 2005) and antinociceptive (Cejas et al., 2000; Eaton et al., 2002) effects following a peripheral nerve injury. These studies indicate that in order to establish that a molecular change within the dorsal root ganglia contribute to neuropathic pain requires more than a simple correlation between the observed molecular change and the presence of neuropathic pain.

As stated above peripheral nerve injuries result in alterations of the properties for generating afferent impulses (action potentials) in primary sensory neurons which in turn are believed to contribute to the initiation of central sensitization which underlies the development of chronic pain. Therefore, one approach to prevent the development of chronic pain has been to block excitability of primary sensory neurons. Interestingly, blocking the excitability of the nerve prior to its injury and for a period following the injury (~week) eliminates the development of sustained neuropathic pain when the injury involves sciatic nerve ligation (Kim and Nabekura, 2011) but not when it involves cutting branches of the sciatic nerve (Suter et al., 2003). This suggests that the injury-evoked alterations of nerve discharges (ectopic and stimuli-evoked) differ whether the nerve is cut or not. The outcome observed in the model involving partial cut of the sciatic nerve (Suter et al., 2003) closely resembles the clinical outcome of many surgical patients that endure peripheral nerve injuries (Perkins and Kehlet, 2000). For these patients, another approach for treatment could be to pharmacologically modulate (rather than block) the activity of dorsal root ganglia sensory neurons even at the early stages following nerve injury. Such pharmacological modulation should be designed to prevent or compensate for their functional alterations evoked by the nerve injury and in this way prevent/limit central sensitization and in turn the level of sustained neuropathic pain. Such modulation could be potentially mediated by altering the excitability of the dorsal root ganglia neuronal somata. The apparent complexity of the role in neuropathic pain of various molecules in part may reflect our lack of understanding in their overall role in chronic pain. Some of the expression changes (and/or their magnitude) could actually reflect a protective response that would limit the level of sustained pain rather than promote the level of sustained pain. Hence, there is a need to use experimental approaches to distinguish between the peripheral nerve injury-induced changes (within the dorsal root ganglia or at any level of the sensory pathway) that contribute to the development of chronic neuropathic pain from those that represent a protective response and hence limit the development and the level of chronic neuropathic pain.

3. An approach to distinguish injury-induced changes that contribute to the development of chronic pain from those that limit the development of neuropathic pain

As summarized above, multiple studies have identified either increases or decreases in a large number of parameters at the molecular level (protein expression/function) and at the cellular level (morphological/functional) in neuropathic pain states. Some of those changes have also been shown to contribute to neuropathic pain. However, the contribution of many of the observed changes is less clear. In fact not all the changes that take place in conditions leading to neuropathic pain are necessarily contributing to neuropathic pain. Most likely some of them could actually represent protective responses that decrease the level of sustained neuropathic pain. One approach to facilitate the distinction between whether a change contributes to or limits the level of neuropathic pain will be use a model in which two levels of neuropathic pain can be induced, and in one of the modalities there is a partial reversal of the level of neuropathic pain. We have found that one such model is the Spared Nerve Injury (SNI). This model has been extensively used but usually by using only one of the modalities. Here we describe the advantage of the simultaneous use of two modalities of the SNI. One modality the Tibial-SNI, displays a transient-strong (low threshold) mechanical allodynia followed by sustained-mild allodynia (Figure 2A green line); while the other modality the Sural-SNI displays sustained strong mechanical allodynia (higher threshold) (Figure 2A blue line). We have used these two modalities of the SNI to help identify the role of injury-evoked changes at the dorsal root ganglia that contribute to the initiation and maintenance of strong mechanical allodynia (transition from acute to chronic pain), compared to injury-evoked changes that could limit the level of sustained mechanical allodynia (compensatory/protective responses). Basically, changes that are found to be proportional to the level of sustained mechanical allodynia would be identified as contributing to long term mechanical allodynia (to the transition from acute to chronic pain) and changes that are inversely proportional to the level of sustained mechanical allodynia would be identified as limiting the sustained level of mechanical allodynia (protective responses) (Figure 2B). The simultaneous use of these two SNI modalities would allow one to more easily identify changes that could help limit the level of sustained neuropathic pain.

By using this approach we have analyzed changes in mRNA in L4 DRG at about 3 months post injury, by doing so we have identified four groups of mRNA: (1) A group of mRNAs that showed the same expression level in Tibial-SNI, Sural-SNI and Sham; (2) A group of mRNAs that showed changes in expression only in Tibial-SNI as compared to Sham and Sural-SNI; (3) A group of mRNAs that showed changes in expression only in Sural-SNI as compared to Sham and Tibial-SNI; and (4) A group of mRNAs that displayed changes in expression in both Sural- and Tibial-SNI, but not always in the same magnitude or direction (↑ or ↓) (not shown). As expected when comparisons were done only between one of the SNI groups (Sural-SNI or Tibial-SNI) and Sham it resulted in a large number of genes that displayed changes in their expression in that SNI group; however, when comparisons were done by selecting the genes that their expression changed in one of the SNI groups but not in the Sham and in the other SNI group; the number of genes that changed was highly reduced. Some genes of interest that changed only in the dorsal root ganglia from Tibial-SNI (presumably genes that could be involved in limiting the level of sustained mechanical allodynia) include a reduction in Hcn2 which encodes a hyperpolarization activated cyclic nucleotide-gated K channel 2 that has been shown to contribute to spontaneous rhythmic activity in both heart and brain (Dibbens et al., 2010; Lin et al., 2009); an increase in Map3k10 a kinase that functions preferentially on the JNK signaling pathway, and that has been reported to be involved in nerve growth factor (NGF) induced neuronal apoptosis (NGF is increased following nerve injury) (see ref in (Castillo et al., 2011)). A decrease in Rbm9, a gene that encodes an RNA binding protein that is believe to be a key regulator of alternative exon splicing in the nervous system. Using this approach will facilitate the identification of additional molecules that are involved in nerve-injured evoked neuropathic pain. Including genes/proteins whose alterations correlate with the initiation and/or maintenance of mechanical allodynia (hence correlating with the transition from acute to chronic pain); as well as with the recuperation from mechanical allodynia (correlating with recuperation from acute pain).

It is well accepted that chronic pain, ultimately reflects functional changes in the brain, in particular in the thalamocortical connections/interactions (Cauda et al., 2009; Cheong et al., 2011; Walton et al., 2010). With respect to structural cortical changes, most of those that have been found to be associated with neuropathic pain have been observed in animals and patients that have been experiencing neuropathic pain for a long period. Such structural changes are believed to underlie the changes in cortical activity observed in patients with long term neuropathic pain (Peyron et al., 2004; Walton et al., 2010). And it has been concluded that such cortical structural changes take place at latter phases of neuropathic pain, and are believed to be a consequence (rather than a cause), of chronic pain. However, a couple of observations support the involvement of early cortical alterations in synaptic plasticity in brain following peripheral nerve injury. One week after Sural-SNI, pyramidal neurons in the contralateral medial prefrontal cortex display an increase in the number of branches and length of basal dendrites, an increase in the spine density and an increase in the NMDA component of synaptic currents (Metz et al., 2009). And recently it was shown that remodeling of cortical connections in the primary sensory cortex is transiently affected early on following sciatic nerve ligation and those changes correlated with the presence of mechanical allodynia (Kim and Nabekura, 2011). The simultaneous use of both SNI models could also help clarify the role of those early cortical structural changes in the initiation of chronic pain.

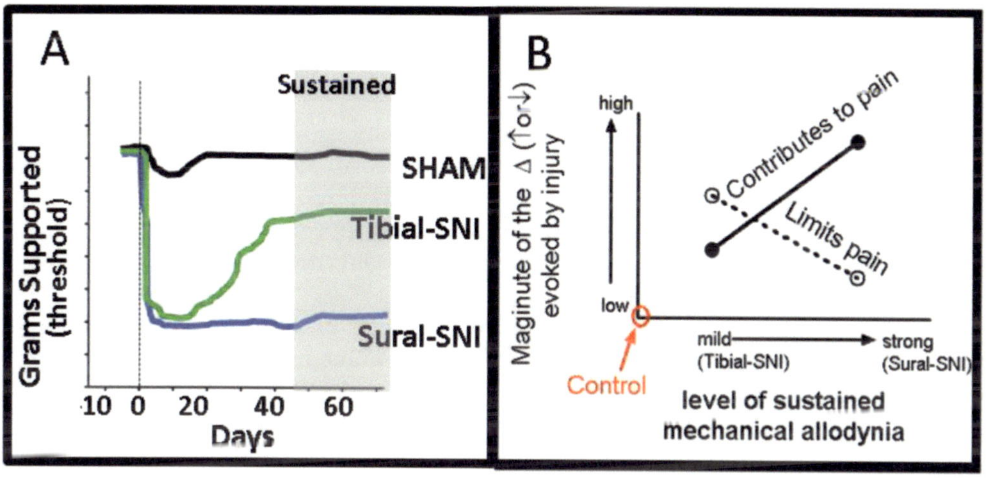

Fig. 2.

4. Conclusion

In summary, peripheral nerve injuries including those occurring during surgery correlate with the development of chronic pain states. Moreover, blocking the nerve impulses during the injury and for a short period following the injury does not prevent the development of chronic pain states in a large number of patients. Hence, there is a need to develop treatments that can be used before and during the early phases of nerve injury (resulting from either surgery or trauma) that will prevent the development of chronic pain in these patients. Most studies have been directed towards the understanding of the changes in the sensory pathway that contribute to the initiation and development of central sensitization. However, equally important but much less studied, are the protective injury-induced functional changes in the sensory pathway in general, and in the dorsal root ganglia in particular that could limit the development of neuropathic pain. Here we describe that the simultaneous use of two of the SNI modalities of the sciatic nerve could facilitate the identification of changes that contribute to the transition from acute to chronic pain as well as those involved in the recovery from acute pain (less than 3 weeks) and that would limit the level of sustained chronic pain; that are involved following a peripheral nerve injury.

5. References

Abdulla, F.A., Smith, P.A., 2001. Axotomy- and autotomy-induced changes in Ca2+ and K+ channel currents of rat dorsal root ganglion neurons. J Neurophysiol. 85, 644-58.

Abram, S.E., Yi, J., Fuchs, A., Hogan, Q.H., 2006. Permeability of injured and intact peripheral nerves and dorsal root ganglia. Anesthesiology. 105, 146-53.

Ali, Z., Ringkamp, M., Hartke, T.V., Chien, H.F., Flavahan, N.A., Campbell, J.N., Meyer, R.A., 1999. Uninjured C-fiber nociceptors develop spontaneous activity and alpha-adrenergic sensitivity following L6 spinal nerve ligation in monkey. J Neurophysiol. 81, 455-66.

Amir, R., Michaelis, M., Devor, M., 2002. Burst discharge in primary sensory neurons: triggered by subthreshold oscillations, maintained by depolarizing afterpotentials. J Neurosci. 22, 1187-98.

Amir, R., Devor, M., 2003a. Electrical excitability of the soma of sensory neurons is required for spike invasion of the soma, but not for through-conduction. Biophys J. 84, 2181-91.

Amir, R., Devor, M., 2003b. Extra spike formation in sensory neurons and the disruption of afferent spike patterning. Biophys J. 84, 2700-8.

Amir, R., Argoff, C.E., Bennett, G.J., Cummins, T.R., Durieux, M.E., Gerner, P., Gold, M.S., Porreca, F., Strichartz, G.R., 2006. The role of sodium channels in chronic inflammatory and neuropathic pain. J Pain. 7, S1-29.

Apfelbaum, J.L., Chen, C., Mehta, S.S., Gan, T.J., 2003. Postoperative pain experience: results from a national survey suggest postoperative pain continues to be undermanaged. Anesth Analg. 97, 534-40, table of contents.

Austin, P.J., Moalem-Taylor, G., The neuro-immune balance in neuropathic pain: involvement of inflammatory immune cells, immune-like glial cells and cytokines. J Neuroimmunol. 229, 26-50.

Berger, J.V., Knaepen, L., Janssen, S.P., Jaken, R.J., Marcus, M.A., Joosten, E.A., Deumens, R., 2011. Cellular and molecular insights into neuropathy-induced pain hypersensitivity for mechanism-based treatment approaches. Brain Res Rev. 67, 282-310.

Birder, L.A., Perl, E.R., 1999. Expression of alpha2-adrenergic receptors in rat primary afferent neurones after peripheral nerve injury or inflammation. J Physiol. 515 (Pt 2), 533-42.

Brazda, V., Klusakova, I., Svizenska, I., Veselkova, Z., Dubovy, P., 2009. Bilateral changes in IL-6 protein, but not in its receptor gp130, in rat dorsal root ganglia following sciatic nerve ligature. Cell Mol Neurobiol. 29, 1053-62.

Castillo, C., Norcini, M., Baquero-Buitrago, J., Levacic, D., Medina, R., Montoya-Gacharna, J.V., Blanck, T.J., Dubois, M., Recio-Pinto, E., 2011. The N-methyl-D-aspartate-evoked cytoplasmic calcium increase in adult rat dorsal root ganglion neuronal somata was potentiated by substance P pretreatment in a protein kinase C-dependent manner. Neuroscience. 177, 308-20.

Cauda, F., Sacco, K., D'Agata, F., Duca, S., Cocito, D., Geminiani, G., Migliorati, F., Isoardo, G., 2009. Low-frequency BOLD fluctuations demonstrate altered thalamocortical connectivity in diabetic neuropathic pain. BMC Neurosci. 10, 138.

Cejas, P.J., Martinez, M., Karmally, S., McKillop, M., McKillop, J., Plunkett, J.A., Oudega, M., Eaton, M.J., 2000. Lumbar transplant of neurons genetically modified to secrete brain-derived neurotrophic factor attenuates allodynia and hyperalgesia after sciatic nerve constriction. Pain. 86, 195-210.

Chen, X., Pang, R.P., Shen, K.F., Zimmermann, M., Xin, W.J., Li, Y.Y., Liu, X.G., 2011. TNF-alpha enhances the currents of voltage gated sodium channels in uninjured dorsal root ganglion neurons following motor nerve injury. Exp Neurol. 227, 279-86.

Cheong, E., Kim, C., Choi, B.J., Sun, M., Shin, H.S., 2011. Thalamic ryanodine receptors are involved in controlling the tonic firing of thalamocortical neurons and inflammatory pain signal processing. J Neurosci. 31, 1213-8.

Chien, L.Y., Cheng, J.K., Chu, D., Cheng, C.F., Tsaur, M.L., 2007. Reduced expression of A-type potassium channels in primary sensory neurons induces mechanical hypersensitivity. J Neurosci. 27, 9855-65.

Chung, J.H., Lee, E.Y., Jang, M.H., Kim, C.J., Kim, J., Ha, E., Park, H.K., Choi, S., Lee, H., Park, S.H., Leem, K.H., Kim, E.H., 2007. Acupuncture decreases ischemia-induced apoptosis and cell proliferation in dentate gyrus of gerbils. Neurol Res. 29 Suppl 1, S23-7.

Decosterd, I., Woolf, C.J., 2000. Spared nerve injury: an animal model of persistent peripheral neuropathic pain. Pain. 87, 149-58.

Devor, M., 1999. Unexplained peculiarities of the dorsal root ganglion. Pain. Suppl 6, S27-35.

Dib-Hajj, S.D., Cummins, T.R., Black, J.A., Waxman, S.G., 2010. Sodium channels in normal and pathological pain. Annu Rev Neurosci. 33, 325-47.

Dibbens, L.M., Reid, C.A., Hodgson, B., Thomas, E.A., Phillips, A.M., Gazina, E., Cromer, B.A., Clarke, A.L., Baram, T.Z., Scheffer, I.E., Berkovic, S.F., Petrou, S., 2010. Augmented currents of an HCN2 variant in patients with febrile seizure syndromes. Ann Neurol. 67, 542-6.

Dubovy, P., Jancalek, R., Klusakova, I., Svizenska, I., Pejchalova, K., 2006. Intra- and extraneuronal changes of immunofluorescence staining for TNF-alpha and TNFR1 in the dorsal root ganglia of rat peripheral neuropathic pain models. Cell Mol Neurobiol. 26, 1205-17.

Dubovy, P., Tuckova, L., Jancalek, R., Svizenska, I., Klusakova, I., 2007. Increased invasion of ED-1 positive macrophages in both ipsi- and contralateral dorsal root ganglia following unilateral nerve injuries. Neurosci Lett. 427, 88-93.

Dubovy, P., Klusakova, I., Svizenska, I., Brazda, V., 2010a. Spatio-temporal changes of SDF1 and its CXCR4 receptor in the dorsal root ganglia following unilateral sciatic nerve injury as a model of neuropathic pain. Histochem Cell Biol. 133, 323-37.

Dubovy, P., Klusakova, I., Svizenska, I., Brazda, V., 2010b. Satellite glial cells express IL-6 and corresponding signal-transducing receptors in the dorsal root ganglia of rat neuropathic pain model. Neuron Glia Biol. 6, 73-83.

Eaton, M.J., Blits, B., Ruitenberg, M.J., Verhaagen, J., Oudega, M., 2002. Amelioration of chronic neuropathic pain after partial nerve injury by adeno-associated viral (AAV) vector-mediated over-expression of BDNF in the rat spinal cord. Gene Ther. 9, 1387-95.

Gahm, J., Wickman, M., Brandberg, Y., 2010. Bilateral prophylactic mastectomy in women with inherited risk of breast cancer--prevalence of pain and discomfort, impact on sexuality, quality of life and feelings of regret two years after surgery. Breast. 19, 462-9.

Gosselin, R.D., Suter, M.R., Ji, R.R., Decosterd, I., 2010. Glial cells and chronic pain. Neuroscientist. 16, 519-31.

Hains, B.C., Klein, J.P., Saab, C.Y., Craner, M.J., Black, J.A., Waxman, S.G., 2003. Upregulation of sodium channel Nav1.3 and functional involvement in neuronal hyperexcitability associated with central neuropathic pain after spinal cord injury. J Neurosci. 23, 8881-92.

Hains, B.C., Saab, C.Y., Klein, J.P., Craner, M.J., Waxman, S.G., 2004. Altered sodium channel expression in second-order spinal sensory neurons contributes to pain after peripheral nerve injury. J Neurosci. 24, 4832-9.

Hanani, M., 2005. Satellite glial cells in sensory ganglia: from form to function. Brain Res Brain Res Rev. 48, 457-76.

Harris, J.A., Corsi, M., Quartaroli, M., Arban, R., Bentivoglio, M., 1996. Upregulation of spinal glutamate receptors in chronic pain. Neuroscience. 74, 7-12.

He, X.H., Zang, Y., Chen, X., Pang, R.P., Xu, J.T., Zhou, X., Wei, X.H., Li, Y.Y., Xin, W.J., Qin, Z.H., Liu, X.G., 2010. TNF-alpha contributes to up-regulation of Nav1.3 and Nav1.8 in DRG neurons following motor fiber injury. Pain. 151, 266-79.

Hirakawa, H., Okajima, S., Nagaoka, T., Kubo, T., Takamatsu, T., Oyamada, M., 2004. Regional differences in blood-nerve barrier function and tight-junction protein expression within the rat dorsal root ganglion. Neuroreport. 15, 405-8.

Hu, P., McLachlan, E.M., 2002. Macrophage and lymphocyte invasion of dorsal root ganglia after peripheral nerve lesions in the rat. Neuroscience. 112, 23-38.

Jang, J.H., Kim, K.H., Nam, T.S., Lee, W.T., Park, K.A., Kim, D.W., Leem, J.W., 2007. The role of uninjured C-afferents and injured afferents in the generation of mechanical hypersensitivity after partial peripheral nerve injury in the rat. Exp Neurol. 204, 288-98.

Kehlet, H., Jensen, T.S., Woolf, C.J., 2006. Persistent postsurgical pain: risk factors and prevention. Lancet. 367, 1618-25.

Kim, D.S., Choi, J.O., Rim, H.D., Cho, H.J., 2002. Downregulation of voltage-gated potassium channel alpha gene expression in dorsal root ganglia following chronic constriction injury of the rat sciatic nerve. Brain Res Mol Brain Res. 105, 146-52.

Kim, S.K., Nabekura, J., 2011. Rapid Synaptic Remodeling in the Adult Somatosensory Cortex following Peripheral Nerve Injury and Its Association with Neuropathic Pain. J Neurosci. 31, 5477-82.

Krekoski, C.A., Parhad, I.M., Clark, A.W., 1996. Attenuation and recovery of nerve growth factor receptor mRNA in dorsal root ganglion neurons following axotomy. J Neurosci Res. 43, 1-11.

Lee, D.H., Iyengar, S., Lodge, D., 2003. The role of uninjured nerve in spinal nerve ligated rats points to an improved animal model of neuropathic pain. Eur J Pain. 7, 473-9.

Lee, Y.J., Zachrisson, O., Tonge, D.A., McNaughton, P.A., 2002. Upregulation of bradykinin B2 receptor expression by neurotrophic factors and nerve injury in mouse sensory neurons. Mol Cell Neurosci. 19, 186-200.

Li, L., Xian, C.J., Zhong, J.H., Zhou, X.F., 2002. Effect of lumbar 5 ventral root transection on pain behaviors: a novel rat model for neuropathic pain without axotomy of primary sensory neurons. Exp Neurol. 175, 23-34.

Lin, H., Xiao, J., Luo, X., Chen, G., Wang, Z., 2009. Transcriptional control of pacemaker channel genes HCN2 and HCN4 by Sp1 and implications in re-expression of these genes in hypertrophied myocytes. Cell Physiol Biochem. 23, 317-26.

Lindia, J.A., Kohler, M.G., Martin, W.J., Abbadie, C., 2005. Relationship between sodium channel NaV1.3 expression and neuropathic pain behavior in rats. Pain. 117, 145-53.

Liu, C.N., Wall, P.D., Ben-Dor, E., Michaelis, M., Amir, R., Devor, M., 2000a. Tactile allodynia in the absence of C-fiber activation: altered firing properties of DRG neurons following spinal nerve injury. Pain. 85, 503-21.

Liu, M., Wood, J.N., 2011. The roles of sodium channels in nociception: implications for mechanisms of neuropathic pain. Pain Med. 12 Suppl 3, S93-9.

Liu, X., Chung, K., Chung, J.M., 1999. Ectopic discharges and adrenergic sensitivity of sensory neurons after spinal nerve injury. Brain Res. 849, 244-7.

Liu, X., Eschenfelder, S., Blenk, K.H., Janig, W., Habler, H., 2000b. Spontaneous activity of axotomized afferent neurons after L5 spinal nerve injury in rats. Pain. 84, 309-18.

Liu, X.J., Salter, M.W., 2010. Glutamate receptor phosphorylation and trafficking in pain plasticity in spinal cord dorsal horn. Eur J Neurosci. 32, 278-89.

Lu, H., Huang, D., Ransohoff, R.M., Zhou, L., 2011. Acute skeletal muscle injury: CCL2 expression by both monocytes and injured muscle is required for repair. FASEB J.

Luo, Z.D., Chaplan, S.R., Higuera, E.S., Sorkin, L.S., Stauderman, K.A., Williams, M.E., Yaksh, T.L., 2001. Upregulation of dorsal root ganglion (alpha)2(delta) calcium channel subunit and its correlation with allodynia in spinal nerve-injured rats. J Neurosci. 21, 1868-75.

Macrae, W.A., 2001. Chronic pain after surgery. Br J Anaesth. 87, 88-98.

Matsuda, S., Baluk, P., Shimizu, D., Fujiwara, T., 1996. Dorsal root ganglion neuron development in chick and rat. Anat Embryol (Berl). 193, 475-80.

McMahon, S.B., Malcangio, M., 2009. Current challenges in glia-pain biology. Neuron. 64, 46-54

Metz, A.E., Yau, H.J., Centeno, M.V., Apkarian, A.V., Martina, M., 2009. Morphological and functional reorganization of rat medial prefrontal cortex in neuropathic pain. Proc Natl Acad Sci U S A. 106, 2423-8.

Milligan, E.D., Watkins, L.R., 2009. Pathological and protective roles of glia in chronic pain. Nat Rev Neurosci. 10, 23-36.

Murphy, P.G., Borthwick, L.S., Johnston, R.S., Kuchel, G., Richardson, P.M., 1999. Nature of the retrograde signal from injured nerves that induces interleukin 6 mRNA in neurons. J Neurosci. 19, 3791-800.

Nassar, M.A., Stirling, L.C., Forlani, G., Baker, M.D., Matthews, E.A., Dickenson, A.H., Wood, J.N., 2004. Nociceptor-specific gene deletion reveals a major role for Nav1.7 (PN1) in acute and inflammatory pain. Proc Natl Acad Sci U S A. 101, 12706-11.

Nassar, M.A., Levato, A., Stirling, L.C., Wood, J.N., 2005. Neuropathic pain develops normally in mice lacking both Na(v)1.7 and Na(v)1.8. Mol Pain. 1, 24.

Nathan, J.D., Pappas, T.N., 2003. Inguinal hernia: an old condition with new solutions. Ann Surg. 238, S148-57.

Newton, R.A., Bingham, S., Case, P.C., Sanger, G.J., Lawson, S.N., 2001. Dorsal root ganglion neurons show increased expression of the calcium channel alpha2delta-1 subunit following partial sciatic nerve injury. Brain Res Mol Brain Res. 95, 1-8.

Obata, K., Yamanaka, H., Fukuoka, T., Yi, D., Tokunaga, A., Hashimoto, N., Yoshikawa, H., Noguchi, K., 2003. Contribution of injured and uninjured dorsal root ganglion neurons to pain behavior and the changes in gene expression following chronic constriction injury of the sciatic nerve in rats. Pain. 101, 65-77.

Obata, K., Yamanaka, H., Kobayashi, K., Dai, Y., Mizushima, T., Katsura, H., Fukuoka, T., Tokunaga, A., Noguchi, K., 2006. The effect of site and type of nerve injury on the expression of brain-derived neurotrophic factor in the dorsal root ganglion and on neuropathic pain behavior. Neuroscience. 137, 961-70.

Osamura, N., Ikeda, K., Ito, T., Higashida, H., Tomita, K., Yokoyama, S., 2005. Induction of interleukin-6 in dorsal root ganglion neurons after gradual elongation of rat sciatic nerve. Exp Neurol. 195, 61-70.

Pannese, E., 1981. The satellite cells of the sensory ganglia. Adv Anat Embryol Cell Biol. 65, 1-111.

Pannese, E., Ledda, M., Arcidiacono, G., Rigamonti, L., 1991. Clusters of nerve cell bodies enclosed within a common connective tissue envelope in the spinal ganglia of the lizard and rat. Cell Tissue Res. 264, 209-14.

Pannese, E., 2002. Perikaryal surface specializations of neurons in sensory ganglia. Int Rev Cytol. 220, 1-34.

Perkins, F.M., Kehlet, H., 2000. Chronic pain as an outcome of surgery. A review of predictive factors. Anesthesiology. 93, 1123-33.

Peyron, R., Schneider, F., Faillenot, I., Convers, P., Barral, F.G., Garcia-Larrea, L., Laurent, B., 2004. An fMRI study of cortical representation of mechanical allodynia in patients with neuropathic pain. Neurology. 63, 1838-46.

Pokorny, H., Klingler, A., Schmid, T., Fortelny, R., Hollinsky, C., Kawji, R., Steiner, E., Pernthaler, H., Fugger, R., Scheyer, M., 2008. Recurrence and complications after laparoscopic versus open inguinal hernia repair: results of a prospective randomized multicenter trial. Hernia. 12, 385-9.

Ringkamp, M., Meyer, R.A., 2005. Injured versus uninjured afferents: Who is to blame for neuropathic pain? Anesthesiology. 103, 221-3.

Romero-Sandoval, E.A., Horvath, R.J., DeLeo, J.A., 2008. Neuroimmune interactions and pain: focus on glial-modulating targets. Curr Opin Investig Drugs. 9, 726-34.

Schafers, M., Sorkin, L.S., Geis, C., Shubayev, V.I., 2003. Spinal nerve ligation induces transient upregulation of tumor necrosis factor receptors 1 and 2 in injured and adjacent uninjured dorsal root ganglia in the rat. Neurosci Lett. 347, 179-82.

Scholz, J., Woolf, C.J., 2007. The neuropathic pain triad: neurons, immune cells and glia. Nat Neurosci. 10, 1361-8.

Seijffers, R., Allchorne, A.J., Woolf, C.J., 2006. The transcription factor ATF-3 promotes neurite outgrowth. Mol Cell Neurosci. 32, 143-54.

Sun, Q., Tu, H., Xing, G.G., Han, J.S., Wan, Y., 2005. Ectopic discharges from injured nerve fibers are highly correlated with tactile allodynia only in early, but not late, stage in rats with spinal nerve ligation. Exp Neurol. 191, 128-36.

Suter, M.R., Papaloizos, M., Berde, C.B., Woolf, C.J., Gilliard, N., Spahn, D.R., Decosterd, I., 2003. Development of neuropathic pain in the rat spared nerve injury model is not prevented by a peripheral nerve block. Anesthesiology. 99, 1402-8.

Takeda, M., Takahashi, M., Matsumoto, S., 2009. Contribution of the activation of satellite glia in sensory ganglia to pathological pain. Neurosci Biobehav Rev. 33, 784-92.

Tal, M., Eliav, E., 1996. Abnormal discharge originates at the site of nerve injury in experimental constriction neuropathy (CCI) in the rat. Pain. 64, 511-8.

Vadivelu, N., Schreck, M., Lopez, J., Kodumudi, G., Narayan, D., 2008. Pain after mastectomy and breast reconstruction. Am Surg. 74, 285-96.

Van Steenwinckel, J., Reaux-Le Goazigo, A., Pommier, B., Mauborgne, A., Dansereau, M.A., Kitabgi, P., Sarret, P., Pohl, M., Melik Parsadaniantz, S., 2011. CCL2 released from neuronal synaptic vesicles in the spinal cord is a major mediator of local inflammation and pain after peripheral nerve injury. J Neurosci. 31, 5865-75.

Wall, P.D., Gutnick, M., 1974a. Ongoing activity in peripheral nerves: the physiology and pharmacology of impulses originating from a neuroma. Exp Neurol. 43, 580-93.

Wall, P.D., Gutnick, M., 1974b. Properties of afferent nerve impulses originating from a neuroma. Nature. 248, 740-3.

Wall, P.D., Devor, M., 1983. Sensory afferent impulses originate from dorsal root ganglia as well as from the periphery in normal and nerve injured rats. Pain. 17, 321-39.

Walton, K.D., Dubois, M., Llinas, R.R., 2010. Abnormal thalamocortical activity in patients with Complex Regional Pain Syndrome (CRPS) type I. Pain. 150, 41-51.

Wang, C.H., Zou, L.J., Zhang, Y.L., Jiao, Y.F., Sun, J.H., 2010. The excitatory effects of the chemokine CCL2 on DRG somata are greater after an injury of the ganglion than after an injury of the spinal or peripheral nerve. Neurosci Lett. 475, 48-52.

Wang, X.C., Qiu, Y.H., Peng, Y.P., 2007. Interleukin-6 protects cerebellar granule neurons from NMDA-induced neurotoxicity. Sheng Li Xue Bao. 59, 150-6.

Wang, X.Q., Peng, Y.P., Lu, J.H., Cao, B.B., Qiu, Y.H., 2009. Neuroprotection of interleukin-6 against NMDA attack and its signal transduction by JAK and MAPK. Neurosci Lett. 450, 122-6.

Watkins, L.R., Milligan, E.D., Maier, S.F., 2001. Glial activation: a driving force for pathological pain. Trends Neurosci. 24, 450-5.

Watkins, L.R., Maier, S.F., 2002. Beyond neurons: evidence that immune and glial cells contribute to pathological pain states. Physiol Rev. 82, 981-1011.

Wu, G., Ringkamp, M., Murinson, B.B., Pogatzki, E.M., Hartke, T.V., Weerahandi, H.M., Campbell, J.N., Griffin, J.W., Meyer, R.A., 2002. Degeneration of myelinated efferent fibers induces spontaneous activity in uninjured C-fiber afferents. J Neurosci. 22, 7746-53.

Xiao, H.S., Huang, Q.H., Zhang, F.X., Bao, L., Lu, Y.J., Guo, C., Yang, L., Huang, W.J., Fu, G., Xu, S.H., Cheng, X.P., Yan, Q., Zhu, Z.D., Zhang, X., Chen, Z., Han, Z.G., 2002. Identification of gene expression profile of dorsal root ganglion in the rat peripheral axotomy model of neuropathic pain. Proc Natl Acad Sci U S A. 99, 8360-5.

Xu, J.T., Xin, W.J., Zang, Y., Wu, C.Y., Liu, X.G., 2006. The role of tumor necrosis factor-alpha in the neuropathic pain induced by Lumbar 5 ventral root transection in rat. Pain. 123, 306-21.

Xu, Q., Yaksh, T.L., 2011. A brief comparison of the pathophysiology of inflammatory versus neuropathic pain. Curr Opin Anaesthesiol. 24, 400-7.

Yajima, Y., Narita, M., Matsumoto, N., Suzuki, T., 2002. Involvement of a spinal brain-derived neurotrophic factor/full-length TrkB pathway in the development of nerve injury-induced thermal hyperalgesia in mice. Brain Res. 958, 338-46.

Yajima, Y., Narita, M., Usui, A., Kaneko, C., Miyatake, M., Yamaguchi, T., Tamaki, H., Wachi, H., Seyama, Y., Suzuki, T., 2005. Direct evidence for the involvement of brain-derived neurotrophic factor in the development of a neuropathic pain-like state in mice. J Neurochem. 93, 584-94.

Zhao, J., Seereeram, A., Nassar, M.A., Levato, A., Pezet, S., Hathaway, G., Morenilla-Palao, C., Stirling, C., Fitzgerald, M., McMahon, S.B., Rios, M., Wood, J.N., 2006. Nociceptor-derived brain-derived neurotrophic factor regulates acute and inflammatory but not neuropathic pain. Mol Cell Neurosci. 31, 539-48.

Zhou, X.F., Chie, E.T., Deng, Y.S., Zhong, J.H., Xue, Q., Rush, R.A., Xian, C.J., 1999. Injured primary sensory neurons switch phenotype for brain-derived neurotrophic factor in the rat. Neuroscience. 92, 841-53.

11

Neuropathic Pain Following Nerve Injury

Stanislava Jergova[1,2]
[1]*University of Miami, Florida*
[2]*Institute of Neurobiology, Slovak Academy of Science*
[1]*USA*
[2]*Slovakia*

1. Introduction

Pain is essential for our wellbeing as it warns us from possible injuries. After injury, pain sensations around injured tissue lead to protective behavior and so indirectly contribute to a faster healing process. Physiological pain is usually acute or subchronic, it progressively diminishes in the process of healing and responds to conventionally used analgesics. However, injury to the somatosensory system may give rise to ongoing pain that persists beyond the healing process of the original injury and is refractory to analgesics. Such pain is termed neuropathic. Neuropathic pain negatively influences quality of life of patients and often interferes with the rehabilitation strategies after nerve injury. Pharmacological treatment or surgical intervention provide only short term alleviation, since adverse effects such as drug tolerance and addictions, motor deficit and worsening pain may emerge over time. Therefore there is a need to identify novel, more effective long term therapies. Cell transplantation and gene therapy present target-oriented therapies minimizing side effects of medication due their local action. Therefore they are promising way to manage chronic neuropathic pain.

2. Anatomy of pain

Stimuli coming from our environment are perceived by peripheral receptors. Each receptor is highly specialized to recognize specific range of mechanical, thermal and chemical stimuli and their intensity. Receptors transform stimuli into a membrane depolarization of primary sensory neurons and the information is propagated by afferent fibers as a train of action potentials to the spinal cord. Depolarization of primary afferent fibers terminations in the spinal cord induce release of neurotransmitters that influence excitability of second order neurons and the information is transferred to the supraspinal centers. Noxious sensations were originally explained as an intensity-dependent activation of primary afferent fibers encoding non-noxious stimuli. The existence of specific receptors activated only by the noxious stimuli was first suggested by Sherington in 1906 (Sherington, 1906, as cited in (McMahon & Koltzenburg, 2005)) and later validated by Perl (1967) (Burges & Perl, 1967, as cited in (McMahon & Koltzenburg, 2005)).

Primary afferent fibers are classified into several groups based on their myelin ensheatment, size and the conduction velocity. Large, myelinated and rapid conducting $A\alpha/\beta$ are activated by non-noxious mechanical stimuli, Aδ fibers mediates thermal and noxious sensations. Small, unmyelinated, slow conducting C fibers are primarily nociceptive. Nociceptors as specialized receptors of noxious stimuli are free nerve endings of C and Aδ fibers. However, low threshold mechanoreceptors Aβ are suggested to play a role in the development of chronic pain. The neuronal bodies of the primary afferent fibers are located in dorsal root ganglia (DRGs). Morphologically they are divided into three groups: large diameter and medium diameter myelinated cells, and small diameter unmyelinated cells presumptive to Aδ, Aβ and Aδ/C fibers respectively. Small and medium diameter cells are classified as nociceptors and therefore have been extensively studied in pain research. These cells can be subdivided into two broad classes based on their neurochemical properties; peptidergic neurons contain neuropeptides as substance P and calcitonin gene-related peptide and express receptors for nerve growth factor. Nonpeptidergic are responsive to glial cell line-derived neurotrophic factors and have binding site for isolectin IB4 obtained from *Bandeiraea simplicifolia.* However, it is not clear if such morphological differences correspond to different functional types, as for example heat activated capsaicin receptor is expressed in both peptidergic and nonpeptidergic neuronal classes (Guo et al., 1999; Michael & Priestley, 1999). Primary afferent fibers terminate in the various levels of dorsal horn. Termination reflects physiological property of a stimulus and its anatomical location. Superficial laminae are primary termination of the nociceptive primary afferents. However neurons in deeper laminae also play a role in the pain processing, especially during chronic pain states.

3. Mechanisms of neuropathic pain

Neuropathic pain presents a paradox outcome of the injury to the somatosensory nervous system, as one could expect reduction of sensations coming from the denervated area. However, there are substantial qualitative changes in the processing of nociceptive information after nerve injury that lead to a persistent pain. The prevalence of neuropathic pain is around 5-8 % in the general population (Daousi et al., 2004) and with insufficient pharmacological treatment it represents a serious medical problem. There is a wide range of injuries and diseases causing neuropathic pain, such as diabetic neuropathy, surgical lesions, multiple sclerosis, spinal cord injury and a stroke. This diversity of clinical conditions related to the neuropathic pain makes it difficult to identify a common mechanism. Moreover, neuropathic pain does not necessarily develop in every patient even when the etiology is very similar, and symptoms within the same etiology may vary substantially between patients.

The major hallmark of neuropathic pain is presence of mechanical and cold hyperalgesia and allodynia. Heat hyperalgesia is reported in fewer cases. *Mechanical allodynia* as a touch evoked pain is the major reason for suffering of neuropathic pain patients. This pain accompanies inflammatory and neuropathic conditions. There are evidences that under both conditions this extreme sensitivity is not elicited by nociceptors but by myelinated low threshold Aβ mechanoreceptors, that normally encode non-painful stimuli. The ability of Aβ fibers to evoke painful sensations is caused by profound alterations of central pain processing (Klede et al., 2003; Koppert et al., 2001). The other disturbances in sensitivity to mechanical stimuli are caused by an excitation of Aδ fibers (pin-prick hyperalgesia) (Ziegler et al., 1999) or the expansion of the receptive field of nociceptors (blunt pressure hyperalgesia) (Reeh et al., 1987). *Hypersensitivity to cold* is prominent after traumatic nerve injuries (Wahren & Torebjork, 1992). The mechanisms of cold hyperalgesia involve changes in the peripheral and central processing of thermal stimuli. A mechanism of *heat hyperalgesia* is assumed to involve sensitized unmyelinated nociceptors.

3.1 Peripheral changes in neuropathic pain

The mechanisms underlying neuropathic pain involve complex pathophysiological changes in the processing of sensory signals. Changes in the neuronal excitability, discharges generated along the nerve fiber, changes in the gene expression and up- or down-regulation of neurotransmitter release, all those contribute to the prolonged hypersensitivity after nerve injury. A brief characteristic of these changes and their impact on the chronic pain development are outlined below.

3.1.1 Ectopic discharges

When the axon loses the connection with the target tissue after traumatic nerve injury or a disease, retrograde transport of vital growth factors (such as fibroblast growth factor and nerve growth factor) to the cell body is disrupted. While in neonates this leads to the death of sensory neurons, in adults a disruption of neurotrophic support causes changes in the neurochemical and electrical properties of sensory neurons. The most important consequence of this phenotypic switch is the development of spontaneous discharges. Spontaneous discharges are generated not at the usual place, i.e. at the termination of primary afferent fibers in the dorsal horn, but rather in the injured area-in the stump of injured nerve, in the corresponding sensory neurons in DRG and the neighboring intact afferents. Stump is formed at the proximal end of transected axon. It gives rise to fine sprouting fibers in the process of regeneration. These sprouts may elongate and reach the target tissue or, in the case of blocked growth (such as after limb amputation), the sprouts form end-bulb neuroma. The presence of spontaneous discharges arising from the neuroma was reported in 1974 by Wall and Gutnic (Wall & Gutnick, 1974, as cited in (McMahon & Koltzenburg, 2005)) in the model of sciatic nerve axotomy and later it was confirmed in other forms of nerve injury, including diabetic polyneuropathy (Dobretsov et al., 2001) and viral infection (Kress & Fickenscher, 2001).

Ectopic discharges may arise not only from axotomized fibers but also from partially injured nerves. The local inflammation and demyelination after nerve injury has been shown to contribute to spontaneous firing in the spared nerve fibers after incomplete axotomy (Kajander & Bennett, 1992; Tal & Eliav, 1996). Other sources of firing are intact axons in close proximity of the injured ones. In the experiments where spinal nerve L5 was transected, ectopic discharges have been recorded from uninjured L4 nerve. These uninjured axons are exposed to a soup of inflammatory mediators such as cytokines and growth factors released by degenerating axon and surrounding tissue. Although there is no direct evidence that such firing elicit hypersensitivity in the area innervated by uninjured axons, their increased excitability may contribute to the development of central sensitization (Ali et al., 1999; Wu et al., 2001). The sensory neurons in the DRG affected by the nerve injury are another source of ectopic activity, especially if the injury is proximal to dorsal root ganglia (Liu et al., 2000) such as during intervertebrae disc herniation. Clinical studies showed that ectopic discharges are correlated with the manifestation of spontaneous pain states and that both are transiently reduced by drugs that eliminate discharges (Campero et al., 1998; Orstavik et al., 2003). The ectopic firing also causes a neurogenic inflammation seen in patients with complex regional pain syndrome. The antidromic propagation of a signal in a nerve fiber during ectopic firing causes stimulation of peripheral nerve endings and subsequent release of neurotransmitter such as SP and calcitonin gene-related peptide. Their vasodilatation activity causes swelling and redness of the innervated tissue, characteristic for causalgia (McMahon & Koltzenburg, 2005).

3.1.2 Relationship of ectopic discharges to hypersensitivity

When the intensity of peripheral stimulus reaches a certain threshold, peripheral receptors respond with discharges and the signal is propagated to the central nervous system (CNS). In the presence of ectopic activity, discharges are elicited by subthreshold stimulus in the process of peripheral sensitization. Moreover, discharges may persist beyond the end of the stimulation. The afterdischarges are generated due to self-sustained activity of ectopic sites and act as signal amplifiers. The subthreshold stimulus can therefore elicit greater-than-normal response.

Peripheral nerves with ectopic sites are hypersensitive to wide range of mechanical, thermal and chemical stimuli. Gentle mechanical pressure or brushing may evoke ongoing firing in the injured nerve. When the spot with ectopic activity develop close to tendons or joints, movements and weight bearing may trigger an ongoing pain accompanying various muscoskeletal disorders. Cold allodynia, a common symptom in neuropathy, is related to increased ectopic discharges in unmyelinated C fibers after cold stimulation. Electrophysiological and immunohistochemical studies demonstrated that it could be caused by an altered expression of thermoresponsive vanilloid receptors (Caterina et al., 1997). Chemical stimuli that depolarize sensory neurons may also excite ectopic discharges. Inflammatory and regeneration processes following nerve injury are mediated by cytokines, peptides, neurotrophins and all of these substances have been shown to contribute to development of ectopic discharges. Moreover, local metabolic changes at the site of injury such as tissue ischemia and elevated blood glucose also contribute to the generation of ectopic discharges (Devor et al., 1992; Levy et al., 2000; Noda et al., 1997; Rivera et al., 2000).

The electrophysiological recordings from DRG cells have shown that afterdischarges are present in a form of oscillation, when the burst of responses is followed by hyperpolarization. During this period the activity is suppressed and can not be elicited by another stimulation. The hyperpolarization may be caused by the activation of potassium channels (Amir & Devor, 1997). The clinical manifestation of this phenomenon is probably the refractory period during paroxysms in trigeminal neuralgia or pain relief by transcutaneous electrical nerve stimulation (Rappaport & Devor, 1994).

3.1.3 Peripheral sensitization

3.1.3.1 Sodium channels

The ability of the injured nerve to generate discharges at various sites may arise from changed expression and trafficking of voltage dependent sodium channels. Nine types of voltage-gated sodium channels have been recognized so far in mammals. They are present throughout the nervous system with the most abundant expression in DRG neurons. They are expressed differently during the development when for example NaV1.3 is present only during embryonic stages. Several studies suggest that the ectopic discharges are evoked by an altered expression and distribution of sodium channels. Experimental axotomy in adult animals reduces the level of RNA of NaV1.6, NaV1.7, NaV1.8 and NaV1.9 but upregulates Nav1.3 which is normally not expressed by adult DRGs. Based on the whole-cell patch-clamp recordings it is suggested that NaV1.3 may be a key player in neuropathic pain and the neurons expressing this channel may exhibit reduced threshold or a high firing frequency (Dib-Hajj et al., 2009; Dib-Hajj et al., 2007). There are also changes in the redistribution of sodium channels, particularly of NaV1.8, increased immunoreactivity of which was observed at the site of nerve injury. This translocation may contribute to the generation of ectopic discharges (Black et al., 2008; Wood et al., 2004). Recent clinical data demonstrated the link between mutation of human Nav1.7 gene and serious neuropathic disorders, like insensitivity to pain or erythermalgia (Dib-Hajj et al., 2007; Drenth & Waxman, 2007).

3.1.3.2 Transient receptor potential channels

Transient receptor potential (TRP) channels is a group of cation channels involved in sensory signaling that undergo changes after nerve injury and during inflammation. The most profound changes have been observed in the expression of capsaicin-activated channel TRPV1 after nerve injury. Sciatic nerve section or spinal nerve ligation cause reduced expression of TRPV1 in all damaged DRG neurons while its increase has been observed in the spared undamaged DRG neurons (Baron, 2000; Caterina, 2007, 2008). The involvement of TRPV1 in the development of heat hyperalgesia was demonstrated in experiments where TRPV1 knockout mice did not develop heat hyperalgesia after inflammation. On the other hand, no changes in the level of heat hyperalgesia were observed in knockout mice compared to wild types after nerve injury. These observations point to different molecular mechanisms of heat hyperalgesia during inflammatory and neuropathic pain. The antinociceptive effect of TRPV1 antagonist further supports the idea of crucial role of TRPV1 in the development of neuropathic pain (Baron, 2000; Hudson et al., 2001; Staaf et al., 2009).

3.1.3.3 Cytokines

Among inflammatory mediators that could contribute to the peripheral sensitization, cytokines IL-1β and TNFα have drawn the most attention. The increased expression of both in the DRGs is closely correlated with the reduced mechanical and thermal withdrawal threshold in animals (Schafers et al., 2003; Sorkin & Doom, 2000). Clinical studies showed that patients with mechanical allodynia have higher levels of serum soluble TNFα receptor. Injection of TNFα or IL-1β receptor antagonists reduced pain-related behavior in experimental animals (Cunha et al., 2000; Sommer & Kress, 2004).

3.2 Central changes in neuropathic pain

The resistance of neuropathic pain to pharmacotherapy suggests that the changes in the pain processing take place also in the central nervous system. In fact, electrophysiological studies showed an increased activity of dorsal horn neurons after peripheral nerve injury (Chapman et al., 1998; Laird & Bennett, 1993; Palecek et al., 1992). However, no correlation was found between responses of the dorsal horn neurons to heat stimuli and the presence of heat hyperalgesia (Laird & Bennett, 1993; Palecek et al., 1992). Also the threshold of dorsal horn neurons to mechanical stimulation was unchanged after peripheral nerve injury. On the other hand, innocuous stimuli evoked activity in the majority of wide dynamic range neurons and the afterdischarges were more prominent in nerve injured animals (Palecek et al., 1992). The underlying mechanisms for increased activity of dorsal horn neurons after peripheral nerve injury are related to the enhanced release of excitatory amino acids and the attenuation of inhibitory signaling.

3.2.1 Disinhibition

The sensory input into the spinal cord is under regulation of inhibitory circuitry maintained by sensory afferents, spinal interneurons and descending inhibition. This regulatory circuitry is disrupted after peripheral nerve injury that leads to misinterpretation of peripheral inputs that could underlie chronic pain development. The main inhibitory neurotransmitters in central nervous system are γ-aminobutyric acid (GABA) and glycin. The importance of GABA signaling for normal pain processing has been shown in experiments where the blockade of spinal GABAergic neurotransmission by intrathecal antagonists produced hypersensitivity to innocuous tactile stimuli (Gwak et al., 2006; Hao et al., 1994; Malan et al., 2002) and where transgenic mice lacking specific subunits of GABA receptors developed hyperalgesia and allodynia (Schuler et al., 2001; Ugarte et al., 2000). The hyperexcitability of dorsal horn neurons in neuropathic pain has been explained by a disruption of inhibitory tone in the spinal cord. In fact, a reduction of GABA and GABA-synthesizing enzyme GAD has been reported after spinal cord injury and peripheral nerve injury. Also the electrophysiological recordings showed reduced spinal inhibitory tone in the injured animals (Castro-Lopes et al., 1993; Eaton et al., 1998; Gwak et al., 2006; Ibuki et al., 1997; Moore et al., 2002). There still a debate about what is the direct cause of reduced GABA production in the dorsal horn. Histological examinations showed a presence of apoptotic cells in the dorsal horn after constriction injury. It was suggested that they are GABAergic inhibitory interneurons; however, detailed stereological investigation doubted this possibility. The study also showed there is no significant loss of GABAergic or glycinergic neurons in animals with neuropathic pain and that the proportion of GABA immunoreactive neurons was similar to control animals without nerve injury (Polgar et al., 2004; Polgar et al., 2003). However, although dysfunction of spinal inhibition seems to be a major factor in persistent pain syndromes, pharmacological targeting of the GABAergic system has not shown satisfactory outcomes. This is in part likely due to the widespread distribution and actions of GABA throughout the CNS.

3.2.2 Enhanced release of excitatory neurotransmitters

There are ample of evidences showing that an activation of glutamate NMDA receptors is involved in the development of neuropathic pain. Recordings from spinal slide preparations of animals with peripheral nerve injury showed enhanced NMDA receptor current, suggesting increased release of glutamate after stimulation (Isaev et al., 2000). The amount of glutamate released from primary afferent fibers into a dorsal horn is controlled by glutamate transporters. Their downregulation after nerve injury contribute to the excess of glutamate in the spinal cord, overactivation of glutamate receptors and hyperexcitability of neurons. Although initial response after nerve injury presents upregulation of glutamate transporters, their expression is reduced later on (Sung et al., 2003).

The upregulation of dynorphin in the spinal cord after nerve injury has been reported in rats and mice (Gardell et al., 2004; Malan et al., 2000). A strain of mouse that does not develop the signs of neuropathic pain does not show increased level of dynorphin, therefore this protein is a suitable marker associated with nerve injury-induced pain (Gardell et al., 2004). Dynorphin may increase a release of excitatory neurotransmitters from primary afferent fibers as suggested from studies showing that release of calcitonin gene-related peptide, substance P and excitatory amino acids into dorsal horn is potentiated by dynorphin (Arcaya et al., 1999; Gardell et al., 2003; Koetzner et al., 2004). Also, the pharmacological inhibition of dynorphin abolished the development of mechanical and thermal hypersensitivity in rats and mice after nerve injury; genetic knockout of dynorphin led to only transient hypersensitivity after nerve injury (Gardell et al., 2004). Those studies point to the important role of spinal dynorphin in the persistent pain.

3.2.3 Reorganization

Several studies suggested that the nerve injury cause an anatomical reorganization in the spinal dorsal horn allowing the signal from non-nociceptive Aβ fibers to reach and activate nociceptive neurons (Woolf et al., 1992). This idea was based on the observation of positive labeling of superficial dorsal horn laminae with retrograde tracer choleratoxin B (CTB) after nerve injury. This tracer, when injected into peripheral nerve, is uptaken by myelinated neurons expressing GM1 receptor and transported into the spinal cord. CTB labeling in the spinal cord thus identify termination of myelinated fibers. In the normal animals, labeling is found in the deeper dorsal horn laminae. Its presence in the superficial area in the vicinity of nociceptive neurons was explained by sprouting of Aβ fibers from deeper laminae. The non-nociceptive input signaled by Aβ fibers may thus excite nociceptive neurons and underlie development of mechanical allodynia. However, subsequent studies showed that there is a phenotypic switch in DRG neurons after axotomy as the expression of GM1 receptors was found also on the unmyelinated nociceptive DRG neurons. Therefore, CTB is transported by both myelinated and unmyelinated afferents which explains its appearance in upper dorsal horn laminae, termination of unmyelinated fibers (Bao et al., 2002; Shehab et al., 2003). Although the structural reorganization does not seems to be a case for abnormal Aβ signal processing, electrophysiological experiments showed the increased Aβ input into the dorsal horn.

3.2.4 Ascending projections-the role of Aβ fibers

The role of Aβ fibers in development of tactile allodynia is further supported by evidences showing that injection of sodium channel blocker lidocain into the supraspinal termination of Ab fibers- nucleus gracilis - block tactile allodynia. An interesting finding in this study was that thermal allodynia was not changed by this treatment (Ossipov et al., 2002; Sun et al., 2001). The expression of neuropeptide Y in DRG neurons after peripheral or spinal nerve injury seems to be related to the activity of Aβ fibers. This protein is not present in DRGs during physiological conditions. After nerve injury its expression is found in DRGs and spinal cord in the area of termination of Aβ fibers (Wakisaka et al., 1991). Neuropeptide Y is also upregulated in the ipsilateral nucleus gracilis after nerve injury (Ossipov et al., 2002). It has been shown that its presence originates from the DRG since neither dorsal rhizotomy nor lesion of the dorsal column blocked its appearance in nucleus gracilis. The significance of this supraspinal center for the development of pain was demonstrated in experiments where injection of neuropeptide Y into nucleus gracilis evoked tactile allodynia. Interestingly, thermal sensitivity was not changed. The findings of these studies indicate that the tactile hypersensitivity is mediated by Aβ input through upregulation of neuropeptide Y in the DRGs and that the development of tactile hypersensitivity can be modulated from supraspinal areas. Also the modulation of tactile hypersensitivity without affecting thermal sensitivity points out to a different processing of mechanical and thermal nociceptive input.

3.2.5 Descending modulation

The spinal processing of nociceptive information is influenced by a descending input that could facilitate or inhibit propagation of the nociceptive signal. The rostral ventromedial medulla (RVM) and periaqueductal gray are the most important sources of the descending control. The electrical stimulation of RVM may elicit both the facilitation or inhibition of nociceptive reflexes and can enhance or inhibit responses of WDR neurons to noxious stimuli (Walker et al., 1999).The facilitatory input from these structures is believed to be critical for the maintenance of neuropathic pain. Spinal transection or hemisection has been shown to abolish development of neuropathic pain signs after peripheral nerve injury (Kauppila et al., 1998) and the lesion of the major pathways connecting RMV to spinal cord, dorsolateral funiculus, also abolished development of neuropathic pain (Burgess et al., 2002). Electrophysiological experiments demonstrated that specific population of RVM cells expressing μ-opioid receptor are directly related to the descending facilitatory input (Heinricher & Neubert, 2004). The selective ablation of these cells prevented the development of neuropathic pain (Burgess et al., 2002; Porreca et al., 2001).

3.2.6 The integration of ascending and descending modulation

The integration of ascending and descending modulation of nociception in the spinal cord was shown in a series of experiments targeting dorsal horn projection neurons. Using ribosome inhibitor protein saporin conjugated with substance P, a specific population of dorsal horn neurons expressing substance P receptor NK1 was eliminated (Nichols et al., 1999; Suzuki et al., 2002). This procedure led to a reduction of tactile and thermal hypersensitivity in rats after peripheral nerve injury or inflammation, suggesting the essential role of those neurons in the development of neuropathic pain. Further experiment revealed that the ablation of NK1 receptor neurons reduced hyperexcitability of wide dynamic range neurons in deeper dorsal horn laminae to mechanical and thermal stimulation (Suzuki et al., 2002). Since the wide dynamic range neurons receive the facilitatory input from RVM by the action of serotonin, a relationship between NK1 neurons and serotonergic pathway was studied. Using serotonin receptor antagonist onadsetron, an effect similar to SP-saporin treatment on wide dynamic range neurons responses was observed (Suzuki et al., 2002). These results demonstrate that the peripheral nerve injury causes an activation of descending facilitatory pathway by signals from ascending fibers arising (at least partially) from NK1 neurons in dorsal horn. The integration of ascending and descending nociceptive signaling contribute to neuropathic pain.

4. Animal models of neuropathic pain

Animal models of acute pain where responses to various mechanical, thermal or electrical stimulations are evaluated provide a good source of our knowledge about basic mechanisms of pain. These models are widely use for the development of analgesic drugs as they provide a reliable outcome comparable to clinical states. However, chronic pain following peripheral or central nerve injury present more difficult task as the drugs successfully used in an acute pain are usually inefficient for neuropathic pain. Our recent knowledge on the mechanisms of neuropathic pain is based on animal models partially mimic some of the clinically observed symptoms of neuropathic pain. The most used models in neuropathic pain research involve injury of the sciatic nerve and specific forms of spinal cord injury. The advantage of sciatic nerve in pain research is based on its anatomical location allowing easy access without extensive surgery and the fact that its branches innervate hind limbs accessible for sensory testing.

4.1 Sciatic nerve axotomy

One of the first chronic pain model based on the injury of the sciatic nerve is frank transection of the sciatic nerve (Wall et at., 1979 as cited in (McMahon & Koltzenburg, 2005)). The painful sensations developed in the denervated area illustrate the paradox of neuropathic pain and mimic clinical state of phantom limb pain. The procedure consists of 5mm section of sciatic and saphenous nerve. The complete anesthesia in the affected area is confirmed by the absence of flexion reflex after strong pinch. The various degree of autotomy behavior develops within 5 weeks post injury. The model was further characterized by variations of nerve injuries, when either saphenous or sciatic nerve was transected alone or at different time points and the degree of autotomy behavior was evaluated. The variations in behavioral outcome between different strains of rats and mice were also studied. These experiments showed that sciatic nerve injury alone is sufficient to evoke autotomy behavior and that degree of autotomy varies considerably between different strains of rats and mice. This model showed to be a useful tool to predict clinical efficacy of drugs to relieve phantom limb pain. Drugs such as sodium channel blockers, tricyclic antidepressant and anticonvulsant, which successfully reduced autotomy, also reduced phantom limb pain in patients (Chabal et al., 1989). It also provides a good tool to study electrophysiological changes after nerve transaction, formation of neuroma and development of ectopic discharges. However, since the limb is denervated, one cannot assess pain related behavior, as the animal lack proper motoric function in the affected paw. Therefore there is a controversy about how much this model and autotomy behavior is related to possible pain sensation. Another arguments point to strain variability of autotomy and provide evidences, that such behavior may be modulated by environment. To address these problems, other models of neuropathic pain were developed based on the various degree of sciatic nerve injury.

4.2 Partial ligation

Ligation of 1/3 to 1/2 of the sciatic nerve is used to mimic causalgia symptoms after nerve trauma (Seltzer et al., 1990; Shir & Seltzer, 1990). Rats display no autotomy and develop the signs of spontaneous pain, tactile, mechanical and thermal hyperesthesia. Pain-related behavior is sympathetically maintained as it is abolished after sympathectomy. The disadvantage of the model is variability of the degree of nerve injury between animals, resulting in different ratio of injured versus uninjured fibers and random distribution of their termination in the spinal cord.

4.3 Chronic constriction injury

Chronic constriction injury present another model of sciatic nerve injury, where four loose ligatures are placed around the nerve, causing swelling and constriction of nerve at the site of ligation (Bennett & Xie, 1988). Within 1 day post injury the constriction caused by edema reduces diameter of sciatic nerve up to 75%. Histological examination and electron microscopy showed massive reduction of myelinated Aα and Aβ fibers and lesser reduction of Aδ (Munger et al., 1992). Electrophysiological experiments indicate almost 90% loss of myelinated and 30% unmyelinated fibers 3 days post injury additional loss within 14 days (Coggeshall et al., 1993) (Kajander & Bennett, 1992). Due to injury to motor fibers, animals walk with a limb with ventroflexed toes. Injury of the sensory fibers results in the development of neuropathic pain symptoms such as thermal and mechanical hyperesthesia. Animals display guarding behavior, avoiding placing weight on the injured paw. There is also an overgrowing of the claws due to reduced grooming. The pain related behavior usually persists up to 2 months. Hypersensitivity to heat is presented in the reduced paw withdrawal latency to the radiant heat. A light tactile stimulation elicits paw withdrawal and expression of nociceptive marker protein c-Fos in dorsal horn (Catheline et al., 1999). Animals also develop cold allodynia demonstrated by exaggerated reaction to the application of acetone. The pain related behavior observed in this model resemble the clinical state of causalgia. Moreover, overgrowing of claws observed in these animals is suggested to be similar to unwillingness of patients to trim their nails as it painful. Animals also display a signs of spontaneous pain by their abnormal posture, guarding behavior and accidental flinches. Although the development of hypersensitivity was attributed to the loss large myelinated Aβ mechanosensitive fibers (Munger et al., 1992), animals did not display robust pain related behavior 2 months post injury in spite of lingering loss of Aβ fibers. Hypersensitivity is probably mediated by sensitized Aδ and C fibers. The ectopic discharges in myelinated fibers are presented proximal to the injury and those may be responsible for the spontaneous and evoked pain-related behavior observed in this model. The disadvantage of this model is again the various degree of nerve injury. Although the variability is lower that in partial ligation model, it is difficult to provide the same degree of constriction in each animal.

4.4 Spinal nerve ligation

The model of spinal nerve ligation overcomes the issues of the previous models where it is not possible to control the amount of injured fibers. The model was developed by Kim&Chung in 1992 (Kim & Chung, 1992). In this models only spinal L5 and L6 branches of the sciatic nerve are ligated, so the corresponding DRGs and spinal cord segments reflects changes related to nerve injury. Uninjured L4 branch and its DRG help to identify how the nerve injury influences surrounding uninjured nerves. After injury rats show a mild limp with slightly everted paw. The development of pain-related behavior is observed 1-2 days post injury as tactile and thermal allodynia (Chaplan et al., 1994; Ossipov et al., 1999). Those signs persisted up to 10 weeks. Cold allodynia is less pronounced. Electrophysiological studies showed an increased number of neurons responding to light mechanical, thermal or cold stimuli although the threshold of response was similar to control animals (Chapman et al., 1998). The experiment where dorsal rhizotomy was performed on attempt to block signals from an injured and uninjured nerve to reach the spinal cord showed that the spontaneous pain may be mediated through injured fibers while the evoked pain requires input from uninjured fibers (Sheen & Chung, 1993; Yoon et al., 1996).

4.5 Spared nerve injury

In spared nerve injury model peripheral branches of the sciatic nerve are ligated and transected (Decosterd & Woolf, 2000). Peroneal and common tibial branch are injured while sural branch is left intact. Such injury caused tactile thermal and cold allodynia persisting over 9 weeks. The signs of neuropathic pain are most prominent at the areas of the hind paw innervated by an uninjured sural nerve. The design of this model allows studying changes in uninjured nerve fibers sharing the common nerve trunk with injured ones and compared it with uninjured fibers in saphenous nerve innervating basically the same area like the injured nerve branches.

4.6 Other models of peripheral nerve injury

Other models of peripheral nerve inujry include immune or toxin-mediated demyelination that simulates demyelinating neuropathy (Wallace et al., 2003). Vincristine, paclitaxel and cisplatin have been used in animal models to mimic polyneuropathy caused by tumor chemotherapy (Peltier & Russell, 2002). Streptozocin-induced damage to pancreatic insulin-producing cells in rats provides an experimental model of diabetic neuropathy (Rondon et al., 2010).

4.7 Spinal cord injury

Neuropathic pain may also develop as a consequence of spinal cord injury (SCI). Although the loss of function is the primary concern of SCI patient, the presence of pain negatively influences the rehabilitation strategies and reduces the quality of life of SCI patients. The prevalence of SCI pain is about 70-80% (Ravenscroft et al., 1999). Neuropathic pain after SCI is difficult to treat as there are several locations in the neuraxis this pain may arise from; there may be increased activity of neurons around the site of the injury, in the nerve or in the brain. The SCI-induced neuropathic pain is classified as at- level, or below-level pain with an incidence of about 30-40% (Siddall et al., 2003). Below-level pain is usually described as severe pain and may develop months or years after initial injury. In the case of at-level pain, the pain probably arises from the spinal cord above the injury site. Spinal local anesthetics blockade above the level of SCI produce temporary pain relief in SCI patient while the same procedure is ineffective in patient with spinal canal obstruction where sensory blockade can not be produce above SCI level (Loubser & Clearman, 1993). The presence of spinal generator of abnormal neuronal activity underlying SCI neuropathic pain was demonstrated in electrophysiological experiments using animal models of SCI where spontaneous activity of the above- level neurons was found after spinal cord transection (Loeser & Ward, 1967). Following this initial study, a number of SCI pain models have been developed, based on mechanical injury such as transection (Christensen et al., 1996; Levitt &

Heybach, 1981; Vierck & Light, 1999), contusion (Hulsebosch et al., 2000; Lindsey et al., 2000; Siddall et al., 1995), irradiation (Xu et al., 1992) and excitotoxicity (Yezierski & Park, 1993). Although the mechanism is different, the presence of SCI pain in these models is evident within couple of days and persists for several weeks to months. The electrophysiological recordings showed an increased background activity of spinal cord neurons, an increased responsiveness to peripheral stimuli and prolonged afterdischarges. The current explanation of such changes is based on the dysfunction of the inhibitory circuitry in the spinal cord, enhanced excitation of neurons through glutamate receptors and changes in the expression of sodium channels (Hains et al., 2003).

The regeneration strategies after SCI may also be related to the development of neuropathic pain. There are evidences that fibers producing excitatory neurotransmitter calcitonin gene-related peptide grow from the superficial lamine into deeper areas and that this reorganization is related to pain behavior (Christensen & Hulsebosch, 1997).

The ongoing pain sensations have been reported in some SCI patients despite of extensive pharmacological and surgical treatments, including removing a part of the spinal cord. Such observations suggest the pain may arise from supraspinal structures. It is not clear which centers in brain may be involved in such pain, although there are some evidences towards electrophysiological and metabolic changes of thalamic neurons (Defrin et al., 2001).

5. Pharmacotherapy of neuropathic pain

The effective pharmacological treatment of neuropathic pain should target an underlying mechanism of given pain state. Although there are usually numerous changes in the processing of nociceptive input that cause neuropathic pain, the idea is to target the most dominant mechanisms to achieve a reduction of pain. Based on our current knowledges on the underlying mechanisms of neuropathic pain, treatments are being developed to reduce the release of pronociceptive neurotransmitters by opiates or calcium channel-binding drugs, to regulate glutamate signaling by inhibiting postsynaptic NMDA receptors, to potentiate inhibitory neurotransmitter by agonist administration, reuptake inhibitors or sodium channel blockers.

Although the conventional analgesics showed to be ineffective in a relieving of NP symptoms, drugs originally developed to restore a balance in the level of neurotransmitter in CNS or to modulate transmembrane potential and excitability of neurons, have been successfully used to reduce some of the neuropathic pain symptoms. However, none of these drugs are able to produce long lasting pain relief. Moreover, their long term use is often negatively influenced by adverse side effects. Therefore there is still a need for better therapies. The currently used pharmacotherapy includes tricyclic antidepressants, anticonvulsants and opioids.

One of the first group of drugs used in clinical trials for neuropathic pain were tricyclic antidepressants (Watson et al., 1982). They proved to be temporarily efficacious in various neuropathic pain conditions but with many side effects. Newer classes of antidepressant that alter serotonergic and noradrenergic signaling have better tolerability and widely used in NP treatment (Rowbotham et al., 2004; Sawynok & Reid, 2001). Sodium channel blockers such as anticonvulsant and local anesthetic drugs reduce the ectopic discharges originating at the injury site. The high specificity of these drugs for sodium channels allows using them systematically without serious failure of normal sodium channel functioning necessary for impulse propagation in nervous system, although a potential cardiac toxicity is an obstacle for their wider use in NP treatment. Gabapentin, an anticonvulsant originally developed to interact with GABA receptors and to increase inhibitory tone when GABA signaling is impaired, have an analgesic effect in some form of neuropathic pain. Its action is not mediated via GABA receptors though; it is believed it acts through voltage- gated calcium channels (Taylor et al., 1998). Voltage-gated calcium channels (N and T family) regulate the influx of calcium into the cell upon proper stimulus. Increase in the intracellular calcium in the neuromuscular junctions cause the contraction of muscle and release of neurotransmitters from nerves. Expression of one of the N type of calcium channel family, α1B, in the superficial laminae of the dorsal horn after the nerve injury and the correlation with the pain behavior point to their involvement in nociception (Cizkova et al., 2002). Calcium channels are therefore an attractive target for development of novel analgesic drugs (Perret & Luo, 2009). Opioid therapy proved to be effective in various form of neuropathic pain (Foley, 2003; Zochodne & Max, 2003). However, as with every drug used in chronic pain treatment, negative side effects such as cognitive impairment, sedation, tolerance and addiction are a limiting factor.

6. Cell based therapy

In search for novel approaches for neuropathic pain treatment, cell based therapy has potential to overcome issues of traditional pharmacotherapy. Transplantation, either intraspinal or intrathecal, of cells releasing analgesic substances provide targeted delivery of desired drug and thus reducing adverse side effects due to its widespread action after oral or systemic injection. Also, local delivery of drugs via indwelling catheters is often limited by possible infections, especially in chronic implantations.

As one of the major factors in persistent pain syndromes is reduced GABAergic inhibitory control, delivery of GABA via cell based therapy has been extensively studied. Intraspinal grafting of GABAergic cells derived from fetal mouse striatum or fetal human telencephalon reduced tactile allodynia in L5/6 spinal nerve ligation model (Mukhida et al., 2007). Intrathecal or intraspinal injection of GABAergic cells derived from human teratocarcinoma cell line (hNT) has also showed positive effect in reducing spinal cord injury pain and spasticity in experimental models (Eaton et al., 2007; Marsala et al., 2004). Enhanced delivery of GABA via gene therapy approaches have shown promise in preclinical models, notably the administration of GAD65-expressing rAAV2 to sciatic nerve or DRG (Kim et al., 2009) and peripherally delivered HSV-based vectors engineered to produce either GAD65 or GAD67 in DRG (Hao et al., 2005) can reduce peripheral neuropathic or SCI pain. Previous findings in our laboratory have shown that the transplantation of neural progenitor cells expressing GABA into the dorsal horn of animals with excitotoxic spinal cord injury can reduce symptoms of spontaneous pain, and can reduce spinal hyperexcitability (wind-up) and hyperalgesia in animals with chronic constriction injury (Jergova et al., 2009; Lee et al., 2001). To enhance the efficiency of GABAergic cell therapy, several approaches are investigated. Recent study demonstrated increased yield of GABAergic precursor cells under a low concentration of the fibroblast growth factor in a cell culture. Also, genetic modification where specific transcriptional factor was blocked promoted GABAergic and reduced glial differentiation (Furmanski et al., 2009).

7. Gene therapy

The most promising approach in alleviating chronic pain may be the use of genetically modified cells releasing combination of molecules with distinct antinociceptive mechanisms. Research in our laboratory is focused on two potential candidates, serine-histogranin, targeting enhanced glutamatergic signaling and conotoxins targeting increased expression of calcium channels.

7.1 Serine-histogranin

[Ser^1] histogranin (SHG) is synthetic analog of histogranin, peptide produced by adrenal glands, pituitary, brain and other tissues (Lemaire et al., 1993) with inhibitory properties at glutamate NMDA receptors (Shukla et al., 1995). Findings in our laboratory suggest that SHG can produce prolonged inhibition of spinal nociceptive responses to a variety of stimuli, and may interact at unique excitatory amino acid receptive sites in the spinal dorsal horn (Hentall et al., 2007). Intrathecal injection of SHG can block NMDA induced hyperalgesia and allodynia with no apparent adverse motor effects (Siegan & Sagen, 1995) in contrast to findings with another NMDA antagonists, MK-801 (Hama & Sagen, 2002; Hama et al., 2003). Recent results showed potentiation of antinociceptive effect of GABAergic transplant by intrathecally injected SHG in the model of peripheral nerve injury (Jergova et al., 2011b).

Previous experience in our laboratory has demonstrated that neuronal progenitor cells readily express transgenes, and thus make an ideal vehicle for delivery of novel analgesic peptides(Gajavelli et al., 2008). An enhanced GABAergic precursor cells transfected by SHG cDNA were recently developed. After intraspinal transplantation they significantly reduced cold allodynia and mechanical hyperalgesia in models of spinal cord injury and peripheral nerve injury-induced pain (Jergova et al., 2011a).

7.2 Conopeptides

Conotoxins are neurotoxic peptides isolated from the venom of marine snail Conus with selective ion channel blocking activity. There are 5 different classes of conotoxins based on the channel or receptor they target: α-conotoxin inhibit nicotinic acetylcholine receptors, δ-conotoxin target voltage-dependent sodium channels, κ-conotoxin inhibits potassium channels, μ-conotoxin inhibits voltage-dependent sodium channels in muscles, ω-conotoxin inhibits N-type voltage-dependent calcium channels. The analgesic effect of ω-conotoxin MVIIA is 100 to 1000 times more potent that of morphine and its synthetic version ziconotide is used in clinical treatment of neuropathic pain (Malmberg & Yaksh, 1995; Olivera, 2006; Wallace et al., 2008). Another group of conopeptides- conantokins, with NMDA antagonist activity is also very interesting in pain research, as enhanced activity of NMDA receptors is hypothesized to contribute to onoing pain (Teichert et al., 2007).

Clinical use of analgesic peptides is limited by poor CNS penetration and thus need to be delivered via intrathecal pumps. However, conopeptides are ideal candidates for recombinant expression at target sites to spinal cord pain processing centers using cell or molecular based strategies. In our laboratory, the intrathecal administration of N-tpe calcium channel inhibitor ω-conotoxin MVIIA produced marked reduction of neuropathic pain symptoms in animals with compression SCI, a particularly difficult clinical target (Hama & Sagen, 2009). Another conopeptide with NMDA antagonist activity, ConG, was found to be very efficient in reducing allodynia in SCI model. When used in combination with conopeptide MVIIA, more robust analgesic effect was observed. Isobolographic analysis showed synergistic effect of these conopeptides, an important finding considering possible side effects in prolonged administration of drugs. Synergism allows using lower concentration of drugs to achieve analgesic effect comparable to separate administration of those drugs at higher concentration. In addition, combination of conopeptide with GABAergic cell grafts may be particularly potent, as combined intrathecal ziconotide and baclofen have been reported to improve neuropathic pain scores in a recent case report (Saulino et al., 2009).

8. Conclusion

The restoration of inhibitory function in the spinal dorsal horn by neural transplantation is a promising strategy for alleviating persistent pain following injury to the nervous system. The recent availability of stem cells that can be directed towards desired neuronal phenotypes and also can be genetically manipulated to produce additional potent therapeutic agents offers the opportunity for targeted pain management and improved outcomes of chronic pain therapies.

9. References

Ali, Z.; Ringkamp, M.; Hartke, T.V.; Chien, H.F.; Flavahan, N.A.; Campbell, J.N. & Meyer, R.A. (1999). Uninjured C-fiber nociceptors develop spontaneous activity and alpha-adrenergic sensitivity following L6 spinal nerve ligation in monkey. *J Neurophysiol,* Vol.81, No.2, 455-466.

Amir, R. & Devor, M. (1997). Spike-evoked suppression and burst patterning in dorsal root ganglion neurons of the rat. *J Physiol,* Vol.501 (Pt 1), 183-196.

Arcaya, J.L.; Cano, G.; Gomez, G.; Maixner, W. & Suarez-Roca, H. (1999). Dynorphin A increases substance P release from trigeminal primary afferent C-fibers. *Eur J Pharmacol,* Vol.366, No.1, 27-34.

Bao, L.; Wang, H.F.; Cai, H.J.; Tong, Y.G.; Jin, S.X.; Lu, Y.J.; Grant, G.; Hokfelt, T. & Zhang, X. (2002). Peripheral axotomy induces only very limited sprouting of coarse myelinated afferents into inner lamina II of rat spinal cord. *Eur J Neurosci,* Vol.16, No.2, 175-185.

Baron, R. (2000). Capsaicin and nociception: from basic mechanisms to novel drugs. *Lancet,* Vol.356, No.9232, 785-787.

Bennett, G.J. & Xie, Y.K. (1988). A peripheral mononeuropathy in rat that produces disorders of pain sensation like those seen in man. *Pain,* Vol.33, No.1, 87-107.

Black, J.A.; Nikolajsen, L.; Kroner, K.; Jensen, T.S. & Waxman, S.G. (2008). Multiple sodium channel isoforms and mitogen-activated protein kinases are present in painful human neuromas. *Ann Neurol,* Vol.64, No.6, 644-653.

Burgess, S.E.; Gardell, L.R.; Ossipov, M.H.; Malan, T.P., Jr.; Vanderah, T.W.; Lai, J. & Porreca, F. (2002). Time-dependent descending facilitation from the rostral ventromedial medulla maintains, but does not initiate, neuropathic pain. *J Neurosci,* Vol.22, No.12, 5129-5136.

Campero, M.; Serra, J.; Marchettini, P. & Ochoa, J.L. (1998). Ectopic impulse generation and autoexcitation in single myelinated afferent fibers in patients with peripheral neuropathy and positive sensory symptoms. *Muscle Nerve,* Vol.21, No.12, 1661-1667.

Castro-Lopes, J.M.; Tavares, I. & Coimbra, A. (1993). GABA decreases in the spinal cord dorsal horn after peripheral neurectomy. *Brain Res,* Vol.620, No.2, 287-291.

Caterina, M.J. (2007). Transient receptor potential ion channels as participants in thermosensation and thermoregulation. *Am J Physiol Regul Integr Comp Physiol,* Vol.292, No.1, R64-76.

Caterina, M.J. (2008). On the thermoregulatory perils of TRPV1 antagonism. *Pain,* Vol.136, No.1-2, 3-4.

Caterina, M.J.; Schumacher, M.A.; Tominaga, M.; Rosen, T.A.; Levine, J.D. & Julius, D. (1997). The capsaicin receptor: a heat-activated ion channel in the pain pathway. *Nature,* Vol.389, No.6653, 816-824.

Catheline, G.; Le Guen, S.; Honore, P. & Besson, J.M. (1999). Are there long-term changes in the basal or evoked Fos expression in the dorsal horn of the spinal cord of the mononeuropathic rat? *Pain,* Vol.80, No.1-2, 347-357.

Chabal, C.; Jacobson, L.; Russell, L.C. & Burchiel, K.J. (1989). Pain responses to perineuromal injection of normal saline, gallamine, and lidocaine in humans. *Pain,* Vol.36, No.3, 321-325.

Chaplan, S.R.; Bach, F.W.; Pogrel, J.W.; Chung, J.M. & Yaksh, T.L. (1994). Quantitative assessment of tactile allodynia in the rat paw. *J Neurosci Methods,* Vol.53, No.1, 55-63.

Chapman, V.; Suzuki, R. & Dickenson, A.H. (1998). Electrophysiological characterization of spinal neuronal response properties in anaesthetized rats after ligation of spinal nerves L5-L6. *J Physiol,* Vol.507 (Pt 3), 881-894.

Christensen, M.D.; Everhart, A.W.; Pickelman, J.T. & Hulsebosch, C.E. (1996). Mechanical and thermal allodynia in chronic central pain following spinal cord injury. *Pain,* Vol.68, No.1, 97-107.

Christensen, M.D. & Hulsebosch, C.E. (1997). Chronic central pain after spinal cord injury. *J Neurotrauma,* Vol.14, No.8, 517-537.

Cizkova, D.; Marsala, J.; Lukacova, N.; Marsala, M.; Jergova, S.; Orendacova, J. & Yaksh, T.L. (2002). Localization of N-type Ca2+ channels in the rat spinal cord following chronic constrictive nerve injury. *Exp Brain Res,* Vol.147, No.4, 456-463.

Coggeshall, R.E.; Dougherty, P.M.; Pover, C.M. & Carlton, S.M. (1993). Is large myelinated fiber loss associated with hyperalgesia in a model of experimental peripheral neuropathy in the rat? *Pain,* Vol.52, No.2, 233-242.

Cunha, J.M.; Cunha, F.Q.; Poole, S. & Ferreira, S.H. (2000). Cytokine-mediated inflammatory hyperalgesia limited by interleukin-1 receptor antagonist. *Br J Pharmacol,* Vol.130, No.6, 1418-1424.

Daousi, C.; MacFarlane, I.A.; Woodward, A.; Nurmikko, T.J.; Bundred, P.E. & Benbow, S.J. (2004). Chronic painful peripheral neuropathy in an urban community: a controlled comparison of people with and without diabetes. *Diabet Med,* Vol.21, No.9, 976-982.
Decosterd, I. & Woolf, C.J. (2000). Spared nerve injury: an animal model of persistent peripheral neuropathic pain. *Pain,* Vol.87, No.2, 149-158.
Defrin, R.; Ohry, A.; Blumen, N. & Urca, G. (2001). Characterization of chronic pain and somatosensory function in spinal cord injury subjects. *Pain,* Vol.89, No.2-3, 253-263.
Devor, M.; White, D.M.; Goetzl, E.J. & Levine, J.D. (1992). Eicosanoids, but not tachykinins, excite C-fiber endings in rat sciatic nerve-end neuromas. *Neuroreport,* Vol.3, No.1, 21-24.
Dib-Hajj, S.D.; Binshtok, A.M.; Cummins, T.R.; Jarvis, M.F.; Samad, T. & Zimmermann, K. (2009). Voltage-gated sodium channels in pain states: role in pathophysiology and targets for treatment. *Brain Res Rev,* Vol.60, No.1, 65-83.
Dib-Hajj, S.D.; Cummins, T.R.; Black, J.A. & Waxman, S.G. (2007). From genes to pain: Na v 1.7 and human pain disorders. *Trends Neurosci,* Vol.30, No.11, 555-563.
Dobretsov, M.; Hastings, S.L.; Stimers, J.R. & Zhang, J.M. (2001). Mechanical hyperalgesia in rats with chronic perfusion of lumbar dorsal root ganglion with hyperglycemic solution. *J Neurosci Methods,* Vol.110, No.1-2, 9-15.
Drenth, J.P. & Waxman, S.G. (2007). Mutations in sodium-channel gene SCN9A cause a spectrum of human genetic pain disorders. *J Clin Invest,* Vol.117, No.12, 3603-3609.
Eaton, M.J.; Plunkett, J.A.; Karmally, S.; Martinez, M.A. & Montanez, K. (1998). Changes in GAD- and GABA- immunoreactivity in the spinal dorsal horn after peripheral nerve injury and promotion of recovery by lumbar transplant of immortalized serotonergic precursors. *J Chem Neuroanat,* Vol.16, No.1, 57-72.
Eaton, M.J.; Wolfe, S.Q.; Martinez, M.; Hernandez, M.; Furst, C.; Huang, J.; Frydel, B.R. & Gomez-Marin, O. (2007). Subarachnoid transplant of a human neuronal cell line attenuates chronic allodynia and hyperalgesia after excitotoxic spinal cord injury in the rat. *J Pain,* Vol.8, No.1, 33-50.
Foley, K.M. (2003). Opioids and chronic neuropathic pain. *N Engl J Med,* Vol.348, No.13, 1279-1281.
Furmanski, O.; Gajavelli, S.; Lee, J.W.; Collado, M.E.; Jergova, S. & Sagen, J. (2009). Combined extrinsic and intrinsic manipulations exert complementary neuronal enrichment in embryonic rat neural precursor cultures: an in vitro and in vivo analysis. *J Comp Neurol,* Vol.515, No.1, 56-71.
Gajavelli, S.; Castellanos, D.A.; Furmanski, O.; Schiller, P.C. & Sagen, J. (2008). Sustained analgesic peptide secretion and cell labeling using a novel genetic modification. *Cell Transplant,* Vol.17, No.4, 445-455.
Gardell, L.R.; Ibrahim, M.; Wang, R.; Wang, Z.; Ossipov, M.H.; Malan, T.P., Jr.; Porreca, F. & Lai, J. (2004). Mouse strains that lack spinal dynorphin upregulation after peripheral nerve injury do not develop neuropathic pain. *Neuroscience,* Vol.123, No.1, 43-52.
Gardell, L.R.; Vanderah, T.W.; Gardell, S.E.; Wang, R.; Ossipov, M.H.; Lai, J. & Porreca, F. (2003). Enhanced evoked excitatory transmitter release in experimental neuropathy requires descending facilitation. *J Neurosci,* Vol.23, No.23, 8370-8379.

Guo, A.; Vulchanova, L.; Wang, J.; Li, X. & Elde, R. (1999). Immunocytochemical localization of the vanilloid receptor 1 (VR1): relationship to neuropeptides, the P2X3 purinoceptor and IB4 binding sites. *Eur J Neurosci,* Vol.11, No.3, 946-958.

Gwak, Y.S.; Tan, H.Y.; Nam, T.S.; Paik, K.S.; Hulsebosch, C.E. & Leem, J.W. (2006). Activation of spinal GABA receptors attenuates chronic central neuropathic pain after spinal cord injury. *J Neurotrauma,* Vol.23, No.7, 1111-1124.

Hains, B.C.; Klein, J.P.; Saab, C.Y.; Craner, M.J.; Black, J.A. & Waxman, S.G. (2003). Upregulation of sodium channel Nav1.3 and functional involvement in neuronal hyperexcitability associated with central neuropathic pain after spinal cord injury. *J Neurosci,* Vol.23, No.26, 8881-8892.

Hama, A. & Sagen, J. (2002). Selective antihyperalgesic effect of [Ser1] histogranin on complete Freund's adjuvant-induced hyperalgesia in rats. *Pain,* Vol.95, No.1-2, 15-21.

Hama, A. & Sagen, J. (2009). Antinociceptive effects of the marine snail peptides conantokin-G and conotoxin MVIIA alone and in combination in rat models of pain. *Neuropharmacology,* Vol.56, No.2, 556-563.

Hama, A.; Woon Lee, J. & Sagen, J. (2003). Differential efficacy of intrathecal NMDA receptor antagonists on inflammatory mechanical and thermal hyperalgesia in rats. *Eur J Pharmacol,* Vol.459, No.1, 49-58.

Hao, J.X.; Xu, X.J. & Wiesenfeld-Hallin, Z. (1994). Intrathecal gamma-aminobutyric acidB (GABAB) receptor antagonist CGP 35348 induces hypersensitivity to mechanical stimuli in the rat. *Neurosci Lett,* Vol.182, No.2, 299-302.

Hao, S.; Mata, M.; Wolfe, D.; Huang, S.; Glorioso, J.C. & Fink, D.J. (2005). Gene transfer of glutamic acid decarboxylase reduces neuropathic pain. *Ann Neurol,* Vol.57, No.6, 914-918.

Heinricher, M.M. & Neubert, M.J. (2004). Neural basis for the hyperalgesic action of cholecystokinin in the rostral ventromedial medulla. *J Neurophysiol,* Vol.92, No.4, 1982-1989.

Hentall, I.D.; Hargraves, W.A. & Sagen, J. (2007). Inhibition by the chromaffin cell-derived peptide serine-histogranin in the rat's dorsal horn. *Neurosci Lett,* Vol.419, No.1, 88-92.

Hudson, L.J.; Bevan, S.; Wotherspoon, G.; Gentry, C.; Fox, A. & Winter, J. (2001). VR1 protein expression increases in undamaged DRG neurons after partial nerve injury. *Eur J Neurosci,* Vol.13, No.11, 2105-2114.

Hulsebosch, C.E.; Xu, G.Y.; Perez-Polo, J.R.; Westlund, K.N.; Taylor, C.P. & McAdoo, D.J. (2000). Rodent model of chronic central pain after spinal cord contusion injury and effects of gabapentin. *J Neurotrauma,* Vol.17, No.12, 1205-1217.

Ibuki, T.; Hama, A.T.; Wang, X.T.; Pappas, G.D. & Sagen, J. (1997). Loss of GABA-immunoreactivity in the spinal dorsal horn of rats with peripheral nerve injury and promotion of recovery by adrenal medullary grafts. *Neuroscience,* Vol.76, No.3, 845-858.

Isaev, D.; Gerber, G.; Park, S.K.; Chung, J.M. & Randik, M. (2000). Facilitation of NMDA-induced currents and Ca2+ transients in the rat substantia gelatinosa neurons after ligation of L5-L6 spinal nerves. *Neuroreport,* Vol.11, No.18, 4055-4061.

Jergova, S.; Collante, D.; Bartley, S.; Rodriguez, C.; Pamphile, G.; Gajavelli, S. & Sagen, J. (2011a). Intraspinal transplantation of recombinant neuroprogenitor cells in a spinal cord injury model of central neuropathic pain, The 29th Annual National Neurotrauma Society Symposium Fort Lauderdale, Florida

Jergova, S.; Furmanski, O.; Collado, M.; Varghese, M.; Gajavelli, S.; Manoah, L.; Hentall, I. & Sagen, J. (2009). Behavioral and neurophysiological effects of GABAergic neuronal precursor cell transplantation in a rat model of chronic neuropathic pain, Society of Neuroscience Abstracts, Chicago, Illinois

Jergova, S.; Varghese, M.S.; Collante, D.; Gajavelli, S. & Sagen, J. (2011b). Antinociceptive effect of recombinant neuroprogenitor intraspinal transplants in models of peripheral and central neuropathic pain, 30th Annual Sientific Meeting of the American Pain Society, Austin, Texas

Kajander, K.C. & Bennett, G.J. (1992). Onset of a painful peripheral neuropathy in rat: a partial and differential deafferentation and spontaneous discharge in A beta and A delta primary afferent neurons. *J Neurophysiol,* Vol.68, No.3, 734-744.

Kauppila, T.; Kontinen, V.K. & Pertovaara, A. (1998). Influence of spinalization on spinal withdrawal reflex responses varies depending on the submodality of the test stimulus and the experimental pathophysiological condition in the rat. *Brain Res,* Vol.797, No.2, 234-242.

Kim, J.; Kim, S.J.; Lee, H. & Chang, J.W. (2009). Effective neuropathic pain relief through sciatic nerve administration of GAD65-expressing rAAV2. *Biochem Biophys Res Commun,* Vol.388, No.1, 73-78.

Kim, S.H. & Chung, J.M. (1992). An experimental model for peripheral neuropathy produced by segmental spinal nerve ligation in the rat. *Pain,* Vol.50, No.3, 355-363.

Klede, M.; Handwerker, H.O. & Schmelz, M. (2003). Central origin of secondary mechanical hyperalgesia. *J Neurophysiol,* Vol.90, No.1, 353-359.

Koetzner, L.; Hua, X.Y.; Lai, J.; Porreca, F. & Yaksh, T. (2004). Nonopioid actions of intrathecal dynorphin evoke spinal excitatory amino acid and prostaglandin E2 release mediated by cyclooxygenase-1 and -2. *J Neurosci,* Vol.24, No.6, 1451-1458.

Koppert, W.; Dern, S.K.; Sittl, R.; Albrecht, S.; Schuttler, J. & Schmelz, M. (2001). A new model of electrically evoked pain and hyperalgesia in human skin: the effects of intravenous alfentanil, S(+)-ketamine, and lidocaine. *Anesthesiology,* Vol.95, No.2, 395-402.

Kress, M. & Fickenscher, H. (2001). Infection by human varicella-zoster virus confers norepinephrine sensitivity to sensory neurons from rat dorsal root ganglia. *FASEB J,* Vol.15, No.6, 1037-1043.

Laird, J.M. & Bennett, G.J. (1993). An electrophysiological study of dorsal horn neurons in the spinal cord of rats with an experimental peripheral neuropathy. *J Neurophysiol,* Vol.69, No.6, 2072-2085.

Lee, J.W.; Yezierski, R.P. & Sagen, J. (2001). Transplantation of embryonic precursor cells into excitotoxically lesioned adult spinal cord: In vivo survival and differentiation in quisqualic acid-treated spinal cord. . *Soc Neurosci Abs,* Vol.27, 369.

Lemaire, P.; Garrett, N.; Kato, K. & Gurdon, J.B. (1993). Construction of subtracted cDNA libraries enriched for cDNAs for genes expressed in the mesoderm of early Xenopus gastrulae. *C R Acad Sci III,* Vol.316, No.9, 931-944.

Levitt, M. & Heybach, J.P. (1981). The deafferentation syndrome in genetically blind rats: a model of the painful phantom limb. *Pain,* Vol.10, No.1, 67-73.

Levy, D.; Tal, M.; Hoke, A. & Zochodne, D.W. (2000). Transient action of the endothelial constitutive nitric oxide synthase (ecNOS) mediates the development of thermal hypersensitivity following peripheral nerve injury. *European Journal of Neuroscience,* Vol.12, No.7, 2323-2332.

Lindsey, A.E.; LoVerso, R.L.; Tovar, C.A.; Hill, C.E.; Beattie, M.S. & Bresnahan, J.C. (2000). An analysis of changes in sensory thresholds to mild tactile and cold stimuli after experimental spinal cord injury in the rat. *Neurorehabil Neural Repair,* Vol.14, No.4, 287-300.

Liu, C.N.; Wall, P.D.; Ben-Dor, E.; Michaelis, M.; Amir, R. & Devor, M. (2000). Tactile allodynia in the absence of C-fiber activation: altered firing properties of DRG neurons following spinal nerve injury. *Pain,* Vol.85, No.3, 503-521.

Loeser, J.D. & Ward, A.A., Jr. (1967). Some effects of deafferentation on neurons of the cat spinal cord. *Arch Neurol,* Vol.17, No.6, 629-636.

Loubser, P.G. & Clearman, R.R. (1993). Evaluation of central spinal cord injury pain with diagnostic spinal anesthesia. *Anesthesiology,* Vol.79, No.2, 376-378.

Malan, T.P.; Mata, H.P. & Porreca, F. (2002). Spinal GABA(A) and GABA(B) receptor pharmacology in a rat model of neuropathic pain. *Anesthesiology,* Vol.96, No.5, 1161-1167.

Malan, T.P.; Ossipov, M.H.; Gardell, L.R.; Ibrahim, M.; Bian, D.; Lai, J. & Porreca, F. (2000). Extraterritorial neuropathic pain correlates with multisegmental elevation of spinal dynorphin in nerve-injured rats. *Pain,* Vol.86, No.1-2, 185-194.

Malmberg, A.B. & Yaksh, T.L. (1995). Effect of continuous intrathecal infusion of omega-conopeptides, N-type calcium-channel blockers, on behavior and antinociception in the formalin and hot-plate tests in rats. *Pain,* Vol.60, No.1, 83-90.

Marsala, M.; Kakinohana, O.; Yaksh, T.L.; Tomori, Z.; Marsala, S. & Cizkova, D. (2004). Spinal implantation of hNT neurons and neuronal precursors: graft survival and functional effects in rats with ischemic spastic paraplegia. *Eur J Neurosci,* Vol.20, No.9, 2401-2414.

McMahon, S. & Koltzenburg, M. (2005). Wall and Melzack's Textbook of Pain. Elsevier.

Michael, G.J. & Priestley, J.V. (1999). Differential expression of the mRNA for the vanilloid receptor subtype 1 in cells of the adult rat dorsal root and nodose ganglia and its downregulation by axotomy. *J Neurosci,* Vol.19, No.5, 1844-1854.

Moore, K.A.; Kohno, T.; Karchewski, L.A.; Scholz, J.; Baba, H. & Woolf, C.J. (2002). Partial peripheral nerve injury promotes a selective loss of GABAergic inhibition in the superficial dorsal horn of the spinal cord. *J Neurosci,* Vol.22, No.15, 6724-6731.

Mukhida, K.; Mendez, I.; McLeod, M.; Kobayashi, N.; Haughn, C.; Milne, B.; Baghbaderani, B.; Sen, A.; Behie, L.A. & Hong, M. (2007). Spinal GABAergic Transplants Attenuate Mechanical Allodynia in a Rat Model of Neuropathic Pain. *Stem Cells,* Vol.25, No.11, 2874-2885.

Munger, B.L.; Bennett, G.J. & Kajander, K.C. (1992). An experimental painful peripheral neuropathy due to nerve constriction. I. Axonal pathology in the sciatic nerve. *Exp Neurol,* Vol.118, No.2, 204-214.

Nichols, M.L.; Allen, B.J.; Rogers, S.D.; Ghilardi, J.R.; Honore, P.; Luger, N.M.; Finke, M.P.; Li, J.; Lappi, D.A.; Simone, D.A. & Mantyh, P.W. (1999). Transmission of chronic nociception by spinal neurons expressing the substance P receptor. *Science,* Vol.286, No.5444, 1558-1561.

Noda, K.; Ueda, Y.; Suzuki, K. & Yoda, K. (1997). Excitatory effects of algesic compounds on neuronal processes in murine dorsal root ganglion cell culture. *Brain Res,* Vol.751, No.2, 348-351.

Olivera, B.M. (2006). Conus peptides: biodiversity-based discovery and exogenomics. *J Biol Chem,* Vol.281, No.42, 31173-31177.

Orstavik, K.; Weidner, C.; Schmidt, R.; Schmelz, M.; Hilliges, M.; Jorum, E.; Handwerker, H. & Torebjork, E. (2003). Pathological C-fibres in patients with a chronic painful condition. *Brain,* Vol.126, No.Pt 3, 567-578.

Ossipov, M.H.; Bian, D.; Malan, T.P., Jr.; Lai, J. & Porreca, F. (1999). Lack of involvement of capsaicin-sensitive primary afferents in nerve-ligation injury induced tactile allodynia in rats. *Pain,* Vol.79, No.2-3, 127-133.

Ossipov, M.H.; Zhang, E.T.; Carvajal, C.; Gardell, L.; Quirion, R.; Dumont, Y.; Lai, J. & Porreca, F. (2002). Selective mediation of nerve injury-induced tactile hypersensitivity by neuropeptide Y. *J Neurosci,* Vol.22, No.22, 9858-9867.

Palecek, J.; Dougherty, P.M.; Kim, S.H.; Paleckova, V.; Lekan, H.; Chung, J.M., Carlton, S.M. & Willis, W.D. (1992). Responses of spinothalamic tract neurons to mechanical and thermal stimuli in an experimental model of peripheral neuropathy in primates. *J Neurophysiol,* Vol.68, No.6, 1951-1966.

Peltier, A.C. & Russell, J.W. (2002). Recent advances in drug-induced neuropathies. *Curr Opin Neurol,* Vol.15, No.5, 633-638.

Perret, D. & Luo, Z.D. (2009). Targeting voltage-gated calcium channels for neuropathic pain management. *Neurotherapeutics,* Vol.6, No.4, 679-692.

Polgar, E.; Gray, S.; Riddell, J.S. & Todd, A.J. (2004). Lack of evidence for significant neuronal loss in laminae I-III of the spinal dorsal horn of the rat in the chronic constriction injury model. *Pain,* Vol.111, No.1-2, 144-150.

Polgar, E.; Hughes, D.I.; Riddell, J.S.; Maxwell, D.J., Puskar, Z. & Todd, A.J. (2003). Selective loss of spinal GABAergic or glycinergic neurons is not necessary for development of thermal hyperalgesia in the chronic constriction injury model of neuropathic pain. *Pain,* Vol.104, No.1-2, 229-239.

Porreca, F.; Burgess, S.E.; Gardell, L.R.; Vanderah, T.W.; Malan, T.P., Jr.; Ossipov, M.H.; Lappi, D.A. & Lai, J. (2001). Inhibition of neuropathic pain by selective ablation of brainstem medullary cells expressing the mu-opioid receptor. *J Neurosci,* Vol.21, No.14, 5281-5288.

Rappaport, Z.H. & Devor, M. (1994). Trigeminal neuralgia: the role of self-sustaining discharge in the trigeminal ganglion. *Pain,* Vol.56, No.2, 127-138.

Ravenscroft, A.; Ahmed, Y.S. & Burnside, I.G. (1999). Chronic pain after spinal cord injury: a survey of practice in UK spinal injury units. *Spinal Cord,* Vol.37, No.1, 25-28.

Reeh, P.W.; Bayer, J.; Kocher, L. & Handwerker, H.O. (1987). Sensitization of nociceptive cutaneous nerve fibers from the rat's tail by noxious mechanical stimulation. *Exp Brain Res,* Vol.65, No.3, 505-512.

Rivera, L.; Gallar, J.; Pozo, M.A. & Belmonte, C. (2000). Responses of nerve fibres of the rat saphenous nerve neuroma to mechanical and chemical stimulation: an in vitro study. *J Physiol,* Vol.527 Pt 2, 305-313.

Rondon, L.J.; Privat, A.M.; Daulhac, L.; Davin, N.; Mazur, A.; Fialip, J.; Eschalier, A. & Courteix, C. (2010). Magnesium attenuates chronic hypersensitivity and spinal cord

NMDA receptor phosphorylation in a rat model of diabetic neuropathic pain. *J Physiol,* Vol.588, No.Pt 21, 4205-4215.

Rowbotham, M.C.; Goli, V.; Kunz, N.R. & Lei, D. (2004). Venlafaxine extended release in the treatment of painful diabetic neuropathy: a double-blind, placebo-controlled study. *Pain,* Vol.110, No.3, 697-706.

Saulino, M.; Burton, A.W.; Danyo, D.A.; Frost, S.; Glanzer, J. & Solanki, D.R. (2009). Intrathecal ziconotide and baclofen provide pain relief in seven patients with neuropathic pain and spasticity: case reports. *Eur J Phys Rehabil Med,* Vol.45, No.1, 61-67.

Sawynok, J. & Reid, A. (2001). Antinociception by tricyclic antidepressants in the rat formalin test: differential effects on different behaviours following systemic and spinal administration. *Pain,* Vol.93, No.1, 51-59.

Schafers, M.; Sorkin, L.S. & Sommer, C. (2003). Intramuscular injection of tumor necrosis factor-alpha induces muscle hyperalgesia in rats. *Pain,* Vol.104, No.3, 579-588.

Schuler, V.; Luscher, C.; Blanchet, C.; Klix, N.; Sansig, G.; Klebs, K.; Schmutz, M.; Heid, J.; Gentry, C.; Urban, L.; Fox, A.; Spooren, W.; Jaton, A.L.; Vigouret, J.; Pozza, M.; Kelly, P.H.; Mosbacher, J.; Froestl, W.; Kaslin, E.; Korn, R.; Bischoff, S.; Kaupmann, K.; van der Putten, H. & Bettler, B. (2001). Epilepsy, hyperalgesia, impaired memory, and loss of pre- and postsynaptic GABA(B) responses in mice lacking GABA(B(1)). *Neuron,* Vol.31, No.1, 47-58.

Seltzer, Z.; Dubner, R. & Shir, Y. (1990). A novel behavioral model of neuropathic pain disorders produced in rats by partial sciatic nerve injury. *Pain,* Vol.43, No.2, 205-218.

Sheen, K. & Chung, J.M. (1993). Signs of neuropathic pain depend on signals from injured nerve fibers in a rat model. *Brain Res,* Vol.610, No.1, 62-68.

Shehab, S.A.; Spike, R.C. & Todd, A.J. (2003). Evidence against cholera toxin B subunit as a reliable tracer for sprouting of primary afferents following peripheral nerve injury. *Brain Res,* Vol.964, No.2, 218-227.

Shir, Y. & Seltzer, Z. (1990). A-fibers mediate mechanical hyperesthesia and allodynia and C-fibers mediate thermal hyperalgesia in a new model of causalgiform pain disorders in rats. *Neurosci Lett,* Vol.115, No.1, 62-67.

Shukla, V.K.; Lemaire, S.; Dumont, M. & Merali, Z. (1995). N-methyl-D-aspartate receptor antagonist activity and phencyclidine-like behavioral effects of the pentadecapeptide, [Ser1]histogranin. *Pharmacol Biochem Behav,* Vol.50, No.1, 49-54.

Siddall, P.; Xu, C.L. & Cousins, M. (1995). Allodynia following traumatic spinal cord injury in the rat. *Neuroreport,* Vol.6, No.9, 1241-1244.

Siddall, P.J.; McClelland, J.M.; Rutkowski, S.B. & Cousins, M.J. (2003). A longitudinal study of the prevalence and characteristics of pain in the first 5 years following spinal cord injury. *Pain,* Vol.103, No.3, 249-257.

Siegan, J.B. & Sagen, J. (1995). Attenuation of NMDA-induced spinal hypersensitivity by adrenal medullary transplants. *Brain Res,* Vol.680, No.1-2, 88-98.

Sommer, C. & Kress, M. (2004). Recent findings on how proinflammatory cytokines cause pain: peripheral mechanisms in inflammatory and neuropathic hyperalgesia. *Neurosci Lett,* Vol.361, No.1-3, 184-187.

Sorkin, L.S. & Doom, C.M. (2000). Epineurial application of TNF elicits an acute mechanical hyperalgesia in the awake rat. *J Peripher Nerv Syst,* Vol.5, No.2, 96-100.

Staaf, S.; Oerther, S.; Lucas, G.; Mattsson, J.P. & Ernfors, P. (2009). Differential regulation of TRP channels in a rat model of neuropathic pain. *Pain,* Vol.144, No.1-2, 187-199.

Sun, H.; Ren, K.; Zhong, C.M.; Ossipov, M.H.; Malan, T.P.; Lai, J. & Porreca, F. (2001). Nerve injury-induced tactile allodynia is mediated via ascending spinal dorsal column projections. *Pain,* Vol.90, No.1-2, 105-111.

Sung, B.; Lim, G. & Mao, J. (2003). Altered expression and uptake activity of spinal glutamate transporters after nerve injury contribute to the pathogenesis of neuropathic pain in rats. *J Neurosci,* Vol.23, No.7, 2899-2910.

Suzuki, R.; Morcuende, S.; Webber, M.; Hunt, S.P. & Dickenson, A.H. (2002). Superficial NK1-expressing neurons control spinal excitability through activation of descending pathways. *Nat Neurosci,* Vol.5, No.12, 1319-1326.

Tal, M. & Eliav, E. (1996). Abnormal discharge originates at the site of nerve injury in experimental constriction neuropathy (CCI) in the rat. *Pain,* Vol.64, No.3, 511-518.

Taylor, C.P.; Gee, N.S.; Su, T.Z.; Kocsis, J.D.; Welty, D.F.; Brown, J.P.; Dooley, D.J.; Boden, P. & Singh, L. (1998). A summary of mechanistic hypotheses of gabapentin pharmacology. *Epilepsy Res,* Vol.29, No.3, 233-249.

Teichert, R.W.; Jimenez, E.C.; Twede, V.; Watkins, M.; Hollmann, M.; Bulaj, G. & Olivera, B.M. (2007). Novel conantokins from Conus parius venom are specific antagonists of N-methyl-D-aspartate receptors. *J Biol Chem,* Vol.282, No.51, 36905-36913.

Ugarte, S.D.; Homanics, G.E.; Firestone, L.L. & Hammond, D.L. (2000). Sensory thresholds and the antinociceptive effects of GABA receptor agonists in mice lacking the beta3 subunit of the GABA(A) receptor. *Neuroscience,* Vol.95, No.3, 795-806.

Vierck, C.J., Jr. & Light, A.R. (1999). Effects of combined hemotoxic and anterolateral spinal lesions on nociceptive sensitivity. *Pain,* Vol.83, No.3, 447-457.

Wahren, L.K. & Torebjork, E. (1992). Quantitative sensory tests in patients with neuralgia 11 to 25 years after injury. *Pain,* Vol.48, No.2, 237-244.

Wakisaka, S.; Kajander, K.C. & Bennett, G.J. (1991). Increased neuropeptide Y (NPY)-like immunoreactivity in rat sensory neurons following peripheral axotomy. *Neurosci Lett,* Vol.124, No.2, 200-203.

Walker, K.; Fox, A.J. & Urban, L.A. (1999). Animal models for pain research. *Mol Med Today,* Vol.5, No.7, 319-321.

Wallace, M.S.; Rauck, R.; Fisher, R.; Charapata, S.G.; Ellis, D. & Dissanayake, S. (2008). Intrathecal ziconotide for severe chronic pain: safety and tolerability results of an open-label, long-term trial. *Anesth Analg,* Vol.106, No.2, 628-637, table of contents.

Wallace, V.C.; Cottrell, D.F.; Brophy, P.J. & Fleetwood-Walker, S.M. (2003). Focal lysolecithin-induced demyelination of peripheral afferents results in neuropathic pain behavior that is attenuated by cannabinoids. *J Neurosci,* Vol.23, No.8, 3221-3233.

Watson, C.P.; Evans, R.J.; Reed, K.; Merskey, H.; Goldsmith, L. & Warsh, J. (1982). Amitriptyline versus placebo in postherpetic neuralgia. *Neurology,* Vol.32, No.6, 671-673.

Wood, J.N.; Boorman, J.P.; Okuse, K. & Baker, M.D. (2004). Voltage-gated sodium channels and pain pathways. *J Neurobiol,* Vol.61, No.1, 55-71.

Woolf, C.J.; Shortland, P. & Coggeshall, R.E. (1992). Peripheral nerve injury triggers central sprouting of myelinated afferents. *Nature,* Vol.355, No.6355, 75-78.

Wu, G.; Ringkamp, M.; Hartke, T.V.; Murinson, B.B.; Campbell, J.N.; Griffin, J.W. & Meyer, R.A. (2001). Early onset of spontaneous activity in uninjured C-fiber nociceptors after injury to neighboring nerve fibers. *J Neurosci,* Vol.21, No.8, RC140.

Xu, X.J.; Hao, J.X.; Aldskogius, H.; Seiger, A. & Wiesenfeld-Hallin, Z. (1992). Chronic pain-related syndrome in rats after ischemic spinal cord lesion: a possible animal model for pain in patients with spinal cord injury. *Pain,* Vol.48, No.2, 279-290.

Yezierski, R.P. & Park, S.H. (1993). The mechanosensitivity of spinal sensory neurons following intraspinal injections of quisqualic acid in the rat. *Neurosci Lett,* Vol.157, No.1, 115-119.

Yoon, Y.W.; Na, H.S. & Chung, J.M. (1996). Contributions of injured and intact afferents to neuropathic pain in an experimental rat model. *Pain,* Vol.64, No.1, 27-36.

Ziegler, E.A.; Magerl, W.; Meyer, R.A. & Treede, R.D. (1999). Secondary hyperalgesia to punctate mechanical stimuli. Central sensitization to A-fibre nociceptor input. *Brain,* Vol.122 (Pt 12), 2245-2257.

Zochodne, D.W. & Max, M.B. (2003). An old acquaintance: opioids in neuropathic pain. *Neurology,* Vol.60, No.6, 894-895.

12

Contribution of Inflammation to Chronic Pain Triggered by Nerve Injury

S. Echeverry, S.H. Lee, T. Lim and J. Zhang
The Alan Edwards Centre for Research on Pain, McGill University
Canada

1. Introduction

An injury to a peripheral nerve can be a slight stretch, a compression or a severe laceration. Such damage usually leads to an acute phase response characterized by nociceptive pain, inflammation and restriction of normal function. However, in about 7%-18% of the general population, pain persists, even after the injury healing, producing a state of chronic neuropathic pain. This type of hypersensitivity is debilitating and refractory to the majority of available analgesics. It adversely affects quality of life and bears a substantial cost to society. In the last two decades, compelling evidence strongly suggested that, in addition to changes in neuronal system, pathogenesis of neuropathic pain involves the interaction between the immune system and the nervous system. Inflammatory process alters local homeostasis and impairs neuronal function. In this chapter, we primarily focus on the evidence with experimental animal models obtained from our laboratory and from literature to highlight inflammatory reaction along the pain pathway (from damaged nerve to the spinal cord), and the critical role of this reaction in the development and maintenance of neuropathic pain. We also discuss the current progress and challenges of translating the inflammation related new targets into therapeutics.

2. Peripheral nerve

2.1 Infiltration of immune cells into injured peripheral nerves

Peripheral nerve injury triggers not only the activation of Schwann's cells and resident immune cells, but also the recruitment of circulating inflammatory cells. The two main cell types that enter the nerves after injury are neutrophils and macrophages. Neutrophils are the first immune cells migrating towards the injury site. Their numbers peak at 24 hours following peripheral nerve injury and decrease progressively after three days post-injury, but still remain significant for at least one week (Nadeau et al, 2011). Infiltrated neutrophils in injured nerves play an important role at the very early stages of neuropathic pain through the release of pro-inflammatory mediators, such as cytokines TNF-α, IL-1β and IL-6 and reactive oxygen species, which are involved in regulating neuronal excitability (Schafers et al., 2003). In addition, neutrophils have a significant impact on subsequent macrophage infiltration to the injured nerves by secreting chemokines/cytokines MIP-1α, MIP-1β and IL-1β (Scapini et al., 2000).

Macrophages from peripheral circulation enter the injured nerve starting about 3 days and persist for several months post-injury (Frisen et al., 1993). Infiltrated macrophages exhibit different functional phenotypes in which they promote both injury and repair. The first important characteristic of macrophages is to be able to secrete pro-inflammatory mediators including TNF-α, IL-1β, IL-6, MIP-1α, MIP-1β and MCP-1. These cytokine/chemokine expressing macrophages show high levels of MAC-1 and low levels of ED-1 antigens (personal unpublished data). Many of these immune molecules detected in damaged nerves at different time points post-injury are directly or indirectly involved in pain hypersensitivity. For instance, MCP-1 plays an important role in macrophage recruitment and the establishment of pain hypersensitivity. It has been observed that MCP-1 mRNA expression is markedly increased in the injured rat sciatic nerves in parallel with an increase of macrophage recruitment (Toews et al., 1998). However, the development of mechanical allodynia is totally abrogated in CCR2 (MCP-1 receptor) knockout mice while macrophage recruitment is attenuated (Abbadie et al., 2003). Furthermore, pro-inflammatory mediators including IL-1β, TNF-α, IL-6 and MIP-1α are directly implicated in pain hypersensitivity (Kiguchi et al., 2010; Sommer & Kress, 2004) through synergistic effects to amplify the inflammatory signals. It has been shown that direct injection of IL-1β and TNF-α into peripheral nerves causes potent mechanical and thermal hyperalgesia in rats (Zelenka et al., 2005) whereas the application of neutralizing antibodies for IL-1β or IL-1 receptor antagonist effectively attenuates tactile allodynia and thermal hyperalgesia in animal models of neuropathic pain (Kawasaki et al., 2008). The use of siRNA against CCR1 and/or CCR5 (MIP-1α receptor) also effectively prevents the induction of tactile allodynia and thermal hyperalgesia through down-regulation of IL-1β (Kiguchi et al,. 2010). Infiltrated macrophages also exhibit powerful phagocytic phenotypes. High level of ED1 antigen was found on the cell surface and membranes of cytoplasmic granules such as phagolysosomes, which indicates a close correlation with macrophage phagocytic activity (Damoiseaux et al., 1994). They engulf cellular debris such as injured Schwann cells and axotomised axons (Bruck, 1997) and promote repair process. However, whether and how these phagocytic macrophages contribute to the pain behaviour needs further investigation.

2.2 Depletion of neutrophils or monocytes/macrophages impairs neuropathic pain behavior associated with nerve injury

Systemic treatment of sciatic nerve injured mice with a monoclonal antibody against the Ly6G antigen specifically expressed by neutrophils demonstrated that depletion of neutrophils attenuates the development of neuropathic pain behaviour (Nadeau et al, 2011). Furthermore, using molecular and pharmacological approaches, partial or complete depletion of macrophages yield beneficial effects in alleviating nerve injury associated chronic pain. For instance, the depletion of circulating macrophages by liposome-encapsulated clodronate results in decreased macrophage recruitment to the injury site, alleviated thermal hyperalgesia and reduced degeneration of axons (Liu et al., 2000) as well as attenuates pain hypersensitivity in diabetic animals (Mert et al., 2009). In addition, Wallerian degeneration (WLD) in response to nerve injury is delayed in genetically deficient mice which delays macrophage recruitment (Araki et al., 2004). Hyperalgesia is also delayed in this type of mice (WLD mice) suggesting that macrophages contribute to the development of neuropathic pain following peripheral nerve injury (Myers et al., 1996).

3. Dorsal Root Ganglia (DRG)

The dorsal root ganglia (DRG) are nodules containing cell bodies of afferent sensory neurons, which lie just outside of the spinal cord, in the intraforaminal spaces of the vertebral column. The nociceptive neurons of the DRG are classified into two groups depending on nerve fiber type: myelinated Aδ-fibers which are fast conducting, or unmyelinated C-fibers which are slow conducting. Like most neurons, sensory neurons in DRG are supported by a cast of other cells. In the DRG these supportive cells are satellite glial cells (SGC), dendritic cells, macrophages, and endothelial cells.

SGCs encapsulate each neuronal cell body, and a basement lamina separates neighbouring engcapsulated neurons (Hanani, 2005). The SGCs in DRG perform many similar functions to the astrocytes of the CNS, as they perform many regulatory and immune functions. For example, SGCs regulate extracellular amounts of glutamate and aspartate (Duce & Keen, 1983). In addition, they supply the glutamate precursor glutamine (Kai-Kai & Howe, 1991), and are a reservoir of the nitric oxide precursor L-arginine (Aoki et al., 1991). In addition, like many other glia, SGCs communicate with each other using gap junctions Normal DRG are also home for a population of resident macrophages. Most of these resident macrophages contact the neuron-satellite cell complex, and there are a smaller number which reside perivascularly (Hanani, 2005). The DRG neurons are very well perfused, and the blood supply is much denser than in peripheral nerve or dorsal root. In fact, each DRG neuron soma is in close proximity to an extensive network of capillaries. The blood supply to the DRG is supplied by fenestrated capillaries which have no blood-nerve barrier, and the vessels allow large molecules to pass easily.

Sensory ganglia do not have dendrites and chemical synapses, and thus each neuron within the ganglia was thought to be an independent communication pathway. However, this turns out not to be the case, and in fact, neighboring DRG neurons have the ability to cross-excite one another. Thus after peripheral nerve injury, cross-excitation is one possible mechanism by which sensory signals can be altered in time, space, and modality to result in neuropathic pain (Devor & Wall, 1990). Inflammation, which increases the excitability of DRG neurons, enhances cross-excitation. For example this mechanism is further influenced by interactions with SGCs.

Following peripheral nerve injury or inflammation, SGCs in DRG activate, and undergo proliferation (Lu et al., 1991). This process is thought to be mediated through release of ATP from damaged neurons, which stimulate purinergic receptors on SCGs (Filippov et al., 2004). Activation of SGCs results in increased glial fibrillary acidic protein (GFAP) expression and release of pro-inflammatory cytokines, for example, TNFα and IL-1β (Ohara et al., 2009). These cytokines released by activated SGCs have excitatory actions on nociceptive neurons (Takeda et al., 2009). In spinal nerve ligation (SNL) injured rats, GFAP expression peaks at one day after nerve injury, and is still present 10 days after (Xie et al., 2009). Gap junctions in SGCs, are also increased after nerve injury (Jeon et al., 2009). These junctions seem to be involved with the generation and maintenance of neuropathic pain, as RNA interference targeting connexin 43, one of the major structural components of gap junctions in SGCs, prevents experimental neuropathic pain (Ohara et al., 2008). Gap junctions allow the redistribution of K^+ ions though SGCs. K^+ ion concentration regulation is another mechanism by which SCGs regulate the excitability of DRG neurons (Takeda et al., 2009).

Peripheral nerve injury or inflammation also recruits resident macrophages of the DRG and circulating macrophages (Hu & McLachlan, 2002). Monocyte chemoattractant protein (MCP)-1 becomes upregulated at the DRG in injured neurons following nerve injury, and this has been found to be a critical event in the recruitment of macrophages (Jeon et al., 2009). The number of macrophages in the DRG peaks at 3 to 7 days after the trigger, and increased macrophages persist for weeks (Xie et al., 2006). The increase in macrophages at the DRG can occur even without any phagocytic events (Milligan & Watkins, 2009). The activated macrophages contribute to the persistence of neuropathic pain, and respond to numerous molecules, such as neurotransmitters, growth factors, and cytokines (Schreiber et al., 2002; Xie et al., 2006).

DRG neurons increase excitability in response to a number of inflammatory compounds, and can do so in a manner that sometimes does not require changes in protein expression. For instance, perfusion of DRG *in vitro* with TNFα results in an increase of A- and C-fiber discharge, as well as increased calcitonin gene related peptide (CGRP) release from nociceptor terminals at the spinal cord (Oprée & Kress, 2000). TNFα can act on TNFR1, one of the receptor subtypes for TNFα which is expressed exclusively by neurons (Li et al., 2004). The electrophysiological effects of TNFα on DRG neurons include a profound enhancement of tetrodotoxin (TTX)-resistant Na^+ channels within a minute of application (Jin & Gereau, 2006), and an increase of vanilloid receptor 1 (TRPV1) function and expression (Hensellek et al., 2007). This increase in excitability of the DRG neurons by TNFα is thought to be mediated through p38 phosphorylation of TTX-resistant sodium channel subunits, and upregulation of TRPV1 protein expression (Jin & Gereau, 2006). Additionally other cytokines can also produce excitatory changes on DRG neurons, such as IL-1β and IL-6. DRG neurons can respond to IL-1β, sensitizing TRPV1 also (Obreja et al., 2002). Similarly, it seems IL-6 has effects on TRPV1 as well. IL-6 sensitizes the ion channel to heat, resulting in increased CGRP release from DRG neurons (Obreja et al., 2005).

Following injury to peripheral nerve, subsets of injured neurons will spontaneously ectopically discharge (Kim et al., 1993). This can result in a chronic sensitization of nociceptive neurons in both the PNS and CNS, resulting in pathological pain. While the exact mechanisms for the development of these changes are unknown, it is clear that inflammatory events at the DRG are critical (Miller et al., 2009). Such events at the DRG may include the cross-excitation of DRG neurons, activation of SGCs, recruitment and activation of macrophages, and the production of chemokines and cytokines.

4. Spinal cord

Central sensitization refers to the process through which a state of hyperexcitability is established in the central nervous system, leading to enhanced processing of nociceptive messages (Perl, 2007). Numerous mechanisms have been implicated in central sensitization, including alteration in glutamatergic neurotransmission/NMDA receptor-mediated hypersensitivity and loss of tonic inhibitory controls (disinhibition) (Basbaum et al., 2009). However, a remarkable series of findings in recent years has demonstrated a previously unrecognized role for inflammation in the initiation and maintenance of central sensitization. The involvement of non-neuronal cells, mainly astrocytes and microglia has been elucidated, to a degree that they appear now as reasonable future therapeutic targets.

4.1 Activation of spinal glial cells following peripheral nerve injury

Glia represent, by far, the most abundant cells in the nervous system, largely outnumbering neurons. Astrocytes and microglia have been shown to undergo structural and functional modifications in the spinal cord in models of chronic pain (Colburn et al., 1999; Inoue & Tsuda, 2009; Moss et al., 2007). The data supporting a crucial role for these glial cells in the pathophysiology of neuropathic pain is ample (Gosselin et al., 2010). The long-lasting changes occurring in glia include structural alterations, cell proliferation, loss of neurotransmitter and release of proinflammatory mediators among other cellular processes. Several models of chronic pain investigated so far result in such glial phenotypic changes, essentially in the spinal cord (the first synaptic relay of the nociceptive pathway). Additionally, the involvement of glia in chronic pain has been remarkably validated by the prevention and reversal of behavioral manifestations of pain following treatments with molecules bearing glia-inhibitory properties (Hua et al., 2005; Milligan et al., 2003; Raghavendra et al., 2003; Tsuda et al., 2003). This suggests that glial alteration could be a crucial mechanism accounting for the persistence of hypersensitivity. In addition to resident glial cells, blood-borne monocytes and macrophages have the ability to infiltrate the spinal cord, where they proliferate and differentiate into activated microglia (Zhang et al., 2007). Activation of different glial/immune cells occurs along a complex temporal pattern. The contribution of each cell population to the modulation of nociceptive processing in pathological conditions follows a well-organized sequence of reciprocal communication between neurons and glia and among glial cells themselves (Inoue & Tsuda, 2009; Vallejo et al,, 2010; Watkins & Maier, 2002).

The events triggering astrocytic and microglial activation as well as the signals resulting from this activation producing pain hypersensitivity are currently under intense investigation. An increasing number of studies have proposed some mechanisms that seem to be consistently involved. Among them, the extracellular activating events, especially in neuropathic pain arising from peripheral damage, are very likely originating from sensory neuronal terminals reaching the spinal cord. Of special interest it's been the discovery of the critical role of several chemokines released by damaged neurons such as fractalkine (Clark et al., 2009; Milligan et al., 2004; Verge et al., 2004) and monocyte chemoatractant protein (MCP-1). The MCP-1 has raised a special interest in neuron-glia communication as its spatial profile of expression in the spinal cord dorsal horn matches that of activated microglia (Beggs & Salter, 2007; Thacker et al., 2009; Zhang & De Koninck, 2006). Peripheral nerve injury not only induces up-regulation of MCP-1 and its receptor CCR2 (Abbadie et al., 2003; Zhang & De Koninck, 2006) but also activation of spinal microglia (Zhang et al., 2007). Microgliosis in the spinal cord was prevented by spinal injection of MCP-1 neutralizing antibody or in mice lacking CCR2 (Zhang et al., 2007). Furthermore blockade of MCP-1/CCR2 signaling successfully prevents the infiltration of blood-borne monocytes into the spinal cord (Zhang et al., 2007). Taken together, these data suggest that spinal MCP-1/CCR2 signaling is critical for spinal microglial activation and the development of neuropathic pain after peripheral nerve damage.

Once activated, it is generally believed that the actions of glia in the context of neuropathic pain rely on their abilities to undergo drastic cellular changes and release of immune molecules including cytokines, chemokines and growth factors (Wieseler-Frank et al., 2005). The role of pro-inflammatory cytokines IL-6, IL-1β and TNF-α has been extensively studied. Blockers of these cytokines have been shown to reduce neuroinflammatory responses (Gomez-Nicola et al., 2008; Kiguchi et al., 2010) reduce neuronal hyperexcitability (Milligan et al., 2001) and block pain in animal models of neuropathy (Cuellar et al., 2004).

4.2 Peripheral nerve injury alters blood spinal cord barrier integrity

The blood spinal cord barrier (BSCB) constitutes a physical/biochemical barrier between the central nervous system (CNS) and the systemic circulation, which serves to protect the microenvironment of the spinal cord. However, several studies (Beggs et al., 2010; Gordh et al., 2006) have reported an important increase in BCSB permeability after peripheral nerve injury. A recent observation from our laboratory revealed that peripheral nerve injury disrupted the integrity of the BSCB and inflammatory mediators are key regulators of BSCB function. MCP-1 released by damaged neurons is an endogenous trigger for the BSCB leakage. BSCB permeability can also be impaired by circulating IL-1β. In contrast, anti-inflammatory cytokines TGF-β1 and IL-10 were able to shut down the openings of the BSCB following nerve injury. The compromised BSCB allows penetration of both inflammatory molecules (e.g., cytokine IL-1β) and immune cells (monocytes/macrophages, lymphocytes) into the spinal cord, participating in the central inflammatory response, a critical process for the development of neuropathic pain (Echeverry et al., 2011). In addition, endothelial cells have the capacity to secrete immune mediators, for example, IL-6 (Vallejo et al., 2010) and bear a series of surface molecules, such as chemokines, to modulate the entrance of immune cells which are known to have an impact on pain hypersensitivity. For a summary of the described kinetics see Fig 1.

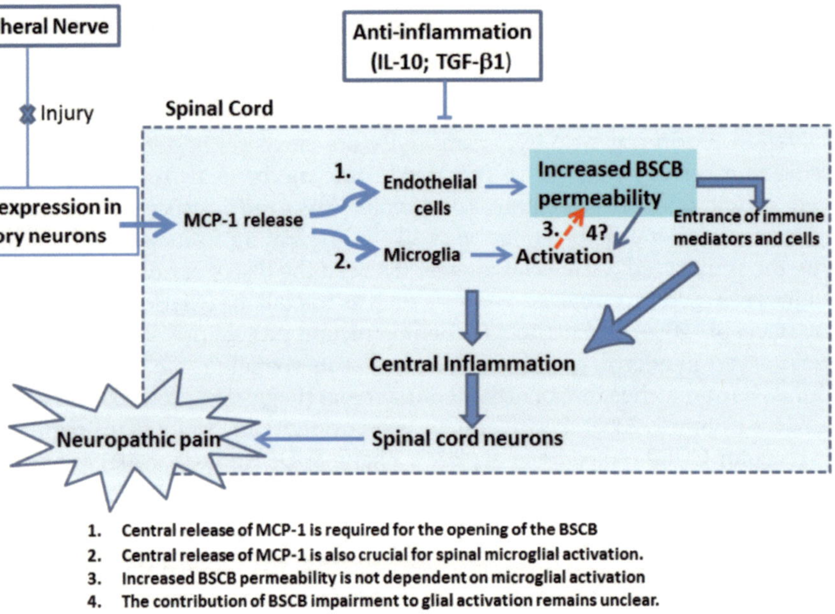

Fig. 1. Neuronal MCP-1 released into the spinal cord not only activated its receptor CCR2 in endothelial cells (1) to impair the integrity of the BSCB, but also activated CCR2 in microglia (2) to trigger microglial activation. Microglial activation is not required for the increase of BSCB permeability (3), although due to the lack of a selective BBB/BSCB blocker without affecting the inflammatory response, it is not clear whether the opening of BSCB can promote microglial activation (4). Central inflammation resulted from the opening of BSCB and microglial activation was necessary for the development of neuropathic pain, since anti-inflammatory cytokines IL-10 and TGF-β1, which were able to shut-down the nerve injury induced BSCB disruption and microglial activation, attenuated neuropathic pain

4.3 Inhibition of the spinal inflammatory reaction can alleviate neuropathic pain

In addition to the fact that following nerve injury, many non-neuronal cells are activated and engaged in an inflammatory reaction, functional investigations using pharmacological or genetic approaches support the roles of spinal inflammation in chronic pain, especially the facilitation of neuropathic pain. Activated microglia release pain enhancing substances such as pro-inflammatory cytokines, nitric oxide, and prostaglandins, that excite spinal pain responsive neurons either directly or indirectly, and promote the release of other transmitters that can act on nociceptive neurons. Drugs that target glial activation have successfully controlled enhanced nociceptive states in animal models either by: inhibiting the synthesis of cytokines, blocking pro-inflammatory cytokine receptors or neutralizing endogenous cytokines, or disrupting pro-inflammatory cytokine signaling pathway with inhibitors of the p38MAP kinase. Anti-inflammatory molecules have been used to validate the concept in different nerve injury models associated with chronic pain. IL-10, secreted by monocytes and TH2 cells, reverses neuropathic pain behavior in animal studies (Sloane et al., 2009; Soderquist et al., 2010). Enhancement of the TGF-β1 pathway through administration of exogenous recombinant ligand (Echeverry et al., 2009) or through transgenic approaches prevents and reverses neuropathic pain induced by peripheral nerve injury (Tramullas et al., 2010). The importance of inflammation in chronic pain is also highlighted by the correlation between the pro- and anti-inflammatory balance and the outcomes of pain states in humans: Patients presenting painful neuropathies or CRPS show elevated levels pro-inflammatory cytokines (Davies et al., 2007) while patients with painless neuropathies have elevated levels of anti-inflammatory cytokines (Uceyler et al., 2007).

5. Current advances and challenges in knowledge translation

In summary, following nerve injury, the communication between the immune and the nervous systems has been enhanced, which is observed not only at the sites of damage (peripheral nerve or DRGs), but also within the spinal cord. Such inflammatory reaction can be a critical underlying mechanism in generating neuropathic pain. The role of immune/glial cells in the development and the persistence of pain after nerve injury challenge conventional concepts that focus on neural activity being solely responsible for the changes that drive neuropathic pain. This shift in our understanding provides an incredible opportunity to progress to a new therapeutic approach that will be beneficial for the millions of people suffering of neuropathic pain. However, translation of such knowledge into clinical use for human has been largely underexplored. To date, very limited evidence is available for the roles of inflammation in persistent neuropathic pain states in human (McMahon & Malcangio, 2009). Only few clinical studies have tested immunosuppressive drugs or drugs interfering with glial functions for neuropathic pain (Scholz & Woolf, 2007). The effectiveness of some anti-inflammatory compounds, such as Anakinra (Kineret®) (recombinant human IL-1 receptor antagonist), Etanercept (Enbrel®) and Infliximab (Remicade®) (TNF inhibitors), was also limited to pain associated with rheumatoid arthritis and other inflammatory conditions. Considering the fact that current treatments for neuropathic pain offer only moderated pain relief with the severe side effects of sedation, tolerance and the risk of dependence, there are enormous needs to develop new therapeutics for which we think targeting one or multiple inflammatory pathways involved in the development of neuropathic pain can be a very exciting strategy. Large sizes, high quality randomized clinical trials with different anti-inflammatory molecules are needed to determine whether glial/immune cell mediated inflammation can be useful for the treatment of neuropathic pain.

6. References

Abbadie, C., Lindia, J., Cumiskey, A. M., Peterson, L. B., Mudgett, J. S., Bayne, E. K., DeMartino, J.A. (2003). Impaired neuropathic pain responses in mice lacking the chemokine receptor CCR2. *Proceedings of the National Academy of Sciences of the United States of America, 100*(13), 7947-52. doi:10.1073/pnas.1331358100

Aoki, E., Semba, R., & Kashiwamata, S. (1991). Evidence for the presence of L-arginine in the glial components of the peripheral nervous system. *Brain research, 559*(1), 159-62.

Araki, T., Sasaki, Y., & Milbrandt, J. (2004). Increased nuclear NAD biosynthesis and SIRT1 activation prevent axonal degeneration. *Science (New York, N.Y.), 305*(5686), 1010-3. doi:10.1126/science.1098014

Basbaum, A. I., Bautista, D. M., Scherrer, G., & Julius, D. (2009). Cellular and molecular mechanisms of pain. *Cell, 139*(2), 267-84. doi:10.1016/j.cell.2009.09.028

Beggs, S., & Salter, M. W. (2007). Stereological and somatotopic analysis of the spinal microglial response to peripheral nerve injury. *Brain, behavior, and immunity, 21*(5), 624-33. doi:10.1016/j.bbi.2006.10.017

Beggs, S., Liu, X. J., Kwan, C., & Salter, M. W. (2010). Peripheral nerve injury and TRPV1-expressing primary afferent C-fibers cause opening of the blood-brain barrier. *Molecular pain, 6*(1), 74. BioMed Central Ltd. doi:10.1186/1744-8069-6-74

Clark, A. K., Yip, P. K., & Malcangio, M. (2009). The liberation of fractalkine in the dorsal horn requires microglial cathepsin S. *The Journal of Neuroscience, 29*(21), 6945-54. doi:10.1523/JNEUROSCI.0828-09.2009

Colburn, R. W., Rickman, A. J., & DeLeo, J. A. (1999). The effect of site and type of nerve injury on spinal glial activation and neuropathic pain behavior. *Experimental neurology, 157*(2), 289-304. doi:10.1006/exnr.1999.7065

Cuellar, J. M., Montesano, P. X., & Carstens, E. (2004). Role of TNF-alpha in sensitization of nociceptive dorsal horn neurons induced by application of nucleus pulposus to L5 dorsal root ganglion in rats. *Pain, 110*(3), 578-87. doi:10.1016/j.pain.2004.03.029

Damoiseaux, J. G., Döpp, E. A., Calame, W., Chao, D., MacPherson, G. G., & Dijkstra, C. D. (1994). Rat macrophage lysosomal membrane antigen recognized by monoclonal antibody ED1. *Immunology, 83*(1), 140-7.

Davies, A. L., Hayes, K. C., & Dekaban, G. A. (2007). Clinical correlates of elevated serum concentrations of cytokines and autoantibodies in patients with spinal cord injury. *Archives of physical medicine and rehabilitation, 88*(11), 1384-93.

Devor, M., & Wall, P. D. (1990). Cross-excitation in dorsal root ganglia of nerve-injured and intact rats. *Journal of neurophysiology, 64*(6), 1733-46.

Duce, I. R., & Keen, P. (1983). Selective uptake of [3H]glutamine and [3H]glutamate into neurons and satellite cells of dorsal root ganglia in vitro. *Neuroscience, 8*(4), 861-6. Retrieved from http://www.ncbi.nlm.nih.gov/pubmed/6866267

Echeverry, S., Shi, X. Q., Rivest, S., & Zhang, J. (2011). Peripheral Nerve Injury Alters Blood-Spinal Cord Barrier Functional and Molecular Integrity through a Selective Inflammatory Pathway. *Journal of Neuroscience, 31*(30), 10819-10828. doi:10.1523/JNEUROSCI.1642-11.2011

Echeverry, S., Shi, X. Q., Haw, A., Liu, H., Zhang, Z.-wei, & Zhang, J. (2009). Transforming growth factor-beta1 impairs neuropathic pain through pleiotropic effects. *Molecular pain, 5*, 16. doi:10.1186/1744-8069-5-16

Filippov, A. K., Fernández-Fernández, J. M., Marsh, S. J., Simon, J., Barnard, E. A, & Brown, D. A. (2004). Activation and inhibition of neuronal G protein-gated inwardly rectifying K(+) channels by P2Y nucleotide receptors. *Molecular pharmacology, 66*(3), 468-77. doi:10.1124/mol.66.3.

Frisén, J., Risling, M., & Fried, K. (1993). Distribution and axonal relations of macrophages in a neuroma. *Neuroscience, 55*(4), 1003-13.

Gordh, T., Chu, H., & Sharma, H. S. (2006). Spinal nerve lesion alters blood-spinal cord barrier function and activates astrocytes in the rat. *Pain, 124*(1-2), 211-21. doi:10.1016/j.pain.2006.05.020

Gosselin, R.-D., Suter, M. R., Ji, R.-R., & Decosterd, I. (2010). Glial cells and chronic pain. *The Neuroscientist, 16*(5), 519-31. doi:10.1177/1073858409360822

Gómez-Nicola, D., Valle-Argos, B., Suardíaz, M., Taylor, J. S., & Nieto-Sampedro, M. (2008). Role of IL-15 in spinal cord and sciatic nerve after chronic constriction injury: regulation of macrophage and T-cell infiltration. *Journal of neurochemistry, 107*(6), 1741-52. doi:10.1111/j.1471-4159.2008.05746.x

Hanani, M. (2005). Satellite glial cells in sensory ganglia: from form to function. *Brain research. Brain research reviews, 48*(3), 457-76. doi:10.1016/j.brainresrev.2004.09.001

Hensellek, S., Brell, P., Schaible, H.-G., Bräuer, R., & Segond von Banchet, G. (2007). The cytokine TNFalpha increases the proportion of DRG neurones expressing the TRPV1 receptor via the TNFR1 receptor and ERK activation. *Molecular and cellular neurosciences, 36*(3), 381-91. doi:10.1016/j.mcn.2007.07.010

Hu, P., & McLachlan, E. M. (2002). Macrophage and lymphocyte invasion of dorsal root ganglia after peripheral nerve lesions in the rat. *Neuroscience, 112*(1), 23-38. Retrieved from http://www.ncbi.nlm.nih.gov/pubmed/12044469

Hua, X.-Y., Svensson, C. I., Matsui, T., Fitzsimmons, B., Yaksh, T. L., & Webb, M. (2005). Intrathecal minocycline attenuates peripheral inflammation-induced hyperalgesia by inhibiting p38 MAPK in spinal microglia. *The European Journal of Neuroscience, 22*(10), 2431-40. doi:10.1111/j.1460-9568.2005.04451.x

Inoue, K., & Tsuda, M. (2009). Microglia and neuropathic pain. *Glia, 57*(14), 1469-79. doi:10.1002/glia.20871

Jeon, S.-M., Lee, K.-M., & Cho, H.-J. (2009). Expression of monocyte chemoattractant protein-1 in rat dorsal root ganglia and spinal cord in experimental models of neuropathic pain. *Brain research, 1251*(Cci), 103-11. Elsevier B.V. doi: 10.1016/j.brainres.2008.11.046

Jin, X., & Gereau, R. W. (2006). Acute p38-mediated modulation of tetrodotoxin-resistant sodium channels in mouse sensory neurons by tumor necrosis factor-alpha. *The Journal of Neuroscience, 26*(1), 246-55. doi:10.1523/JNEUROSCI.3858-05.2006

Kai-Kai, M. A., & Howe, R. (1991). Glutamate-immunoreactivity in the trigeminal and dorsal root ganglia, and intraspinal neurons and fibres in the dorsal horn of the rat. *The Histochemical Journal, 23*(4), 171-179. doi:10.1007/BF01046588

Kawasaki, Y., Zhang, L., Cheng, J.-K., & Ji, R.-R. (2008). Cytokine mechanisms of central sensitization: distinct and overlapping role of interleukin-1beta, interleukin-6, and tumor necrosis factor-alpha in regulating synaptic and neuronal activity in the superficial spinal cord. *The Journal of Neuroscience, 28*(20), 5189-94. doi:10.1523/JNEUROSCI.3338-07.2008

Kiguchi, N., Maeda, T., Kobayashi, Y., Fukazawa, Y., & Kishioka, S. (2010). Macrophage inflammatory protein-1 a mediates the development of neuropathic pain following peripheral nerve injury through. *Pain, 149*(2), 305-315. doi: 10.1016/j.pain.2010.02.025

Kim, S. H., Na, H. S., Sheen, K., & Chung, J. M. (1993). Effects of sympathectomy on a rat model of peripheral neuropathy. *Pain, 55*(1), 85-92.

Li, Y., Ji, A., Weihe, E., & Schäfer, M. K.-H. (2004). Cell-specific expression and lipopolysaccharide-induced regulation of tumor necrosis factor alpha (TNFalpha) and TNF receptors in rat dorsal root ganglion. *The Journal of Neuroscience, 24*(43), 9623-31. doi:10.1523/JNEUROSCI.2392-04.2004

Liu, T., van Rooijen, N., & Tracey, D. J. (2000). Depletion of macrophages reduces axonal degeneration and hyperalgesia following nerve injury. *Pain, 86*(1-2), 25-32. Retrieved from http://www.ncbi.nlm.nih.gov/pubmed/10779657

Lu, X., & Richardson, P. M. (1991). Inflammation near the Nerve Cell Body enhances Axonal regeneration. *The Journal of Neuroscience*, 11(4):972-978.

McMahon, S. B., & Malcangio, M. (2009). Current challenges in glia-pain biology. *Neuron, 64*(1), 46-54. Elsevier Inc. doi:10.1016/j.neuron.2009.09.033

Mert, T., Gunay, I., Ocal, I., Guzel, a I., Inal, T. C., Sencar, L., & Polat, S. (2009). Macrophage depletion delays progression of neuropathic pain in diabetic animals. *Naunyn-Schmiedeberg's archives of pharmacology, 379*(5), 445-52. doi:10.1007/s00210-008-0387-3

Miller, R. J., Jung, H., Bhangoo, S. K., & White, F. A. (2009). Cytokine and Chemokine Regulation of Sensory Neuron Function. *Sensory Neuron*, 417-449. doi:10.1007/978

Milligan, E D, O'Connor, K a, Armstrong, C. B., Hansen, M. K., Martin, D, Tracey, K. J., Maier, S F, et al. (2001). Systemic administration of CNI-1493, a p38 mitogen-activated protein kinase inhibitor, blocks intrathecal human immunodeficiency virus-1 gp120-induced enhanced pain states in rats. *The journal of Pain, 2*(6), 326-33. Retrieved from http://www.ncbi.nlm.nih.gov/pubmed/14622812

Milligan, E D, Zapata, V., Chacur, M., Schoeniger, D., Biedenkapp A., J, O'Connor, K .A., Verge, G M. (2004). Evidence that exogenous and endogenous fractalkine can induce spinal nociceptive facilitation in rats. *The European journal of neuroscience, 20*(9), 2294-302. doi:10.1111/j.1460-9568.2004.03709.x

Milligan, E. D., & Watkins, L.R. (2009). Pathological and protective roles of glia in chronic pain. *Nature reviews. Neuroscience, 10*(1), 23-36. doi:10.1038/nrn2533

Milligan, E. D., Twining, C., Chacur, Marucia C., Biedenkapp A., Joseph, O'Connor, Kevin, Poole, S., Tracey, K., et al. (2003). Spinal glia and proinflammatory cytokines mediate mirror-image neuropathic pain in rats. *The Journal of Neuroscience, 23*(3), 1026-40. Retrieved from http://www.ncbi.nlm.nih.gov/pubmed/12574433

Moss, A., Beggs, S., Vega-Avelaira, D., Costigan, M., Hathway, G. J., Salter, M. W., & Fitzgerald, M. (2007). Spinal microglia and neuropathic pain in young rats. *Pain, 128*(3), 215-24. doi:10.1016/j.pain.2006.09.018

Myers, R. R., Heckman, H. M., & Rodriguez, M. (1996). Reduced hyperalgesia in nerve-injured WLD mice: relationship to nerve fiber phagocytosis, axonal degeneration, and regeneration in normal mice. *Experimental neurology, 141*(1), 94-101. doi:10.1006/exnr.1996.0142

Obreja, O, Biasio, W., Andratsch, M., Lips, K. S., Rathee, P K, Ludwig, A., Rose-John, S. (2005). Fast modulation of heat-activated ionic current by proinflammatory interleukin 6 in rat sensory neurons. *Brain: a journal of neurology, 128*(Pt 7), 1634-41. doi:10.1093/brain/awh490

Obreja O., Rathee P. K., Lips, K. S., Distler, C., & Kress, M. (2002). IL-1 beta potentiates heat-activated currents in rat sensory neurons: involvement of IL-1RI, tyrosine kinase, and protein kinase C. *The FASEB journal, 16*(12), 1497-503. doi:10.1096/fj.02-0101com

Ohara, P. T., Vit, J.-P., Bhargava, A., & Jasmin, L. (2008). Evidence for a role of connexin 43 in trigeminal pain using RNA interference in vivo. *Journal of neurophysiology, 100*(6), 3064-73. doi:10.1152/jn.90722.2008

Ohara, P. T., Vit, J.-P., Bhargava, A., Romero, M., Sundberg, C., Charles, A. C., & Jasmin, L. (2009). Gliopathic pain: when satellite glial cells go bad. *The Neuroscientist, 15*(5), 450-63. doi:10.1177/1073858409336094

Oprée, A., & Kress, M. (2000). Involvement of the proinflammatory cytokines tumor necrosis factor-alpha, IL-1 beta, and IL-6 but not IL-8 in the development of heat hyperalgesia: effects on heat-evoked calcitonin gene-related peptide release from rat skin. *The Journal of Neuroscience, 20*(16), 6289-93. Retrieved from http://www.ncbi.nlm.nih.gov/pubmed/10934280

Perl, E. R. (2007). Ideas about pain, a historical view. *Nature reviews. Neuroscience, 8*(1), 71-80. doi:10.1038/nrn2042

Raghavendra, V., Tanga, F., & Deleo, J. A. (2003). Inhibition of Microglial Activation Attenuates the Development but Not Existing Hypersensitivity in a Rat Model of Neuropathy. *Journal of Experimental Pharmacology, 306*(2), 624-630. doi:10.1124/jpet.103.052407.2003

Nadeau, S., Filali, M., Zhang, J., Bradley, K., Rivest, S., Soulet, D., Iwakura, Y., de Rivero Vaccari, J.P., Keane, R.W., & Lacroix, S. (2011). Functional Recovery after Peripheral Nerve Injury is Dependent on the Pro-Inflammatory Cytokines IL-1a and TNF-a: Implications for Neuropathic Pain. *The Journal of Neuroscience, In press.*

Scapini, P., Lapinet-Vera, J. A., Gasperini, S., Calzetti, F., Bazzoni, F., & Cassatella, M. A. (2000). The neutrophil as a cellular source of chemokines. *Immunological reviews, 177*(4), 195-203. Retrieved from http://www.ncbi.nlm.nih.gov/pubmed/11138776

Scholz, J., & Woolf, C. J. (2007). The neuropathic pain triad: neurons, immune cells and glia. *Nature neuroscience, 10*(11), 1361-8. doi:10.1038/nn1992

Schreiber, R. C., Vaccariello, S. A., Boeshore, K., Shadiack, A. M., & Zigmond, R. E. (2002). A comparison of the changes in the non neuronal cell populations of the superior cervical ganglia following decentralization and axotomy. *Journal of neurobiology, 53*(1), 68-79. doi:10.1002/neu.10093

Sloane, E. M., Soderquist, R. G., Maier, S. F., Mahoney, M. J., Watkins, L. R., & Milligan, E. D. (2009). Long-term control of neuropathic pain in a non-viral gene therapy paradigm. *Gene therapy, 16*(4), 470-5. doi:10.1038/gt.2009.21

Soderquist, R.G., Sloane, E.M., Loram, L.C., Harrison, J A., Dengler, E.C., Johnson, S. M., Amer, L.D., Young, C.S., Makenzie, T.L., Poole, S., Frank, M.G., Watkins, L.R., Milligan, E.D., & Mahoney, M.J. (2010). Release of plasmid DNA-encoding IL-10 from PLGA microparticles facilitates long-term reversal of neuropathic pain following a single intrathecal administration. *Pharmaceutical research, 27*(5), 841-54. doi:10.1007/s11095-010-0077-y

Sommer, C., & Kress, M (2004). Recent findings on how proinflammatory cytokines cause pain: peripheral mechanisms in inflammatory and neuropathic hyperalgesia. *Neuroscience letters, 361*(1-3), 184-7. doi:10.1016/j.neulet.2003.12.007

Takeda, M., Takahashi, M., & Matsumoto, S. (2009). Contribution of the activation of satellite glia in sensory ganglia to pathological pain. *Neuroscience and biobehavioral reviews, 33*(6), 784-92. doi:10.1016/j.neubiorev.2008.12.005

Thacker, M. A., Clark, A. K., Bishop, T., Grist, J., Yip, P. K., Moon, L. F., Thompson, S. N., Marchand, F., McMahon, S.B. (2009). CCL2 is a key mediator of microglia activation in neuropathic pain states. *European journal of pain, 13*(3), 263-72. doi:10.1016/j.ejpain.2008.04.017

Tramullas, M., Lantero, A., Díaz, A., Morchón, N., Merino, D., Villar, A., Buscher, D., et al. (2010). BAMBI (bone morphogenetic protein and activin membrane-bound inhibitor) reveals the involvement of the transforming growth factor-beta family in pain modulation. *The Journal of neuroscience, 30*(4), 1502-11. doi: 10.1523/JNEUROSCI.2584-09.2010

Tsuda, M., Shigemoto-Mogami, Y., & Koizumi, S. (2003). P2X 4 receptors induced in spinal microglia gate tactile allodynia after nerve injury. *Nature, 424*(August), 1-6. doi:10.1038/nature01859.1.

Uçeyler, N., Eberle, T., Rolke, R., Birklein, F., & Sommer, C. (2007a). Differential expression patterns of cytokines in complex regional pain syndrome. *Pain, 132*(1-2), 195-205. doi:10.1016/j.pain.2007.07.031

Uçeyler, N., Tscharke, A., & Sommer, C. (2007b). Early cytokine expression in mouse sciatic nerve after chronic constriction nerve injury depends on calpain. *Brain, behavior, and immunity, 21*(5), 553-60. doi:10.1016/j.bbi.2006.10.003

Vallejo, R., Tilley, D. M., Vogel, L., & Benyamin, R. (2010). The role of glia and the immune system in the development and maintenance of neuropathic pain. *Pain practice, 10*(3), 167-84. doi:10.1111/j.1533-2500.2010.00367.x

Verge, G.M., Milligan, E.D., Maier, S.F., Watkins, L.R., Naeve, G. S., & Foster, A. C. (2004). Fractalkine (CX3CL1) and fractalkine receptor (CX3CR1) distribution in spinal cord and dorsal root ganglia under basal and neuropathic pain conditions. *The European journal of neuroscience, 20*(5), 1150-60. doi:10.1111/j.1460-9568.2004.03593.x

Bruck, W. (1997). The role of macrophages in Wallerian degeneration. *Brain Pathology, 7*(2), 741-52.

Watkins, L.R., & Maier, S.F. (2002). Beyond neurons: evidence that immune and glial cells contribute to pathological pain states. *Physiological reviews, 82*(4), 981-1011. doi:10.1152/physrev.00011.2002

Wieseler-Frank, J., Maier, S.F., & Watkins, L.R. (2005). Immune-to-brain communication dynamically modulates pain: physiological and pathological consequences. *Brain, behavior, and immunity, 19*(2), 104-11. doi:10.1016/j.bbi.2004.08.004

Xie, W., Strong, J. A., & Zhang, J. M. (2009). Early blockade of injured primary sensory afferents reduces glial cell activation in two rat neuropathic pain models. *Neuroscience, 160*(4), 847-57. IBRO. doi:10.1016/j.neuroscience.2009.03.016

Xie, W.-R., Deng, H., Li, H., Bowen, T. L., Strong, J. A., & Zhang, J.-M. (2006). Robust increase of cutaneous sensitivity, cytokine production and sympathetic sprouting in rats with localized inflammatory irritation of the spinal ganglia. *Neuroscience, 142*(3), 809-22. doi:10.1016/j.neuroscience.2006.06.045

Zelenka, M., Schäfers, M., & Sommer, C. (2005). Intraneural injection of interleukin-1beta and tumor necrosis factor-alpha into rat sciatic nerve at physiological doses induces signs of neuropathic pain. *Pain, 116*(3), 257-63. doi:10.1016/j.pain.2005.04.018

Zhang, J., & De Koninck, Y. (2006). Spatial and temporal relationship between monocyte chemoattractant protein-1 expression and spinal glial activation following peripheral nerve injury. *Journal of Neurochemistry, 97*(3), 772-83. doi:10.1111/j.1471-4159.2006.03746.x

Zhang, J., Shi, X.Q., Echeverry, S., Mogil, J. S., De Koninck, Y., & Rivest, S. (2007). Expression of CCR2 in both resident and bone marrow-derived microglia plays a critical role in neuropathic pain. *The Journal of Neuroscience, 27*(45), 12396-406. doi: 10.1523/JNEUROSCI.3016-07.2007

13

Neuropathy Secondary to Chemotherapy: A Real Issue for Cancer Survivors

Esther Uña Cidón
Oncology Department, Clinical University Hospital and Faculty of Medicine of Valladolid Spain

1. Introduction

Cancer is still a major public health problem worldwide, being one of the leading causes of population mortality. In 2000, malignant tumours were responsible for 12 percent of the nearly 56 million deaths worldwide from all causes. In many countries, more than a quarter of deaths were attributable to cancer (Parkin et al., 2005). According to the World Cancer Report, which is the most comprehensive global examination of the disease to date, cancer rates are expected to further increase by 50% to 15 million new cases by 2020. Absolute deaths from cancer worldwide are projected to continue to rise to over 11 million by 2030 (Parkin et al., 2005). However, due to advances in multimodal treatment, screening and therefore early detection, as well as chemoprevention, the number of cancer survivors are also expected to increase in the near future (Parkin et al., 2005). This fact highlights the relevance of fostering and maintaining survivors´ quality of life (QOL).

Most patients diagnosed with cancer will receive chemotherapy over the course of the disease with a neoadjuvant, adjuvant, or palliative. Several major classes of chemotherapeutic agents can be grouped by their underlying mechanism of action (Hausheer et al., 2006). All these drugs can also have different profiles of toxicity according to their mechanism, some very serious. One of the most common and distressing adverse event is peripheral neuropathy whose incidence is now growing. In fact many chemotherapeutic agents belonging to different groups associate a dose-limiting chemotherapy-induced peripheral neuropathy (CIPN). The different properties of these agents are contributing to the pathogenesis of this toxicity, leading to variation in incidence, severity, kind of damage, etc. depending on the agent considered (Hausheer et al., 2006).

CIPN involves sensory and motor nerve damage or dysfunction with a prolonged course, which causes permanent damage in some long-term cancer survivors with the subsequent impairment in their QOL (Hausheer et al., 2006). CIPN affects not only QOL, since toxicity may have an impact on the planned therapy, and such alterations could have negative consequences for the outcome, especially if the patient´s malignancy is responding to treatment (Hausheer et al., 2006). Despite the increasing awareness of this potential toxicity and the improved knowledge of the pathogenic mechanisms, emerging evidence suggests that the incidence of CIPN is substantially under-reported in clinical trials, due mainly to relevant limitations in the available grading scales that are commonly used for assessment (Cavaletti & Marmiroli, 2010).

Agent	Mechanism of anticancer action	Most frequent clinical uses
Cisplatin	Alkylating, crosslink to DNA	Lung cancer, Bladder cancer, Ovarian cancer, Testicular cancer, Gastric cancer, Head and neck cancer, Cervical cancer, Malignant mesothelioma
Carboplatin	Alkylating, crosslink to DNA	Ovarian cancer, Lung cancer
Oxaliplatin	Alkylating, crosslink to DNA	Colorectal cancer
Paclitaxel	Hyperpolymerisation of microtubules	Ovarian cancer, Breast cancer, Kaposi sarcoma, Lung cancer (non-small-cell), Head and neck cancer, Gastric cancer
Docetaxel	Hyperpolymerisation of microtubules	Breast cancer, Gastric cancer, Prostate cancer, Head and neck cancer, Lung cancer (non-small-cell)
Ixabepilone	Hyperpolymerisation of microtubules	Breast cancer
Vincristine	Depolymerisation of microtubules	Acute leukaemia, Hodgkin lymphoma, Non-Hodgkin lymphoma, Rhabdomyo-sarcoma, Neuroblastoma, Wilms tumour
Vinorelbine	Depolymerisation of microtubules	Lung cancer (non-small-cell), Ovarian cancer, Breast cancer, Prostate cancer
Bortezomib	Proteasome inhibition	Multiple myeloma, Mantle cell lymphoma
Thalidomide	Antiangiogenic Immune-modulator	Multiple myeloma

Table 1. Mechanisms of anticancer action and most frequent clinical uses of neurotoxic agents (Cavaletti, G. & Marmiroli, 2006).

The challenges in diagnosing and assessing the extent of functional impairment in a reliable and reproducible manner is a paramount consideration for the clinician to make a clinical decision as well as in clinical trials involving the prospective evaluation of neurotoxic chemotherapy or interventions aimed at the prevention or mitigation of CIPN (Gándara et al., 1991). The drugs most commonly associated with CIPN are platinum analogues, antitubulins, the proteasome inhibitor bortezomib, and thalidomide, which are very commonly used in a wide range of solid and haematological malignancies (Windebank &

Grisold, 2008). In addition, most cases will receive a combination of several chemotherapeutic compounds aiming to enhance the effectiveness of such treatment but with the disadvantage of inducing CIPN more often than individual agents (Cavaletti & Marmiroli, 2010).

The clinical manifestations of CIPN are subjective and predominantly manifest as pure sensory symptoms, most frequently reported as progressive distal symmetrically distributed. The most important symptoms are numbness, tingling, "pins and needles", burning sensations, decreased or altered sensation, or increased sensitivity that may sometimes be painful in the feet and hands (Hilkens & Van den Bent, 1997; Lipton et al., 1989). The primary clinical goal in assessing these patients is to determine the presence of these complications after making a correct differential diagnosis and also to evaluate their severity because sometimes they can interfere with activities of daily living (ADL). These assessments are critical for making decisions related to the continuity, dose-intensity, or dose-density of the anticancer treatment (Cavaletti & Marmiroli, 2010). Although the most important spectrum of CIPN symptoms is sensory in nature, motor weakness may also be reported and when present is observed in patients with more persistent and severe sensory symptoms (American Society of Health-System Pharmacists, 2002). In fact, isolated motor weakness with the complete absence of sensory involvement has not been described, but if observed in a patient, consideration should be given to other conditions that may produce pure motor weakness, including steroid myopathy which is proximal, diabetic, or paraneoplastic motor neuropathy (Hausheer et al., 2006). The onset of CIPN is usually gradually progressive, although in some patients it can appear immediately after the administration of a neurotoxic drug or even during the infusion. This condition may thus pose difficulties for the clinician, especially to diagnose those patients with coexisting problems or disorders that involve the peripheral nervous system (Hausheer et al., 2006). No standard treatment currently exists for the prevention, mitigation, or management of CIPN (Hausheer et al., 2006).

This chapter will focus on all these aspects of CIPN including the clinical manifestation, diagnosis, management, mechanisms underlying its onset, assessment, and current status of neuroprotection. The different agents used in anticancer treatments that might be related to toxicity will also be reviewed.

	Sensory	Sensory and motor
Platinum agents	X	
Bortezomib	X	
Thalidomide	X	
Taxanes		X
Epothilones		X
Vinca alkaloids		X

Table 2. Classification of the most important agents reported in CIPN (Hilkens & Van den Bent, 1997; Lipton et al., 1989).

2. Pathogenic mechanisms and clinical features of CIPN

The underlying pathogenic mechanisms for the development of CIPN have not been fully elucidated. In fact, a variety of mechanisms have been proposed. Different chemotherapeutic agents cause highly similar patterns and spectra of clinical manifestations, which include the length-dependent, symmetrical stocking-glove distribution with predominantly sensory symptoms subjectively reported by the patient (Gregg et al., 1992; McKeage et al., 2001; Verdu et al., 1989). The next sections will review the pathogenic mechanisms clinical features associated with every group of drugs or isolated agents previously mentioned in this chapter.

3. Platinum analogues

The profiles of general toxicity and neurotoxicity differ among the three platinum drugs (Cavaletti & Marmiroli, 2010; Hausheer et al., 2006; McWhinney et al., 2009). Although platinum-based chemotherapies (mainly cisplatin and carboplatin) are a mainstay for the treatment of most solid tumours, their clinical use is severely curtailed by dose-limiting nephro-, oto-, and neurotoxicities (Cavaletti & Marmiroli, 2010; Hausheer et al., 2006; McWhinney et al., 2009). Neurotoxicity induced by platinum agents is characterised by a dose-dependent, cumulative, predominantly painful sensory neuropathy, presenting with symptoms in the distal extremities. These agents are most frequently associated with the development of axonopathy, but platinum-induced neuronopathy may also be observed, especially with higher doses of platinum (McWhinney et al., 2009). Due to the absence of therapies that either cure or prevent platinum-induced CIPN, especially with the advent of newer members of this class of anticancer agents, we need a better understanding of the underlying pathophysiology to develop more-effective therapies or even preventive measures.

Cisplatin, carboplatin, and oxaliplatin differ in solubility, chemical reactivity, oxygenated leaving groups, pharmacokinetics, and toxicology (McKeage, 1995). The leaving groups on each molecule are responsible for the differences in each drug's reactivity with nucleophiles, which is likely to contribute to their differences in toxic profiles (Hah et al., 2006; McWhinney et al., 2009). Despite of these differences, the primary mechanisms involved in their neurotoxicity are likely to be similar.

These agents can enter the DG and peripheral nerves, as opposed to the brain, mainly through passive diffusion, although current data indicates the presence of metal transporters that may also be involved in their entrance into the cell (Krarup-Hansen et al., 1999; Thompson et al., 1984). Current research indicates that after entering the DG cell, these agents will form an adduct with DNA (Cavaletti & Marmiroli et al., 2010). In fact, platinum agents undergo aquation to form a positively charged molecule that interacts with DNA to form crosslinks and finally DNA/platinum adducts (Cavaletti & Marmiroli et al., 2010). These DNA intrastrand adducts and interstrand crosslinks will alter the tertiary structure of DNA leading on the one hand to alterations in cell-cycle kinetics with postmitotic DG neurons trying to reenter the cell cycle and on the other hand to the promotion of apoptosis (Gill & Windebank, 1998).

The level of these compounds in DG neurons at a given cumulative dose has been significantly correlated with the degree of neurotoxicity (Cavaletti et al., 1992; Dzagnidze et al., 2007; Gregg et al., 1992; Meijer et al., 1999). The severity of neurotoxicity, however, involves other factors (Cavaletti et al., 1992; Dzagnidze et al., 2007; Gregg et al., 1992; Meijer et al., 1999; Verdu et al., 1999). The level of hydrolysis of cisplatin and oxaliplatin differs from that of carboplatin, which is higher. This finding may contribute to the difference in the associated neurotoxic severity patterns (McWhinney et al., 2009). In this way, patients from clinical trials treated with these agents have shown that the severity of neurotoxicity is more commonly seen with cisplatin than with oxaliplatin and is much more severe than that observed with carboplatin (McWhinney et al., 2009).

In the case of cisplatin, the differences in the degree of neurotoxicity could also be associated with the different plasma levels of the intermediary products of the aquation to the process of DNA adduct formation (McWhinney et al., 2009). Although these drugs cause the main cellular damage by the formation of these DNA adducts, additional complexes of covalently crosslinked platinum-DNA-protein have been proposed as another mechanism more specifically studied with cisplatin (Chvalova et al., 2007). These complexes lead to disruption of nuclear metabolism and spatial organisation of chromatin, and even inhibit DNA replication and repair (McWhinney et al., 2009). Another suggested underlying mechanism is the involvement of oxidative stress and mitochondrial dysfunction as a trigger of neuronal apoptosis. This process might be mediated by an increased activity of tumour protein p53 and mitochondrial release of cytochrome C (Cavaletti & Marmiroli, 2010).

Even though the exact mechanism of neuronal apoptosis is not fully understood, one proposal has suggested that the machinery of DNA repair is unable to repair the damaged DNA (Gill & Windebank, 1998). Polymorphisms in the DNA-repair genes, including genes for base-excision repair, nucleotide-excision repair, mismatch repair, and double-strand break repair pathways, cause the individuals to be less proficient in repairing carcinogen-induced damage (Cavaletti & Marmiroli, 2010). Moreover, platinum-DNA complexes (Zhu et al., 2005) interfere with the normal function of cellular proteins (i.e. binding or interactions with other proteins), and apoptosis has been observed in DG neurons following treatment with cisplatin, both *in vitro* and *in vivo*, and is correlated with increased platinum-DNA binding in these DG neurons (Cavaletti & Marmiroli, 2010). Finally, all these platinum compounds appear to affect the axons, myelin sheath, neuronal cell body, and the glial structures of the neurons. In support, levels of platinum are significantly higher in the DG than in the brain and spinal cord, which are protected by the blood-brain barrier (Hausheer et al., 2006).

Oxaliplatin and cisplatin differ in their severity of neurotoxicity to the DG, with cisplatin being more neurotoxic. In fact, cisplatin produces about three times more platinum- DNA adducts in the DG than do equimolar doses of oxaliplatin (McWhinney et al., 2009). Acute oxaliplatin neurotoxicity is thought to be caused by transient dysfunction of nodal, axonal, voltage-gated sodium channels, probably owing to an oxalate chelating effect on both calcium and magnesium ions that could interfere with the kinetics of sodium channels (McDonald et al., 2005; Ta et al., 2006). However, the small-conductance Ca(++)-activated K(+) channels, encoded by the SK1-3 genes, are also involved in membrane excitability, playing a role in after-hyperpolarisation at the motor nerve terminal. Because the SK3 gene is characterised in Caucasians by a highly polymorphic CAG motif within exon 1, SK3 gene polymorphism may influence the development of acute nerve hyperexcitability in oxaliplatin-treated patients. The results of the study by Basso et al. (2011) have suggested that oxaliplatin neurotoxicity may be related to distribution of the polymorphic CAG motif of the SK3 gene, which might modulate nerve after-hyperpolarisation. The allele with 13-14 CAG repeats could mark patients susceptible to acute oxaliplatin neurotoxicity.

The platinum drugs all share the 'coasting' phenomenon, which is an increase in the severity of symptoms for weeks, or even months, following the withdrawal of treatment (Cavaletti & Marmiroli, 2010).

Consequently, CIPN induced by platinum agents is a significant factor affecting the efficacy of the platinum drugs, as patients may experience either more negative side effects than benefits from this drug class or be forced to forego further therapy with an active agent.

3.1 Cisplatin

Cisplatin is a widely used chemotherapeutic agent with antitumour activity for a wide range of cancers. Along with its potent anticancer activity, though, cisplatin has also significant toxicities. Cisplatin-induced CIPN is the most common dose-limiting toxic effect. The reported incidence as a single agent ranges from 49-100% depending on the dose, schedule, treatment duration, and the drugs used previously. This toxicity is dose-related and generally appears after cumulative doses in excess of 300 mg/m^2 (Cavaletti & Marmiroli, 2010; Hausheer et al., 2006; McWhinney et al., 2009).

Cisplatin-induced CIPN is first characterised by painful paraesthesias and numbness in symmetrical stocking and glove distribution which typically occurs during the first few drug cycles and is thought to be produced by axonopathy. Sometimes this toxicity can be accompanied by progressively reduced or absent reflexes in the affected extremities. In several cases, loss of vibration sense, paraesthesia, and ataxia can be apparent after several cycles. Motor weakness and other central and autonomic symptoms such as Lhermitte´s sign, myelopathy, bilateral jaw pain, and urinary dysfunctions may also appear (Park et al., 2009).

In most patients, neurotoxicity occurs late along the course of treatment, but some patients report an earlier onset of symptoms after the administration of a single dose of cisplatin, especially with doses as high as 100 mg/m^2 or more. The mechanism proposed for this last toxicity is neuronopathy (Cavaletti & Marmiroli, 2010; Hausheer et al., 2006; McWhinney et al., 2009). In both cases, we must remember that all these symptoms can be progressive even after the end of treatment and in many cases are irreversible. Moreover, if cisplatin is used in combination with other drugs such as taxanes or vinca alkaloids, the appearance of neurotoxicity is more likely (Cavaletti & Marmiroli, 2010; Hausheer et al., 2006; McWhinney et al., 2009).

3.2 Carboplatin

Neurotoxicity secondary to carboplatin is less frequent (4–6%) (American Society of Health-System Pharmacists, n.d.) than that observed with cisplatin or the thirdgeneration platinum, oxaliplatin (15–60%), and is typically less severe (U.S. Food and Drug Administration, n.d.). Risk of CIPN induced by carboplatin increases in patients older than 65 years and in patients previously treated with cisplatin. Additionally, carboplatin does not cause the loss of hearing that is seen in the majority of patients treated with cisplatin (Chaney et al., 2005; Kartalou & Essigmann, 2001; Wang & Lippard, 2005). Carboplatin-induced CIPN is clinically indistinguishable from that induced by cisplatin, and although reported to be less severe, several studies suggest that the severity may be similar for both drugs.

3.3 Oxaliplatin

The more recently developed oxaliplatin has provided a more dramatic reduction of nephro- and ototoxicity than its counterparts (McWhinney et al., 2009). It is structurally different from both cisplatin and carboplatin. The neurotoxicity of oxaliplatin, though, has been described as the most common and dose-limiting toxicity this agent can associate. Oxaliplatin can cause two different types of neurotoxicity.

One type is an acute, transient, dose-related, and painful sensory peripheral neuropathy that is exacerbated by exposure to cold and is very frequent (Becouarn et al., 1998; Gilles-Amar et al., 1999; Grothey, 2003; Grothey & Schomoll, 2001). In fact, at least 90% of patients receiving oxaliplatin will develop symptoms during or soon after its administration, even from the first dose, but the symptoms typically solves within hours to days (Cassidy & Misset, 2002; Gamelin et al., 2002; Giacchetti et al., 2000; Maindrault-Goebel et al., 2001). This acute form consists of paraesthesia, dysaesthesia, and hypoaesthesia in hands, feet, perioral area, or throat and in many cases is precipitated by cold air, cold objects, or cold drinks. Pharyngolaryngeal dysaesthesia is reported by a small number of patients but is very disturbing. It is characterised by a subjective sensation of dyspnea and/or dysphagia accompanied by laryngospasm and stridor (Cavaletti & Marmiroli, 2010; Hausheer et al., 2006; McWhinney et al., 2009). The acute neurotoxicity may appear with notable signs of hyperexcitability similar to an acute myotonia (Hart et al., 1997; Saadati & Saif, 2009). This syndrome is an infrequent condition characterised by the inability to release gripped objects, muscle stiffness, slowed muscle relaxation, increased sweating, and less commonly, paraesthesia. The exact mechanism of myotonia is unknown. It has been postulated that either persistent sodium-channel activity or decreased potassium conductance can be a mechanism for producing axonal hyperexcitability and repetitive discharges in human nerve cells (Hart et al., 1997; Saadati & Saif, 2009; Zielasek et al., 2000). Atypical acute neurotoxicities are sometimes described. One case combined acute motor and sensory hyperexcitability but affected only one hemibody contralateral to the arm of infusion (Uña, 2009). The patient had a history of previous brain ischemic transient attacks, which might have played a role in the atypical presentation of acute neurotoxicity. This asymmetry of symptoms may have been due to the subclinical neurological changes in neurons or axons after ischemia (Uña, 2009).

The second type of neurotoxicity, which is a more chronic, cumulative, sensory form, is persistent and has a gradual onset after multiple exposures to the drug. Although this type of neurotoxicity often decreases with drug discontinuation, it does not disappear (Cavaletti & Marmiroli, 2010; Hausheer et al., 2006; McWhinney et al., 2009). In fact, after stopping the administration of oxaliplatin, the chronic neurotoxicities improve in most patients within 4 6 months and will completely disappear in approximately 40% of patients by 6–8 months. This chronic pattern of sensory neuropathy has been observed in about 50% of patients who received oxaliplatin with infusional 5-FU/LV in a clinical trial but generally appears in approximately 16-21% of patients (Krishnan et al., 2005). It is characterised by paraesthesias, dysaesthesias, and hypoaesthesias that can interfere with ADL (Cavaletti & Marmiroli, 2010; Hausheer et al., 2006; McWhinney et al., 2009).

4. Antitubulins: Taxanes

The two taxanes (paclitaxel and docetaxel) are widely employed in standard anti-neoplastic practice and have demonstrated anticancer activity against many types of malignancies. Although these agents are now well established, they can cause some side effects, including the suppression of bone marrow (mainly neutropaenia), hypersensitive reactions, dermal reactions, edaema, and neurotoxicity, especially a sensory type that is usually persistent and difficult to manage. This toxicity will usually result in dose modification and changes in the planned treatment with the potential impact to the patient´s prognosis.

Taxanes produce a symmetric, axonal, predominantly sensory, distal neuropathy with less-prominent motor involvement. The exact mechanism for CIPN induced by taxanes is still unknown. These drugs target the soma of sensory neurons causing direct damage to cells. On the other hand, a process of "dying back", starting from distal nerve endings followed by effects on Schwann cells, neuronal bodies, or axonal transport. Reduced cytoplasmatic flow in the affected neurons is the most widely accepted mechanism of taxane neurotoxicity. High concentrations of taxanes in the DG, macrophage activation in both the DG and peripheral nerves, and microglial activation within the spinal cord are other mechanisms that can contribute to the genesis of taxane-induced neuropathy (Cavaletti et al., 1995, 1997, 2000; Persohn et al., 2005). The incidence of this peripheral neuropathy is related to several factors, such as single or cumulative dose per course. Risk factors include treatment schedule, prior or concomitant administration of platinum compounds or vinca alkaloids, age, and pre-existing peripheral neuropathy of other causes.

Therapy based on antitubulin drugs usually induces paraesthesias, numbness, and/or pain in a stocking-and-glove distribution. At a clinical examination, neuropathy would be detected as reduced vibration perception or sense of position, pain and temperature sensation, and impaired deep-tendon reflexes. If the treatment continues, muscular weakness can occur, mostly in foot, finger and ankle extensor muscles. Neuropathic pain, usually restricted to the glabrous skin of the fingertips and toes, can be observed in some patients, and myalgias are common following the administration of taxanes.

4.1 Paclitaxel

Paclitaxel-induced CIPN is a schedule- and dose-dependent, cumulative toxicity, with dose being the most important risk factor for developing CIPN. The standard approved doses and schedule of paclitaxel are 135 and 175 mg/m^2 administered every three weeks over three hours of intravenous infusion. A weekly schedule, though, has gained acceptance and is an increasingly widespread practice. Paclitaxel-induced CIPN has been reported for all schedules or doses, although with weekly schedules, the overall reported CIPN ranged from 59-78%. The speed of the infusion has also been correlated with the severity of CIPN. However, a randomised open-label study of weekly one-hour versus three-hour infusions of paclitaxel (100 mg/m^2) has shown that differences in the incidence of induced CIPN between the two schedules were not significant. Although this study was small, the findings suggested that the duration of the paclitaxel infusion by itself does not appear to have a significant effect on the incidence or severity of paclitaxel-induced neuropathy. Weekly schedules may allow less time to neurological recovery, which may underlie the higher incidence of CIPN, probably due to the greater accumulation of paclitaxel in the peripheral nerves and the greater disruption of peripheral axonal transport (Shemesh & Spira, 2010).

This toxicity is manifested by a sensory neuropathy that can associate motor symptoms in some cases. Axonopathies and neuronopathies have also been reported (Lipton et al., 1989; Openshaw et al., 2004; Rowinsky et al., 1990; Sahenk et al., 1994). Clinical features are the following: symmetrical, progressive, length-dependent stocking-glove distribution of paraesthesias; numbness; tingling; burning pain; dysaesthesias; or decreased vibration and proprioception. The loss of deep tendon reflexes might be manifested in latter phases. If the patient receives high doses of paclitaxel, the neuropathy can include motor and autonomic dysfunction and even coma and death secondary to an acute and serious encephalopathy. All these symptoms are not completely reversible. Some researchers suggest that Cremophor (polyoxyethylated castor oil), which is a vehicle used to formulate paclitaxel, is responsible for the CIPN (Henningsson et al., 2001; ten Tije et al., 2003). Several lines of evidence, though, do not support this conclusion (New et al., 1996). In fact, paclitaxel by itself is highly neurotoxic and accumulates in mammalian DG cells in culture leading to a disruption of microtubules. On the other hand, several taxanes are formulated without Cremophor and all have induced neuropathy with similar manifestations and severity (Hausheer et al., 2006). Besides all these data, Cremophor has not demonstrated any neurotoxicity in animals. The available evidence thus does support taxane by itself as the neurotoxic agent (Hausheer et al., 2006).

4.2 Docetaxel

Docetaxel is a semisynthetic analogue of paclitaxel with a different profile of toxicity. Its use as an anticancer treatment has spread in recent years. This agent has activity against different tumours as a single agent or in combinations. Docetaxel-induced CIPN is clinically indistinguishable from paclitaxel-induced CIPN. The most neurotoxic dosages are related to schedules exceeding 36 mg/m^2 per week (Fazio et al., 1999; Tankanow, 1998). The manufacturer reports an incidence of CIPN ranging from 20-58%, and various studies have reported that with doses between 75-100 mg/m^2, the incidence of CIPN varies between 6-59%, being up to 14% in grade 3 and 4 toxicities (Burnstein et al., 2000). Although some studies have suggested a mild neurotoxicity, some patients experience more severe damage and symptoms with cumulative doses over 400 mg/m^2 (Katsumata, 2003; Tankanow, 1998).

4.3 Abraxane

Abraxane is a relatively recent agent approved for anticancer treatment. It is an albumin-stabilised, nanoparticle formulation of paclitaxel designed to overcome poor water solubility and the hypersensitive reactions associated with paclitaxel (Anonymous, 2004). It also has less severe myelo-suppression. When this new taxane appeared, data supported a lower neurotoxicity than conventional paclitaxel with Cremophor. The above study showed that Abraxane at a dosage of 260 mg/m^2 by intravenous infusion every 3 weeks produced a significantly higher incidence of severe neurotoxicity than that observed with conventional paclitaxel infused for 3 hours at a dose of 175 mg/m^2. The data demonstrated that 10% of patients receiving Abraxane versus 2% with paclitaxel experienced severe CIPN.

5. Antitubulins: Epothilones

Epothilones such as ixabepilone are microtubule-targeting anticancer agents. These compounds induce polymerisation of tubulin dimers in microtubules *in vitro* and stabilise preformed microtubules against conditions favouring depolymerisation (Altmann et al., 200; Bollag et al., 1995; Kowalski et al., 1997).

They are very similar to taxanes in their mechanism of anticancer activity and have a common binding site on tubulin, so these two classes of anticancer agents might also share, at least in part, the same mechanism of CIPN (Cavaletti & Marmiroli, 2010). Epothilone-induced CIPN is very similar to that induced by taxanes. A considerably faster recovery in patients receiving epothilones is the most important difference between the two types of CIPN (Cavaletti & Marmiroli, 2010).

6. Antitubulins: Vinca alkaloids

This group of anticancer compounds includes several agents such as vincristine, vinblastine, vinorelbine, vindesine, and most recently vinflunine (Cavaletti & Marmiroli, 2010). In contrast to taxanes and epothilones, these drugs alter the neuronal cytoskeleton. They prevent the polymerisation of tubulin from soluble dimers into microtubules, leading to a loss of axonal microtubules and alterations in their length, arrangement, and orientation. Finally, Wallerian-like axonal degeneration occurs, and axonal transport is also affected (Lobert et al., 1996; Sahenk et al., 1987; Tanner et al., 1998; Topp et al., 2000). The affinity for tubulin differs among all these agents (decreasing in the following order vincristine, vinblastine, vinorelbine, and vinflunine), with affinity being responsible for the distinct severities of neurotoxicity (Lobert et al, 1996).

Vincristine commonly produces isolated sensory CIPN but may be associated with severe motor neuropathy(Postma et al., 1993). This toxicity is very important and is considered a major dose-limiting side effect. An autonomic neuropathy and demyelination are sometimes manifested (Postma et al., 1993). The dose level and the cumulative dose are the most important factors associated with the development of severe vincristine-induced CIPN. The appearance of this toxicity tends to occur two to three weeks after injection (Hausheer, et al., 2006). The most frequent complaints are sensory symptoms such as symmetrical length-dependent paraesthesias, pain, numbness, or tingling in the hands and feet, but muscle cramps or loss of deep-tendon reflexes may also occur (Quasthoff, s. & Hartung, 2002; Tarlaci, 2008). Other symptoms are postural hypotension or urogenital dysfunction related to autonomic alteration, although the most frequent symptoms of this dysfunction are colicky abdominal pain and constipation (92,93). Other dysautonomic manifestations are less common (Quasthoff, s. & Hartung, 2002). In fact, sensory symptoms and loss of ankle stretch reflexes (which is due to muscle spindle toxicity) are the earliest and almost universal signs of neuropathy. A study by Pal (1999) showed that the loss of ankle reflex appears at two weeks, and paraesthesia in four to five weeks. By the end of this study, though, the ankle reflex was absent in all patients, sensory signs and symptoms were present in 75% (impaired vibration detection being the most frequent), and 62.5% presented with constipation.

Weakness in the form of a length-dependent, symmetrical, progressive distal axonopathy is the most common clinical presentation. When this alteration is mild, the patient looses the capacity to walk on the heels, but this neuropathy can become serious enough to render the patient immobile (Hausheer, et al., 2006). Some cases have been also described of vincristine-induced CIPN with neuropathic pain, which are very distressing and painful with very difficult treatments. The study by by Park et al. (2010) investigated the antinociceptive effect of memantine and morphine on a vincristine-induced CIPN model in rats. The authors concluded that systemic morphine and memantine have an antinociceptive effect in animal models. These results suggest that both morphine and memantine may be an alternative approach for the treatment of vincristine-induced, peripheral, neuropathic pain. Other experimental studies have also shown beneficial effects of hydroalcoholic extract of *Acorus calamus* comparable to those obtained with pregabalin. The beneficial effects of the extract are attributed to its anti-oxidative, anti-inflammatory, and calcium-inhibitory properties (Muthuraman et al., 2011). Repeated dosages of imipramine have been considered effective after opioid-analgesic, resistant, mechanical allodynia induced by vincristine in rats (Saika et al., 2009).

The use of vincristine and other vinca alkaloids has also been associated with cranial-nerve palsy, a feature not associated with other neurotoxic antineoplastic drugs.

The toxicity induced by vinca alkaloids usually appears after cumulative doses of 6 to 8 mg, and a severe neurotoxicity occurs after a dose of 30 mg (Trobaugh-Lotrario et al., 2003). This fact must be kept in mind in order to stop the treatment before complications arise. During vincristine treatment, sensory symptoms can even precede the clinical evidence of peripheral nerve damage, but impairment of large sensory-fibres is relatively uncommon.

Recovery generally occurs within one to three months after the cessation of treatment, although symptoms can sometimes persist (Hausheer, et al., 2006). Other vinca-alkaloids have fewer incidences of neurotoxicity than does vincristine, with neutropaenia as the most relevant dose-limiting toxicity.

7. Bortezomib

Bortezomib is a proteasome inhibitor used as a treatment for multiple myeloma (Mohty et al., 2010). The reported mechanism of action involves the reversible inhibition of the 26S proteasome in mammalian cells. This inhibition prevents the targeted proteolysis that affects multiple, cellular, signalling cascades, leading to cytotoxicity (Hausheer, et al., 2006). This agent can also cause a peripheral neuropathy with a particular profile, which makes it easy to diagnose, although its pathophysiology is not well understood despite many results from experimental studies. The neuropathy may be a class effect of proteasome inhibitors.

In rats, bortezomib induces a significant and dose-dependent reduction in the conduction velocities of sensory nerve fibres, with recovery taking several weeks (Cavaletti et al., 2007). Examination of the sciatic nerve showed mild to moderate pathological changes, involving predominantly the Schwann cells and myelin, although axonal degeneration was also observed (Cavaletti et al., 2007). Bortezomib also induces changes in DG neurons such as satellite-cell intracytoplasmatic vacuolisation due to damage to mitochondria and the endoplasmic reticulum, resembling the changes described in Schwann cells of the sciatic nerve (Silverman et al., 2006). In animal models, bortezomib interferes with transcription, nuclear processing and transport, and cytoplasmic translation of messenger RNA in DG neurons (Casafont et al., 2010). The final result is widespread damage of myelinated and unmyelinated axons (Bruna et al., 2010; Meregalli et al., 2009,104).

Some studies indicate that mitochondrial and endoplasmic reticulum-mediated dysregulation of calcium plays an important role in the origin of bortezomib-induced neuropathy (Landowski et al., 2005; Montagut et al., 2006). In fact, bortezomib is able to activate the mitochondrial-based apoptotic pathway according to several findings. The mitochondrial uniporter has been identified as a critical determinant of cytotoxicity, which can be mediated by dysregulation of Ca++ homeostasis (Landowski et al., 2005). Moreover, derangement of the neurotrophin network has also been described, since bortezomib inhibits the activation of NFk-B, thereby blocking the transcription of the trophic Nerve Growth Factor (Cavaletti & Nobile-Orazio, 2007; Montagut et al., 2006). In another study, the DG neuronal cell bodieswere shown to be the primary target for CIPN induced by proteasome inhibitor-. After proteasome inhibition *in vivo*, chromatolysis followed by cytoplasmic accumulation of eosinophilic material and evidence of neurofilaments and juxtanuclear electron-dense cytoplasmic deposits were observed within the DG neurons (Argyriou et al., 2008; Cavaletti & Nobile-Orazio, 2007). These lesions were attributed to the levels of blood and cellular proteasome inhibition. In addition, Poruchynsky et al. (2008) demonstrated that proteasome inhibitors increase tubulin polymerisation and stabilisation in tissue-culture cells. This finding represents a possible mechanism contributing to neuropathy and cellular toxicity. Finally, neurotoxicity may be triggered by some autoimmune or inflammatory factors. In a large randomised study, administration of bortezomib was associated with the development of CIPN in approximately 37% of patients, with 14% experiencing grade 3 neuropathy (Anonymous, 2005). This toxicity is sensory, but motor symptoms have sometimes been associated. The most common symptoms are a burning sensation, hyperaesthesia or hypoaesthesia, paraesthesias, and neuropathic pain. Dose reductions are considered as good management to improve these symptoms leading to a resolution in most patients (Anonymous, 2005).

8. Thalidomide

Thalidomide is an oral immunomodulatory agent used in the treatment of patients with multiple myeloma. Thalidomide-induced CIPN is a common toxicity, sometimes very serious and permanent. The mechanisms of thalidomide-induced CIPN are not well known (Hausheer et al., 2006). Proposals include a reduction in the blood supply to nerves due to thalidomide's anti-angiogeneic properties, direct cytotoxic effects on DG neurons, or dysregulation of neurotrophin activity through effects on NFk-B. In fact, alteration in the usual process of Wallerian degeneration due to a reduction in TNF-a and a secondary inhibition of NFk-B have already been described (Mileshkin & Prince, 2006). Studies based on biopsies of sural nerves were performed to elucidate the exact mechanism, showing that Wallerian degeneration and a selective loss of large-diameter fibres without demyelinisation were lesions underlying this toxicity (Mileshkin & Prince, 2006). A study by Kocer et al. (2009) has suggested that thalidomide-induced CIPN is a dose-dependent, peripheral neuropathy, mainly localised to the peripheral nerves in a length-dependent manner. Another study has shown that variations in genes involved in a drug's neurotoxicity are likely to influence a patient´s risk of developing this adverse effect. In fact, the most significant SNPs (single nucleotide polymorphisms) associated with thalidomide-induced CIPN were seen in the ADME (drug Absorption, Distribution, Metabolism, and Excretion), ABC, cytochrome, and solute-carrier families of genes (Johnson, 2008).

The incidence of thalidomide-induced CIPN is about 30%, often reported as a dose-limiting but not a cumulative problem (Hausheer et al., 2006). This toxicity usually appears after a prolonged period of time receiving this treatment, although some reports have shown that it can occur after a short treatment and sometimes once the treatment has been stopped. The most common symptoms include numbness, tingling, paraesthesias, and/or dysaesthesias with or without sensory loss. They occur in the hands and feet. The symptoms usually do not affect muscle strength, although mild weakness might appear, and deep-tendon reflexes may be reduced or absent. The Lhermitte phenomenon can occur but is very rare

	Thalidomide	**Bortezomib**
Incidence	> 70%	< 40%
Grade 1-2	50%	30 ·
Grade 3-4	20%	< 10%
Main type of neuropathy	Mainly sensory	Mainly sensory
Motor signs	Often	Rare
Painful neuropathy	Rare	Often
Risk factors	Prolonged treatment	Unknown
Consequences	Limits doses and duration of treatment	Managed with dose modifications
Reversibility	No	> 50%

Table 3. Characteristics of CIPN induced by bortezomib and thalidomide (Modified from Mohty et al, 2009).

Several studies have attempted to identify the risk factors and/or predictors of the onset, course, or long-term persistence of this neuropathy; the results, however, have been conflicting and, overall, inconclusive (Hausheer et al., 2006; Mohty et al., 2010). Possible risk factors or predictors for a more severe neuropathy include age, sex, comorbidities, changes in the levels of circulating growth factors or other biological markers, pre-existing peripheral neuropathy (about 15% of patients with multiple myeloma have some degree of disease related peripheral nerve damage before chemotherapy), and previous treatment with potentially neurotoxic antineoplastic drugs (Argyriou et al., 2010; Hausheer et al., 2006; Mohty et al., 2010).None of these factors, though, has been systematically evaluated. Pharmacogenetic studies to evaluate individual susceptibility have failed due to the absence of identified genetic targets. In addition, only a small number of studies have been performed in patients treated with specific classes of neurotoxic antineoplastic agents, and these studies focused exclusively on platinum drugs or taxanes. Controlling and monitoring the patient is very important in order to detect this toxicity as early as possible and to stop treatment immediately to reduce the global damage.

9. Diagnosing CIPN

Several types of criteria are used to assess these patients, such as the National Cancer Institute Common Toxicity Criteria for Adverse Events (NCI-CTCAE), World Health Organization (WHO) guides, Eastern Cooperative Oncology Group (ECOG) scales, Ajani criteria, and quantitative sensory tests (QST) such as vibration-perception threshold (VPT), nerve-conduction velocity tests (NCV), nerve biopsy, or electrophysiologic measurements such as electromyography (EMG), which have usually been applied in combination with neurologic evaluations. However, the assessment of CIPN currently has no gold standard. Many studies have reported that objective assessments of CIPN including neurologic evaluation, QST, electrophysiological testing, and nerve biopsy must be used in an attempt to diagnose and objectively quantify CIPN.

The limitations of these approaches include the lack of standardisation, poor correlation of objective findings with patient-reported symptoms and severity, the additional time and resources consumed during the performance of these tests, and the fact that some are invasive and painful to patients. Also, the expectation that an objective method could reliably diagnose or quantify the severity of a predominantly subjective medical condition may be unreasonable. The clinical assessment of subjective symptoms (assessment of patients) is most commonly and reliably assessed by patient-based questionnaires and scales that have also shown to be convenient for patients and their providers. The use of physician-based methods or objective diagnostic tools seem not to have any clinical advantage in assessing CIPN.

9.1 Neurophysiological evaluation

Nerve-conduction studies (NCS) could be effective in studying CIPN in clinical trials (Bird et al., 2006). In fact, they might be crucial in defining as soon as possible the subclinical changes and in assessing the extent of the damage. Moreover, some evidence indicated that an extremely careful neurophysiological evaluation of the peripheral nerves could discriminate between low and high risk of developing severe CIPN, but the validity of this approach has not been confirmed (Lanzani et al., 2008). These methods have more limitations, such as very poor patient compliance due to the high incidence of discomfort during these procedures, and patients not uncommonly withhold consent to NCV repetitions.

Another major limitation of NCS is the measurement of velocity and amplitude in the largest and fastest-conducting nerves fibres and so cannot provide information about small fibres. Furthermore, NCS and nerve biopsies are applied to regions proximal to CIPN distribution, which may at least partially explain the poor correlation and diagnostic usefulness of these two methods. A normal finding in a NCS cannot exclude the presence of neuropathy. Even if the nerve damage is very intense and extensive, the NCV results can be normal because they only reflect the status of surviving fibres. Besides this theoretical advantage of early recognition of subclinical CIPN, neurophysiological examination of the peripheral nerves is the most effective noninvasive method to assess the pathological features underlying nerve damage (that is, demyelination versus axonopathy). Early recognition of the pathogenic mechanism can be relevant in patients with an atypical course of peripheral neuropathy during chemotherapy or also in patients with other neurologic disorders, such as diabetes, that could coexist. In almost all cases of CIPN, the final event occurring in peripheral nerves is an axonopathy with loss of nerve fibres, indicated by reductions in amplitudes of sensory and compound motor action potentials upon neurophysiological evaluation. In contrast, the hallmark of demyelinating neuropathies is a reduction in the velocity of nerve conduction.

EMG examination of skeletal muscles has rarely been used in the assessment and monitoring of CIPN, possibly because motor impairment is rarely a major feature of CIPN, and needle examination is more invasive than NCS. In addition, EMG scoring and replication are difficult. Somatosensory-evoked potentials have occasionally been used to monitor sensory deterioration in oncologic patients. These studies are mainly used to evaluate preganglionic disorders of nervous system and DG but also postganglionic disorders that could be otherwise evaluated by routine NCS (Hausheer et al., 2006).

Objective measures of assessing CIPN, such as NCS, EMG, nerve biopsy, and detailed neurologic evaluations have not reliably demonstrated their accuracy and are not routinely used to make clinical decisions for managing these patients.

Adverse event	Grade 1	Grade 2	Grade 3	Grade 4	Grade 5
Neuralgia (a)	Mild pain	Moderate pain, L-ADL	Severe pain, sc-ADL		
Dysaesthesia (b)	Mild sensory alteration	Moderate sensory alteration; L-ADL	severe sensory alteration; limiting sc-ADL		
Paraesthesia (c)	Mild symptoms	Moderate symptoms; L-ADL	severe symptoms; limiting self-care ADL		
Peripheral motor neuropathy (d)	Asymptomatic; clinical or diagnostic observations only; intervention not indicated	Moderate symptoms; L-ADL	severe symptoms; assistive device indicated sc-ADL	Life-threatening consequences; urgent intervention indicated	Death
Peripheral sensory neuropathy (e)	Asymptomatic; loss of deep tendon reflexes or paraesthesias	Moderate symptoms; L-ADL	severe symptoms; sc-ADL	Life-threatening consequences; urgent intervention indicated	Death

(a) Intense, painful sensation along a nerve or group of nerves.
(b) Distortion of sensory perception, resulting in an abnormal and unpleasant feeling
(c) Functional disturbances of sensory neurons resulting in abnormal cutaneous sensations of tingling, numbness, pressure, cold, and warmth that are experienced in the absence of a stimulus.
(d) Inflammation or degeneration of the peripheral motor nerves.
(e) Inflammation or degeneration of the peripheral sensory nerves.
Limiting-Activities of Daily Living (L-ADL): preparing meals, shopping, using the telephone, managing money, etc.
Self-care Activities of Daily Living (sc-ADL): bathing, dressing and undressing, feeding self, using the toilet, taking medications, and not being bedridden.

Table 4. Chemotherapy-induced peripheral neurotoxicity-related terms as reported in National Cancer Institute—Common Toxicity Criteria version 4.03 (NCI-CTCAE v4.03).

9.2 Nerve biopsy and histopathological studies

Even though sural nerve biopsy and postmortem examinations of CIPN were very useful in the past, due to most cases being treated with more than one neurotoxic agent and specimens being obtained at different times during or after chemotherapy, the estimation of the impact of these confounding factors or the underlying cancer in these pathological changes was difficult to establish. Consequently, most of the available data on the pathological changes induced by anticancer drugs have been obtained in rodent experimental models(Cavaletti et al., 2008). Generally, except in atypical cases, nerve biopsy in CIPN in clinical practice is not indicated.

Skin biopsy has emerged as an alternative to obtain pathological information in patients with CIPN (Lauria, 2005). It is a minimally invasive procedure that can be repeated in the same patient throughout the course of treatment to measure the density of intra-epidermal fibres. This procedure can be performed very distally and could, therefore, be more sensitive than NCS, particularly in small-fibre neuropathies. Moreover, it allows the investigation of the presence of re-innervation and may provide prognostic information about the long-term course of CIPN, which would be very important. Despite all these potential advantages, skin biopsy is subjectively interpreted, so its value in CIPN evaluation remains to be confirmed.

9.3 The role of neuroimaging

The role of neuroimaging in evaluating CIPN is very limited and so is only considered as an adjunct to research in selected patients. Magnetic Resonance Imaging (MRI) might help to demonstrate the involvement of central-nervous pathways and to verify spinal-cord pathological changes induced by cisplatin (Sghirlanzoni et al., 2005) and thalidomide (Giannini et al., 2003) therapies.

9.4 Assessment of patients

The reported incidence and prevalence of CIPN vary greatly according to different series due to the different methods of assessment and the large number of anticancer agents and schedules used. In most clinical trials, the appearance and severity of CIPN is evaluated by using Common Toxicity Criteria (CTC) scales created by the National Cancer Institute (NCI) in the USA. The latest version of the CTC scale now used is NCI CTCAE 4.0 (4.0.3 version). This scale, however, has several limitations (Cavaletti & Marmiroli, 2010). The interobserver disagreement (Cavaletti & Marmiroli, 2010) seen with the previous versions and the tendency to underestimate the severity of the CIPN are likely to be compounded, because the scale evaluates the occurrence and severity of sensory and motor CIPN by considering almost exclusively the symptoms reported by the patient, graded with the unspecific terms 'mild', 'moderate' and 'severe', and the subjective evaluation of the impact of these symptoms on the patients´ ADL (Postma et al., 1998). This scale also introduces separate definitions to express every symptom, such as dysaesthesia, paraesthesia, etc., instead of just using the generic "peripheral neuropathy". With these data, it a formal neurological evaluation would not be necessary to assess the seriousness of a CIPN, although the lack of validation in large groups of oncological patients makes an accurate grading of CIPN difficult. Moreover, an accurate neurological examination is subject to the cooperation of patients and the skills and interpretations of clinicians (Krarup, 1999).

Another limitation of CTC scales is the narrow scoring range that does not allow accurate and fine graduation of the impairment and could result in a so-called ceiling effect. Also the quality of information they provide on the location, type, and severity of functional impairment is poor (Cavaletti et al., 2006). In fact, these scales are unable to establish the pathological changes underlying CIPN and cannot distinguish between different types of fibres affected or sites of neurotoxic target, resulting in evaluations of sensory impairments located in the same region as having the same score (Hausheer et al., 2006). Aiming to overcome all these limitations and to improve CIPN evaluation and monitoring, other clinical scales have been developed with a higher quality of neurological information. These scales are used for specific drugs or classes of agents but are time-consuming, require special training, and have never been formally validated in comparison with CTC scales (Cavaletti & Marmiroli, 2010; Hausheer et al., 2006). Another major issue in patients with cancer is the appearance of neuropathic pain as a symptom of CIPN. In such cases, an accurate distinction between iatrogenic and cancer pain must be made. Different scales have been used to differentiate between these types of pain, but none has been specifically developed for patients with CIPN (Antonacopoulou et al., 2010; Argyriou et al., 2009).

Despite all these limitations, the use of CTC scales to evaluate CIPN has several advantages such as quick administration, easy generalisation to most antineoplastic agents, ease of learning by oncologists, and technical simplicity (Cavaletti & Marmiroli, 2010; Hausheer et al., 2006) The 'patient-oriented' evaluation of symptoms and functional impairment has become an important priority in the assessment of these oncological patients (Cavaletti & Marmiroli, 2010; Hausheer et al., 2006). This approach has become relevant because the number of long-term survivors and the amountof attention being paid to the quality of life of these patients are increasing. This subjective judgment is very important for all patients but mainly for those with intermediate grades of severity of CIPN, and can be used to properly and quickly manage the CIPN to avoid severe grades (Hausheer et al., 2006).

To meet the above objective, several questionnaires and scales based on the patients' perceptions of their QOL and on functional limitations in daily activities have been created to measure the severity of CIPN (Hausheer et al., 2006). The Functional Assessment of Cancer Therapy/Gynecologic Oncology Group-Neurotoxicity (FACT/GOG-Ntx) and the FACT-Taxane patient-based tools have been studied in patients with CIPN (Cella et al., 2002). These two questionnaires specifically evaluate CIPN and the symptoms related to other neurologic functions such as hearing, sight, etc.These scales, however, do not have a scoring system for establishing the CIPN grade needed for determining the modification of treatment doses or the discontinuation or delay of treatment to avoid severe impairment. The EORTC QlQ-CIPN20 (European Organisation for Research and Treatment of Cancer 20-item module for CIPN) questionnaire is another tool used with the same goal (European Organisation for Research and Treatment of Cancer, 2005). FACT/GOG-Ntx (Cella et al., 2002) and EORTC QlQ-CIPN20 (European Organisation for Research and Treatment of Cancer, 2005) have been described as the most effective tools, but they still need to be formally tested and compared with an objective CIPN evaluation in large oncological series. In recognition of the importance that these questionnaires have gained, the FDA released guidelines in December 2009 for the use of measurements of patient-reported outcomes in the development of medical product to support labelling claims (U.S. Food and Drug Administration, 2009).

9.5 Combining methods: Semi-quantitative assessment and composite scales in CIPN

These methods have been commonly used to evaluate neuropathies other than CIPN but have also been used to examine the CIPN, due to the expertise accumulated (Hausheer et al., 2006; Shy et al., 2003). Among the most sensitive neurological signs of CIPN are the impaired vibration sensation and epicritic (two-point discrimination) touch perception (Cavaletti et al., 2004; Hausheer et al., 2006). The semi-quantitative assessment using thresholds of vibrational and thermal perception has only occasionally been used as an endpoint for clinical trials and is rarely used in clinical practice (Forsyth et al., 1997). These methods, though, are not widely used. They are expensive, their results vary according to the device used, the availability of instrumentation is low, and no formal comparisons have been made with accepted clinical scales for most neurotoxic drugs. These methods are also highly influenced by the examiner's training and expertise and by the patients' cooperation, so their actual advantage over careful clinical examination is still being debated (Cavaletti & Marmiroli, 2010; Hausheer et al., 2006).

Combination methods are being used to enhance the possibility of detecting and scoring CIPN and to characterise the type of sensory impairment (Hausheer et al., 2006). These methods include different combinations of clinical evaluation of symptoms and signs of CIPN, neurophysiological examinations, testing threshold of vibration perception, and sometimes the evaluation of QOL and ADL functions (Cavaletti & Marmiroli, 2010).

Composite scales are methods based on clinical aspects and instrumental techniques. In fact, these methods combine the use of neurophysiological and semi-quantitative evaluations (Cavaletti & Marmiroli, 2010). These scales were assumed to be more accurate for evaluating CIPN but have not been validated on a large scale. Regardless, they have gained acceptance with cancer patients (CI-PERINOMS Study Group, 2009). Composite scales allow a thorough investigation of several features of CIPN and its accurate scoring (Cavaletti & Marmiroli, 2010). These scales are thus potentially useful for clinical trials, but the need to perform instrumental examinations makes their use in daily practice difficult. For this reason, some have proposed that only the clinically based segments should be used. Moreover, when these reduced versions were compared to CTC scales, they showed superior effectiveness in CIPN grading. In addition, their use was feasible (Cavaletti & Marmiroli, 2010; Hausheer et al., 2006). Despite this evidence, the Total Neuropathy Score (TNS), the most commonly used composite scale, and its slightly modified versions used to evaluate the neurotoxicity of various chemotherapy agents were not designed to detect and report the occurrence of neuropathic pain in the course of CIPN (Cavaletti et al., 2003).

10. Prevention of CIPN

The development of CIPN may deteriorate QOL of cancer patients by interfering with ADL such as dressing, eating, or walking, leading finally to a decrease in physical independence.

Though several agents, such as growth factors, antioxidants, anticonvulsants, and antidepressant agents, have been evaluated as potential chemopreventive compounds, no effective treatment exists for preventing or limiting the occurrence and severity of CIPN (Cavaletti & Marmiroli, 2010; Hausheer et al., 2006).

The ideal CIPN chemopreventive agent should prevent or alleviate CIPN without interfering with chemotherapeutic antitumour activity and with no additional toxicity (Albers et al., 2007; Cavaletti & Marmiroli, 2006; Kannarkat et al., 2007; Toyooka & Fujimura, 2009; Wolf et al., 2008).

Most of the available data on neuroprotectants have been obtained using animal models. The most extensively studied drugs are platinum and antitubulin agents.

The earliest attempts to prevent CIPN were based on the use of compounds such as amifostine, diethyldithiocarbamate, and BNP7787, which can protect different tissues from toxic agents. Results, however, were conflicting, and the effectiveness of these agents is inconclusive. Indeed, the use of these agents may actually reduce anticancer activity (Masuda et al., 2011; Moore et al., 2003).

10.1 Growth factors

Neuron development and survival are supported by several growth factors that interact with cognate receptors expressed by neurons and glial cells (Cavaletti & Marmiroli, 2010).

In the earliest preclinical studies, several members of the neurotrophin family, namely nerve growth factor (NGF), brain-derived neurotrophic factor, and neurotrophin 3, were investigated (Aloe et al., 2000; Gao et al., 1995; Tredici et al., 1999). Leukaemia inhibitory factor, which is a cytokine involved in the differentiation of stem cells and the regeneration of neurons, was tested in a randomised, double-blind, placebo-controlled clinical trial in paclitaxel-treated patients. The results were discouraging without any evidence of neuroprotection (Davis et al., 2005).

NGF has been postulated as an effective protectant against cisplatin CIPN. A randomised prospective study was conducted to evaluate the potential safety and efficacy of subcutaneously administered recombinant human (rh) NGF in 1019 patients with diabetic neuropathy (Apfel et al., 2000). Patients were randomised to receive this product or placebo three times weekly for three consecutive months. Changes from baseline neuropathy were examined and compared between the two treatment groups by quantitative sensory tests: Neuropathy Impairment Score, Neuropathy Symptoms and Change, monofilament test, and NCS. The results showed that rhNGF had no significant benefit compared to a placebo.

The ACTH analogue, Org 2766, is a neurotrophic factor studied for the prevention of CIPN. This agent and NGF promote survival of neurons exposed to neurotoxic chemotherapy (Hovestadt et al., 1992). Org 2766 has shown effectiveness in preventing cisplatin-induced CIPN in animal experiments and in cases of impaired velocity of sensory-nerve conduction. A study by van der Hoop et al. (1990) of patients with ovarian cancer confirmed these findings and showed that Org 2766 had no adverse impact on the efficacy of anticancer treatments. Other studies, though, have claimed that the length of the follow-up period in the above study was too short to detect CIPN development. A more prolonged follow-up of the patients included in the Van der Hoop study failed to demonstrate the expected advantage (Roberts et al., 1997).

Erythropoietin has demonstrated promising results in cisplatin and docetaxel models of CIPN (Bianchi et al., 2007; Cervellini et al., 2010). It is considered as a multifunctional trophic factor with potent activity during erythropoiesis and with a neurotrophic action on several neural cells in the central and peripheral nervous systems. In fact, erythropoietin's receptor is upregulated after injury to nervous tissue. The use of erythropoietin as a neuroprotectant in oncological practice, however, is currently prevented by concerns of safety, such as embolic adverse events (Dicato & Plawny, 2010). The efforts to establish a neuroprotective agent against cisplatin-induced CIPN have been unsuccessful, therefore randomised controlled clinical trials are needed for candidates that can prevent this debilitating side effect.

10.2 Antioxidants

Free radicals and oxidative stress are factors implicated in CIPN, although their effects have not been demonstrated beyond doubt (Carozzi et al., 2010). Nevertheless, several antioxidants, such as glutathione, vitamin E, α-lipoic acid, and *N*-acetylcysteine, have been tested as neuroprotectants in different experimental models of CIPN. Due to the tolerability and safety of most of these agents, several have been tested in small clinical trials (Hausheer et al., 2006).

Glutathione and vitamin E have been tested in platinum or taxane treatments, but despite some evidence of activity by these agents, these trials were not adequately powered to offer conclusive evidence of neuroprotection, and their results will require further confirmation (Argyriou et al., 2005; Bove et al., 2001; Cascinu et al., 1995, 2002). Reduced glutathione (GSH) has a high affinity for heavy metals and prevented the accumulation of platinum in the DG (Cascinu et al., 2002; Schmidinger et al., 2000). Several studies with experimental models have shown a preventive role of the administration of GSH in cisplatin-induced CIPN. Moreover, several reports of placebo-controlled trials of GSH to prevent cisplatin and oxaliplatin-induced CIPN have been performed but were underpowered to obtain solid conclusions. In a study by Cascinu et al. (2002), nine of 21 patients in a group treated with GSH and 15 of 19 patients in a placebo group developed oxaliplatin-induced CIPN. The authors used NCI-CTC to assess CIPN with the known interobserver variability, which is considered an important limitation of this study. This study, as previous studies, was too underpowered to obtain a useful conclusion. As a consequence of these data, GSH has not been approved in the US or in most European countries.

10.3 Anticonvulsants and antidepressants

The use of anticonvulsant or antidepressant drugs (such as carbamazepine, lamotrigine, gabapentine or pregabalin, and venlafaxine) has also been attempted in patients with cancer, generally in small groups of individuals. The primary endpoint of these studies was a reduction rather than a prevention of the severity of CIPN-associated sensory symptoms and neuropathic pain (Cavaletti & Marmiroli, 2010; Hausheer et al., 2006). Regardless of the aim of the studies, though, the results were not clinically relevant.

Gabapentine has been examined in phase II and III trials to determine its potential role as a treatment for mitigating pain and other symptoms associated with CIPN. None of these studies have detected any significant benefit in reducing intensity of pain or sensory neuropathy (Wong et al., 2005). Gabapentine has been also evaluated as an agent for lowering the incidence and severity of oxaliplatin-induced CIPN, but this drug has failed to lower either (Mitchell et al., 2005). Carbamazepine antagonises the effect of oxaliplatin in experimental models with rat DG neurons incubated with this anticancer agent (Adelsberger et al., 2000). Oxaliplatin increases the amplitude and duration of compound action potentials and lengthens the refractory period of peripheral nerves, suggesting an interaction with voltage-gated sodium channels. Clinical studies with carbamazepine, though, have given conflicting results for the ability of carbamazepine to prevent oxaliplatin-induced CIPN or mitigate symptoms (Hausheer et al., 2006; Lersh et al., 2002; Wilson et al., 2002). Venlafaxine is an antidepressant with clinical activity against oxaliplatin-induced acute CIPN (Durand et al., 2011). A study by Durand et al. (2011) tested the efficacy of this drug to prevent and relieve oxaliplatin-induced CIPN. From October 2005 to May 2008, 48 patients with oxaliplatin-induced acute CIPN were randomised in a double-blind study to receive either a placebo or 50 mg venlafaxine one hour prior to oxaliplatin infusion followed by an extended release of 37.5 mg venlafaxine twice daily from day 2 to day 11. Neurotoxicity was evaluated using the numeric rating scale (NRS) for pain intensity and experienced relief under treatment, the Neuropathic Pain Symptom Inventory, and the oxaliplatin-specific neurotoxicity scale. The primary endpoint was the percentage of patients with 100% relief under treatment. Twenty of 24 patients in arm A (venlafaxine) and 22 of 24 patients in arm B (placebo) were assessable for neurotoxicity, and based on the NRS, full relief was more frequent in the venlafaxine arm: 31.3% versus 5.3% ($P = 0.03$) without grade 3–4 events (Durand et al., 2011). These findings are very important because this drug has shown clinical activity against the most disturbing and dose-limiting toxicity of oxaliplatin, which is a very common anticancer agent currently used in clinical practice (Durand et al., 2011).

10.4 Amifostine

This product was approved by the FDA in 1996 for reducing the cumulative toxicity of repeated dosages of cisplatin on the kidney. It has been also studied as a potential preventer of CIPN, mainly induced by cisplatin and paclitaxel, but findings were inconsistent. The American Society of Clinical Oncology has developed guidelines for recommending the current clinical use of this agent, although it has generally failed to demonstrate any benefit (Hensley et al., 1999).

A phase II study of patients diagnosed with gynecologic tumours evaluated the potential efficacy of amifostine in the prevention or alleviation of clinically disturbing neuropathy associated with paclitaxel administered every 3 weeks combined with cisplatin (Moore et al., 2003). The baseline and subsequent evaluations were performed with the NCI-CTC scale, the FACT/GOG-Ntx neurotoxicity questionnaire, and the Vibration Perception Threshold (VPT). Twenty-seven patients were evaluated, but the study closed prematurely because the prospectively defined limit for neuropathy was exceeded when four patients developed grade 2-4 CIPN according to the NCI-CTC scale (Moore et al., 2003). Amifostine efficacy was thus insufficient to warrant a phase III clinical trial. Others found that VPT results were less sensitive to detect CIPN than were patients' questionnaires (Moore et al., 2003). One study attempted to evaluate the efficacy of amifostine in preventing CIPN in patients treated with paclitaxel in monotherapy with conventional dosages administered every three weeks or combined with doxorubicin or carboplatin (Leong et al., 2003). Other studies used higher dosages of amifostine (250 mg/m^2 every three weeks) (Gelmon et al., 1999), patients treated with cisplatin as monotherapy at high dosages (120 mg/m^2 every four weeks) (Gradishar et al., 2001), or amifostine combined with docetaxel, but none provided any evidence for a protective or mitigating role of amifostine in CIPN (Makino, 2004).

10.5 Glutamine and glutamate

The administration of glutamate has been evaluated for preventing CIPN induced by paclitaxel, cisplatin, and vindesine. Evidence of a neuroprotective efficacy for glutamate with no negative impact on anticancer activity has been demonstrated in rat models, but the mechanism behind these results is unknown (Hausheer et al., 2006). Glutamine has also been evaluated in experimental and clinical studies. A study by Vahdat et al. (2001) reported a reduction in paclitaxel-induced CIPN but no reduction in numbness or paraesthesias in neurophysiologic evaluations. This study, though, had several limitations to clear results, such as small sample size and absence of a placebo-control arm, among others, which rendered definitive conclusions difficult (Hausheer et al., 2006). All these agents should be tested in a double-blind, placebo-controlled, clinical trial.

10.6 Tavocept (disodium 2,2′-dithiobisethane sulfonate, BNP7787, dimesna)

Tavocept is an investigational agent designed to prevent and mitigate clinically important toxicities associated with taxane and platinum-type chemotherapeutic agents, including CIPN (Hausheer et al., 1998). The mechanism of action, safety, effectiveness, and potential for tumour protection of this agent have been extensively evaluated using *in vitro* and *in vivo* models (Parker et al., 2010).

Preclinical studies conducted in rat models show that, under the applied experimental conditions, this agent exerts a protective effect against the neurotoxicity induced by multiple administration of cisplatin or paclitaxel (Cavaletti et al., 1999; Hausheer et al., 1999). Studies conducted in human tumour xenografts demonstrated that the agent does not interfere with the efficacy of chemotherapy (Boven et al., 2002). Masuda et al. (2011) conducted a phase I trial of BNP7787 (disodium 2,2'-dithio-bis-ethane sulfonate, Tavocept™) primarily to determine its safety and potential efficacy to prevent and mitigate paclitaxel- and cisplatin-induced toxicities. Twenty-two patients with stage IIIB/IV non-small-cell lung cancer (NSCLC) received BNP7787 alone one week before co-administration of BNP7787 with paclitaxel followed by cisplatin. The authors found that the appropriate dose was 18.4 g/m^2 of BNP7787, although no dose-limiting toxicity was observed up to 41.0 g/m^2. Mild discomfort at the intravenous site, thirst, and nausea were the most common symptoms of toxicity. Co-administration of paclitaxel and cisplatin did not appear to influence the pharmacokinetics of BNP7787 and mesna. In conclusion, the authors recommended a dose for phase II/III studies of 18.4 mg/m^2 of BNP7787 in combination with paclitaxel and cisplatin. Further studies are warranted to assess whether BNP7787 prevents and mitigates common and serious paclitaxel- and cisplatin-related side effects.

BioNumerik Pharmaceuticals, Inc. and ASKA Pharmaceutical Co. (Tokyo, Japan) have announced the results of a phase III trial of this agent in patients with advanced NSCLC. The results indicated no statistically significant benefit in preventing or reducing the severity of CIPN (primary endpoint). This study was a multicentre, double-blind, randomised, placebo-controlled phase III trial, conducted by ASKA in Japan, and included

182 patients who received the chemotherapeutic drugs paclitaxel and cisplatin as first-line therapy for advanced NSCLC every 3 weeks. The number of patients reporting either severe sporadic or cumulative neuropathy was approximately 50% lower in the Tavocept arm, compared with placebo, according to BioNumerik, but this result did not reach statistical significance (P = .1565). BioNumerik and ASKA believe the lack of statistical significance is likely due to the relatively small size of the trial. A surprising observation was an increase in median survival of approximately 40 days for patients receiving Tavocept, compared with the placebo group. For patients with adenocarcinoma, the median survival was increased by approximately 138 days in the Tavocept patients, compared with the placebo group. These findings are very encouraging, but more studies are needed to obtain confident conclusions.

10.7 Calcium and magnesium infusions for acute oxaliplatin neuropathy

Infusions of calcium and magnesium have been studied for the management of the acute form of oxaliplatin-induced peripheral neuropathy. A study by Gamelin et al. (2002) on patients diagnosed with advanced colorectal cancer tested the efficacy of calcium/magnesium infusions in patients treated with oxaliplatin. Sixty-three patients were treated and received 1 g calcium gluconate and 1 g magnesium sulfate before and after administration of oxaliplatin, and 38 patients did not receive these treatments. Patients treated with infusions of calcium and magnesium achieved a higher cumulative dose of oxaliplatin, had fewer treatment discontinuations due to CIPN (5% versus 56%), had a lower incidence of CIPN of any grade (27% versus 75%), had a lower incidence of laryngopharyngeal dysaesthesia, and were more likely to endure the treatment compared to the other population. All these positive effects were presented without an adverse impact on anticancer activity.

The N04C7 trial prospectively evaluated the activity of intravenous calcium and magnesium as neuroprotectant agents against cumulative oxaliplatin-related sensory neurotoxicity. Patients with colon cancer undergoing adjuvant therapy with FOLFOX were randomised to intravenous calcium and magnesium treatment (1g calcium gluconate plus 1g magnesium sulfate pre- and post-oxaliplatin) or a placebo in a double-blinded manner. The study was closed in view of preliminary reports from another trial suggesting that calcium and magnesium decreased the efficacy of anticancer treatment (Hochster et al., 2007). Despite the early discontinuation, this study demonstrated the activity of these agents as neuroprotectants against oxaliplatin-induced CIPN in adjuvant colon cancer. Before considering these infusions as standard components of oxaliplatin-based chemotherapies, further studies will be needed to refute the notion that these agents decrease the efficacy of anticancer therapies (Grothey et al., 2011; Nikcevich et al., 2008). In contrast to the previous study, a study by Gamelin et al. (2004) found no differences in objective response rate or in progression-free or overall survival. They also found a significantly lower frequency and severity of oxaliplatin neurotoxicity. The authors continue to propose infusions of calcium and magnesium for reducing oxaliplatin neurotoxicity in FOLFOX regimens, provided that the compounds are delivered sequentially and not concurrently. The temptation to reduce the frequency of infusions for outpatients could lead to the administration of some compounds at the same time and in the same delivery apparatus, which could lead to lower drug stability and thus reduced activity.

10.8 Xaliproden

Xaliproden is a non-peptidic neurotrophic drug that has recently been used in oxaliplatin-treated patients experiencing CIPN. This drug acts as a $5HT_{1A}$ agonist. It has neurotrophic and neuroprotective effects *in vitro* (Appert-Collin et al., 2005; Duong et al., 1999; Labie et al., 1999) and has been proposed for use in the treatment of several neurodegenerative conditions, including amyotrophic lateral sclerosis (Meininger et al., 2004) and Alzheimer's disease (Lemaire et al., 2002).

Xaliproden remains under investigation for treatment of CIPN (Susman, 2006; Wolf et al., 2008). Researchers from Scotland recently conducted a phase III clinical trial to evaluate xaliproden for the prevention of oxaliplatin associated CIPN. They have reported that xaliproden (SR57746A) reduces the risk of grade 3-4 and incidence of oxaliplatin-induced CIPN in patients with colorectal cancer (Cassidy et al., 2006).

10.9 Acetyl-L-carnitine

Acetyl-L-carnitine (ALC) is an additional intervention method used to treat CIPN. A study by Flatters et al. (2006) examined the potential efficacy of ALC to prevent and treat pain induced by paclitaxel. Rats received intraperitoneal injections of paclitaxel with daily administration of ALC. Authors concluded that the association of ALC prevented the development of paclitaxel-induced pain. This effect lasted for at least three weeks after the last dose of ALC. In a separate experiment, daily administration of ALC to rats with established paclitaxel-induced pain produced an analgesic effect which was quickly dissipated after ALC treatment was withdrawn.

10.10 Others

Other compounds with different mechanisms of action, such as carboxypeptidase II inhibitors or calpain inhibitors, have been investigated in preclinical and clinical studies, although their routine use in clinical practice has not been well established (Cavaletti & Marmiroli, 2010). Nimodipine, a calcium-channel antagonist, has been evaluated in conjunction with cisplatin, but the trial stopped prematurely due to significantly increased gastrointestinal toxicity (McWhinney et al., 2009). A cytokine called LIF, or leukaemia inhibiting factor, was shown to have a role in diminishing peripheral neurotoxicity in animal models, but this effect was not confirmed in clinical samples.

11. Future

While the pharmaceutical research industry attempts to discover new, less-neurotoxic analogues of the currently available drugs (such as the thalidomide derivative Lenalidomide) (Cundari & Cavaletti, 2009), treatment modification or withdrawal are the only options currently available to oncologists for reducing neuropathy. Such a limited choice is a worrying issue since symptomatic treatment of CIPN is largely ineffective, particularly on long-lasting or permanent symptoms and signs of impairment that are frequent in platinum- or taxane-treated patients. The unfavourable outcome of CIPN is indeed becoming more worrying due to the increasing incidence of long-term cancer survival. This fact makes patient QOL a key concern since the potential effects of CIPN on the lives of these people can be devastating. Close monitoring of individuals for early signs of CIPN will improve the long-term neurological outcome, highlighting the importance of early recognition that should be achievable through a close collaboration between oncologists and neurologists.With improved long-term survival, however, comes the importance of addressing QOL issues.

11.1 Markers of neurotoxicity

In addition to efforts to identify a successful neuroprotective agent, several studies have attempted to establish the role of various phenotypic markers for CIPN. An accurate marker of neurotoxicity that would enable a quantitative monitoring of the progress of neurotoxicity or provide a prediction of the ultimate severity would prove valuable in controlling this toxicity.

Cavaletti et al. (2004) indicated a highly significant correlation between the decrease in circulating levels of nerve growth factor (NGF) and the severity of CIPN in patients treated with cisplatin and paclitaxel. The correlation, however, did not predict final neurological outcome. In addition, nerve electrophysiological studies have been used to detect the progression of CIPN. Further studies to evaluate the effectiveness of both blood markers and electrophysiology in the detection of neurotoxic progression, though, must be performed to conclude that these provide any sufficient benefit to the patient.

The most recent step in this research is the introduction of genome-wide studies, which are an effective tool for identifying specific regions of the genome that are associated with either drug response or drug toxicity. This research could enhance the identification of putative candidate genes and ultimately the particular genomic signatures related to a drug response and the development of toxicity (Potti et al., 2006). Moreover, genome-wide studies of polymorphisms describe variability between individuals and associate these with response and toxicity.All these efforts are needed to determine genetic linkages as a cause of platinum-based toxicity and the toxicities other anticancer treatments. Ultimately, the goal is to diminish these effects and increase the beneficial antitumour therapies (Mileshkin et al., 2006).

12. Conclusions

CIPN is a common and very serious toxicity secondary to several anticancer agents that presents diagnostic and therapeutic challenges. This distressing complication interferes with the QOL of patients, with the administration of anticancer treatments, and subsequently with prognoses. Thus, much remains to be done to kno better understand the pathogenic mechanisms, clinical features, and the best tools for measuring the severity of neuropathic toxicity. The present situation is very unsatisfactory. Improving our understanding of CIPN is a difficult but achievable goal requiring an effective, open-minded collaborative network of neurologists and medical oncologists to focus on this severe adverse effect of anticancer agents.

13. Acknowledgements

I would like to dedicate this chapter to Dr Valentín Mateos Marcos who taught me all I know about the relevant field of Neurology.

14. References

Adelsberger, H., Quasthoff, S., Grosskreutz, J., Lepier, A., Eckel, F. & Lersch, C. (2000). The chemotherapeutic oxaliplatin alters voltage-gated Na(+) channel kinetics on rat sensory neurons. *European Journal of Pharmacology,* Vol. 406, No. 1, pp. 25-32, ISSN 0014-2999

Albers, J., Chaudhry, V., Cavaletti, G. & Donehower, R. (2007). Interventions for preventing neuropathy caused by cisplatin and related compounds. *Cochrane Database of Systematic Reviews,* Vol., No. 1, pp. CD005228, ISSN 1469-493X

Aloe, L., Manni, L., Properzi, F., De Santis, S. & Fiore, M. (2000). Evidence that nerve growth factor promotes the recovery of peripheral neuropathy induced in mice by cisplatin: behavioral, structural and biochemical analysis. *Autonomic Neuroscience,* Vol. 86, No. 1-2, pp. 84-93, ISSN 1566-0702

Altmann, K.H., Wartmann, M. & O'Reilly, T. (2000). Epothilones and related structures--a new class of microtubule inhibitors with potent in vivo antitumor activity. *Biochimica et Biophysica Acta,* Vol. 1470, No. 3, pp. M79-91, ISSN 0006-3002

American Society of Health-System Pharmacists. (n.d.). Carboplatin. Available from http://www.ashp.org/mngrphs/ahfs/a395017.htm

American Society of Health-System Pharmacists. (2002). Docetaxel. American Hospital Formulary Service (AHFS), p. 927.

Anonymous (2004). Abi 007. *Drugs in R and D,* Vol. 5, No. 3, pp. 155-159, ISSN 1174-5886

Anonymous. (2005). Velcade (package insert). *In* I. Millennium Pharmaceuticals (ed.), Cambridge, MA.

Antonacopoulou, A.G., Argyriou, A.A., Scopa, C.D., Kottorou, A., Kominea, A., Peroukides, S. & Kalofonos, H.P. (2010). Integrin beta-3 L33P: a new insight into the pathogenesis of chronic oxaliplatin-induced peripheral neuropathy? *European Journal of Neurology,* Vol. 17, No. 7, pp. 963-968, ISSN 1468-1331

Apfel, S.C., Schwartz, S., Adornato, B.T., Freeman, R., Biton, V., Rendell, M., Vinik, A., Giuliani, M., Stevens, J.C., Barbano, R. & Dyck, P.J. (2000). Efficacy and safety of recombinant human nerve growth factor in patients with diabetic polyneuropathy: A randomized controlled trial. rhNGF Clinical Investigator Group. *JAMA,* Vol. 284, No. 17, pp. 2215-2221, ISSN 0098-7484

Appert-Collin, A., Duong, F.H., Passilly Degrace, P., Warter, J.M., Poindron, P. & Gies, J.P. (2005). MAPK activation via 5-hydroxytryptamine 1A receptor is involved in the neuroprotective effects of xaliproden. *International Journal of Immunopathology and Pharmacology,* Vol. 18, No. 1, pp. 21-31, ISSN 0394-6320

Argyriou, A.A., Chroni, E., Koutras, A., Ellul, J., Papapetropoulos, S., Katsoulas, G., Iconomou, G. & Kalofonos, H.P. (2005). Vitamin E for prophylaxis against chemotherapy-induced neuropathy: a randomized controlled trial. *Neurology,* Vol. 64, No. 1, pp. 26-31, ISSN 1526-632X

Argyriou, A.A., Iconomou, G. & Kalofonos, H.P. (2008). Bortezomib-induced peripheral neuropathy in multiple myeloma: a comprehensive review of the literature. *Blood,* Vol. 112, No. 5, pp. 1593-1599, ISSN 1528-0020

Argyriou, A.A., Antonacopoulou, A.G., Scopa, C.D., Kottorou, A., Kominea, A., Peroukides, S. & Kalofonos, H.P. (2009). Liability of the voltage-gated sodium channel gene SCN2A R19K polymorphism to oxaliplatin-induced peripheral neuropathy. *Oncology,* Vol. 77, No. 3-4, pp. 254-256, ISSN 1423-0232

Argyriou, A.A., Zolota, V., Kyriakopoulou, O. & Kalofonos, H.P. (2010). Toxic peripheral neuropathy associated with commonly used chemotherapeutic agents. *Journal of BUON,* Vol. 15, No. 3, pp. 435-446, ISSN 1107-0625

Barajon, I., Bersani, M., Quartu, M., Del Fiacco, M., Cavaletti, G., Holst, J.J. & Tredici, G. (1996). Neuropeptides and morphological changes in cisplatin-induced dorsal root ganglion neuronopathy. *Experimental Neurology,* Vol. 138, No. 1, pp. 93-104, ISSN 0014-4886

Basso, M., Modoni, A., Spada, D., Cassano, A., Schinzari, G., Lo Monaco, M., Quaranta, D., Tonali, P.A. & Barone, C. (2011). Polymorphism of CAG motif of SK3 gene is associated with acute oxaliplatin neurotoxicity. *Cancer Chemotherapy and Pharmacology,* Vol. 67, No. 5, pp. 1179-1187, ISSN 1432-0843

Becouarn, Y., Ychou, M., Ducreux, M., Borel, C., Bertheault-Cvitkovic, F., Seitz, J.F., Nasca, S., Nguyen, T.D., Paillot, B., Raoul, J.L., Duffour, J., Fandi, A., Dupont-Andre, G. & Rougier, P. (1998). Phase II trial of oxaliplatin as first-line chemotherapy in metastatic colorectal cancer patients. Digestive Group of French Federation of Cancer Centers. *Journal of Clinical Oncology,* Vol. 16, No. 8, pp. 2739-2744, ISSN 0732-183X

Bianchi, R., Gilardini, A., Rodriguez-Menendez, V., Oggioni, N., Canta, A., Colombo, T., De Michele, G., Martone, S., Sfacteria, A., Piedemonte, G., Grasso, G., Beccaglia, P., Ghezzi, P., D'Incalci, M., Lauria, G. & Cavaletti, G. (2007). Cisplatin-induced peripheral neuropathy: neuroprotection by erythropoietin without affecting tumour growth. *European Journal of Cancer,* Vol. 43, No. 4, pp. 710-717, ISSN 0959-8049

Bird, S. J., Brown, M. J., Spino, C., Watling, S. & Foyt, H. L. (2006). Value of repeated measures of nerve conduction and quantitative sensory testing in a diabetic neuropathy trial. *Muscle Nerve* 34,214–224

Bollag, D.M., McQueney, P.A., Zhu, J., Hensens, O., Koupal, L., Liesch, J., Goetz, M., Lazarides, E. & Woods, C.M. (1995). Epothilones, a new class of microtubule-stabilizing agents with a taxol-like mechanism of action. *Cancer Research,* Vol. 55, No. 11, pp. 2325-2333, ISSN 0008-5472

Bove, L., Picardo, M., Maresca, V., Jandolo, B. & Pace, A. (2001). A pilot study on the relation between cisplatin neuropathy and vitamin E. *Journal of Experimental and Clinical Cancer Research,* Vol. 20, No. 2, pp. 277-280, ISSN 0392-9078

Boven, E., Verschraagen, M., Hulscher, T.M., Erkelens, C.A., Hausheer, F.H., Pinedo, H.M. & van der Vijgh, W.J. (2002). BNP7787, a novel protector against platinum-related toxicities, does not affect the efficacy of cisplatin or carboplatin in human tumour xenografts. *European Journal of Cancer,* Vol. 38, No. 8, pp. 1148-1156, ISSN 0959-8049

Bruna, J., Udina, E., Ale, A., Vilches, J.J., Vynckier, A., Monbaliu, J., Silverman, L. & Navarro, X. (2010). Neurophysiological, histological and immunohistochemical characterization of bortezomib-induced neuropathy in mice. *Experimental Neurology,* Vol. 223, No. 2, pp. 599-608, ISSN 1090-2430

Burstein, H.J., Manola, J., Younger, J., Parker, L.M., Bunnell, C.A., Scheib, R., Matulonis, U.A., Garber, J.E., Clarke, K.D., Shulman, L.N. & Winer, E.P. (2000). Docetaxel administered on a weekly basis for metastatic breast cancer. *Journal of Clinical Oncology,* Vol. 18, No. 6, pp. 1212-1219, ISSN 0732-183X

Carozzi, V.A., Marmiroli, P. & Cavaletti, G. (2010). The role of oxidative stress and anti-oxidant treatment in platinum-induced peripheral neurotoxicity. *Current Cancer Drug Targets,* Vol. 10, No. 7, pp. 670-682, ISSN 1873-5576

Casafont, I., Berciano, M.T. & Lafarga, M. (2010). Bortezomib induces the formation of nuclear poly(A) RNA granules enriched in Sam68 and PABPN1 in sensory ganglia neurons. *Neurotoxicity Research,* Vol. 17, No. 2, pp. 167-178, ISSN 1476-3524

Cascinu, S., Cordella, L., Del Ferro, E., Fronzoni, M. & Catalano, G. (1995). Neuroprotective effect of reduced glutathione on cisplatin-based chemotherapy in advanced gastric cancer: a randomized double-blind placebo-controlled trial. *Journal of Clinical Oncology,* Vol. 13, No. 1, pp. 26-32, ISSN 0732-183X

Cascinu, S., Catalano, V., Cordella, L., Labianca, R., Giordani, P., Baldelli, A.M., Beretta, G.D., Ubiali, E. & Catalano, G. (2002). Neuroprotective effect of reduced glutathione on oxaliplatin-based chemotherapy in advanced colorectal cancer: a randomized, double-blind, placebo-controlled trial. *Journal of Clinical Oncology,* Vol. 20, No. 16, pp. 3478-3483, ISSN 0732-183X

Cassidy, J. & Misset, J.L. (2002). Oxaliplatin-related side effects: characteristics and management. *Seminars in Oncology,* Vol. 29, No. 5 Suppl 15, pp. 11-20, ISSN 0093-7754

Cassidy, J., Bjarnason, G.A., Hickish, T., Topham, C., Provencio, M., Bodoky, G., Landherr, L., Koralewski, P., Lopez-Vivanco, G. & Said, G. (2006). Randomized double blind (DB) placebo (plcb) controlled phase III study assessing the efficacy of xaliproden (X) in reducing the cumulative peripheral neuropathy (PSN) induced by oxaliplatin (Ox) and 5-FU/LV combination (FOLFOX4) in 1st line treatment of patients (pts) with metastatic colorectal cancer. *Journal of Clinical Oncology,* Vol. 24, No. Supplement, pp. Abstract 3507.

Cavaletti, G., Tredici, G., Marmiroli, P., Petruccioli, M.G., Barajon, I. & Fabbrica, D. (1992). Morphometric study of the sensory neuron and peripheral nerve changes induced by chronic cisplatin (DDP) administration in rats. *Acta Neuropathologica,* Vol. 84, No. 4, pp. 364-371, ISSN 0001-6322

Cavaletti, G., Tredici, G., Braga, M. & Tazzari, S. (1995). Experimental peripheral neuropathy induced in adult rats by repeated intraperitoneal administration of taxol. *Experimental Neurology,* Vol. 133, No. 1, pp. 64-72, ISSN 0014-4886

Cavaletti, G., Cavalletti, E., Montaguti, P., Oggioni, N., De Negri, O. & Tredici, G. (1997). Effect on the peripheral nervous system of the short-term intravenous administration of paclitaxel in the rat. *Neurotoxicology,* Vol. 18, No. 1, pp. 137-145, ISSN 0161-813X

Cavalletti, E., Cavaletti, G., Tredici, G., Oggioni, N., Spinelli, S., Reddy, D., Yao, S., Parker, A., Zhao, M., Wu, M., Haridas, K., P., S. & Hausheer, F. (1999). Oral and intravenous BNP7787 protects against paclitaxel-mediated neurotoxicity in Wistar rats. Abstract 2632, 1999 AACR Meeting.

Cavaletti, G., Cavalletti, E., Oggioni, N., Sottani, C., Minoia, C., D'Incalci, M., Zucchetti, M., Marmiroli, P. & Tredici, G. (2000). Distribution of paclitaxel within the nervous system of the rat after repeated intravenous administration. *Neurotoxicology,* Vol. 21, No. 3, pp. 389-393, ISSN 0161-813X

Cavaletti, G., Bogliun, G., Marzorati, L., Zincone, A., Piatti, M., Colombo, N., Parma, G., Lissoni, A., Fei, F., Cundari, S. & Zanna, C. (2003). Grading of chemotherapy-induced peripheral neurotoxicity using the Total Neuropathy Scale. *Neurology*, Vol. 61, No. 9, pp. 1297-1300, ISSN 1526-632X

Cavaletti, G., Bogliun, G., Marzorati, L., Zincone, A., Piatti, M., Colombo, N., Franchi, D., La Presa, M.T., Lissoni, A., Buda, A., Fei, F., Cundari, S. & Zanna, C. (2004). Early predictors of peripheral neurotoxicity in cisplatin and paclitaxel combination chemotherapy. *Annals of Oncology*, Vol. 15, No. 9, pp. 1439-1442, ISSN 0923-7534

Cavaletti, G., Jann, S., Pace, A., Plasmati, R., Siciliano, G., Briani, C., Cocito, D., Padua, L., Ghiglione, E., Manicone, M. & Giussani, G. (2006). Multi-center assessment of the Total Neuropathy Score for chemotherapy-induced peripheral neurotoxicity. *Journal of the Peripheral Nervous System*, Vol. 11, No. 2, pp. 135-141, ISSN 1085-9489

Cavaletti, G. & Marmiroli, P. (2006). The role of growth factors in the prevention and treatment of chemotherapy-induced peripheral neurotoxicity. *Current Drug Safety*, Vol. 1, No. 1, pp. 35-42, ISSN 1574-8863

Cavaletti, G., Gilardini, A., Canta, A., Rigamonti, L., Rodriguez-Menendez, V., Ceresa, C., Marmiroli, P., Bossi, M., Oggioni, N., D'Incalci, M. & De Coster, R. (2007). Bortezomib-induced peripheral neurotoxicity: a neurophysiological and pathological study in the rat. *Experimental Neurology*, Vol. 204, No. 1, pp. 317-325, ISSN 0014-4886

Cavaletti, G. & Nobile-Orazio, E. (2007). Bortezomib-induced peripheral neurotoxicity: still far from a painless gain. *Haematologica*, Vol. 92, No. 10, pp. 1308-1310, ISSN 1592-8721

Cavaletti, G., Nicolini, G. & Marmiroli, P. (2008).Neurotoxic effects of antineoplastic drugs: the lesson of pre-clinical studies. *Front. Biosci.*13, 3506–3524.

Cavaletti, G. & Marmiroli, P. (2010). Chemotherapy-induced peripheral neurotoxicity. *Nature Reviews. Neurology*, Vol. 6, No. 12, pp. 657-666, ISSN 1759-4766

Cella, D., Chang, C.H., Lai, J.S. & Webster, K. (2002). Advances in quality of life measurements in oncology patients. *Seminars in Oncology*, Vol. 29, No. 3 Suppl 8, pp. 60-68, ISSN 0093-7754

Cervellini, I., Bello, E., Frapolli, R., Porretta-Serapiglia, C., Oggioni, N., Canta, A., Lombardi, R., Camozzi, F., Roglio, I., Melcangi, R.C., D'Incalci, M., Lauria, G., Ghezzi, P., Cavaletti, G. & Bianchi, R. (2010). The neuroprotective effect of erythropoietin in docetaxel-induced peripheral neuropathy causes no reduction of antitumor activity in 13762 adenocarcinoma-bearing rats. *Neurotoxicity Research*, Vol. 18, No. 2, pp. 151-160, ISSN 1476-3524

Chaney, S.G., Campbell, S.L., Bassett, E. & Wu, Y. (2005). Recognition and processing of cisplatin- and oxaliplatin-DNA adducts. *Critical Reviews in Oncology/Hematology*, Vol. 53, No. 1, pp. 3-11, ISSN 1040-8428

Chvalova, K., Brabec, V. & Kasparkova, J. (2007). Mechanism of the formation of DNA-protein cross-links by antitumor cisplatin. *Nucleic Acids Research*, Vol. 35, No. 6, pp. 1812-1821, ISSN 1362-4962

CI-PERINOMS Study Group. (2009). CI-PERINOMS: chemotherapy-induced peripheral neuropathy outcome measures study. *Journal of the Peripheral Nervous System*, Vol. 14, No. 2, pp. 69-71, ISSN 1529-8027

Corbo, M. & Balmaceda, C. (2001). Peripheral neuropathy in cancer patients. *Cancer Investigation*, Vol. 19, No. 4, pp. 369-382, ISSN 0735-7907

Cundari, S. & Cavaletti, G. (2009). Thalidomide chemotherapy-induced peripheral neuropathy: actual status and new perspectives with thalidomide analogues derivatives. *Mini Reviews in Medicinal Chemistry,* Vol. 9, No. 7, pp. 760-768, ISSN 1389-5575

Davis, I.D., Kiers, L., MacGregor, L., Quinn, M., Arezzo, J., Green, M., Rosenthal, M., Chia, M., Michael, M., Bartley, P., Harrison, L. & Daly, M. (2005). A randomized, double-blinded, placebo-controlled phase II trial of recombinant human leukemia inhibitory factor (rhuLIF, emfilermin, AM424) to prevent chemotherapy-induced peripheral neuropathy. *Clinical Cancer Research,* Vol. 11, No. 5, pp. 1890-1898, ISSN 1078-0432

Dicato, M. & Plawny, L. (2010). Erythropoietin in cancer patients: pros and cons. *Current Opinion in Oncology,* Vol. 22, No. 4, pp. 307-311, ISSN 1531-703X

Duong, F.H., Warter, J.M., Poindron, P. & Passilly, P. (1999). Effect of the nonpeptide neurotrophic compound SR 57746A on the phenotypic survival of purified mouse motoneurons. *British Journal of Pharmacology,* Vol. 128, No. 7, pp. 1385-1392, ISSN 0007-1188

Durand, J.P., Deplanque, G., Montheil, V., Gornet, J.M., Scotte, F., Mir, O., Cessot, A., Coriat, R., Raymond, E., Mitry, E., Herait, P., Yataghene, Y. & Goldwasser, F. (2011). Efficacy of venlafaxine for the prevention and relief of oxaliplatin-induced acute neurotoxicity: results of EFFOX, a randomized, double-blind, placebo-controlled phase III trial. *Annals of Oncology,* Epub ahead of print, pp., 1569-8041

Dzagnidze, A., Katsarava, Z., Makhalova, J., Liedert, B., Yoon, M.S., Kaube, H., Limmroth, V. & Thomale, J. (2007). Repair capacity for platinum-DNA adducts determines the severity of cisplatin-induced peripheral neuropathy. *Journal of Neuroscience,* Vol. 27, No. 35, pp. 9451-9457, ISSN 1529-2401

European Organisation for Research and Treatment of Cancer (2005). EORTC QOL module for chemotherapy-induced peripheral neuropathy: eORTC QLQ-CIPN20. Available from http://groups.eortc.be/qol/qolg_projects.htm#neuropathy&20(2005)

Fazio, R., Quattrini, A., Bolognesi, A., Bordogna, G., Villa, E., Previtali, S., Canal, N. & Nemni, R. (1999). Docetaxel neuropathy: a distal axonopathy. *Acta Neuropathologica,* Vol. 98, No. 6, pp. 651-653, ISSN 0001-6322

Flatters, S.J., Xiao, W.H. & Bennett, G.J. (2006). Acetyl-L-carnitine prevents and reduces paclitaxel-induced painful peripheral neuropathy. *Neuroscience Letters,* Vol. 397, No. 3, pp. 219-223, ISSN 0304-3940

Forsyth, P.A., Balmaceda, C., Peterson, K., Seidman, A.D., Brasher, P. & DeAngelis, L.M. (1997). Prospective study of paclitaxel-induced peripheral neuropathy with quantitative sensory testing. *Journal of Neuro-Oncology,* Vol. 35, No. 1, pp. 47-53, ISSN 0167-594X

Gamelin, E., Gamelin, L., Bossi, L. & Quasthoff, S. (2002). Clinical aspects and molecular basis of oxaliplatin neurotoxicity: current management and development of preventive measures. *Seminars in Oncology,* Vol. 29, No. 5 Suppl 15, pp. 21-33, ISSN 0093-7754

Gamelin, L., Boisdron-Celle, M., Delva, R., Guerin-Meyer, V., Ifrah, N., Morel, A. & Gamelin, E. (2004). Prevention of oxaliplatin-related neurotoxicity by calcium and magnesium infusions: a retrospective study of 161 patients receiving oxaliplatin combined with 5-Fluorouracil and leucovorin for advanced colorectal cancer. *Clinical Cancer Research,* Vol. 10, No. 12 Pt 1, pp. 4055-4061, ISSN 1078-0432

Gandara, D.R., Perez, E.A., Weibe, V. & De Gregorio, M.W. (1991). Cisplatin chemoprotection and rescue: pharmacologic modulation of toxicity. *Seminars in Oncology,* Vol. 18, No. 1 Suppl 3, pp. 49-55, ISSN 0093-7754

Gao, W.Q., Dybdal, N., Shinsky, N., Murnane, A., Schmelzer, C., Siegel, M., Keller, G., Hefti, F., Phillips, H.S. & Winslow, J.W. (1995). Neurotrophin-3 reverses experimental cisplatin-induced peripheral sensory neuropathy. *Annals of Neurology,* Vol. 38, No. 1, pp. 30-37, ISSN 0364-5134

Gelmon, K., Eisenhauer, E., Bryce, C., Tolcher, A., Mayer, L., Tomlinson, E., Zee, B., Blackstein, M., Tomiak, E., Yau, J., Batist, G., Fisher, B. & Iglesias, J. (1999). Randomized phase II study of high-dose paclitaxel with or without amifostine in patients with metastatic breast cancer. *Journal of Clinical Oncology,* Vol. 17, No. 10, pp. 3038-3047, ISSN 0732-183X

Giacchetti, S., Perpoint, B., Zidani, R., Le Bail, N., Faggiuolo, R., Focan, C., Chollet, P., Llory, J.F., Letourneau, Y., Coudert, B., Bertheaut-Cvitkovic, F., Larregain-Fournier, D., Le Rol, A., Walter, S., Adam, R., Misset, J.L. & Levi, F. (2000). Phase III multicenter randomized trial of oxaliplatin added to chronomodulated fluorouracil-leucovorin as first-line treatment of metastatic colorectal cancer. *Journal of Clinical Oncology,* Vol. 18, No. 1, pp. 136-147, ISSN 0732-183X

Giannini F, Volpi N, Rossi S, Passero S, Fimiani M, Cerase A. (2003). Thalidomide-induced neuropathy: a ganglionopathy? N*eurology* 60, 877–878

Gill, J.S. & Windebank, A.J. (1998). Cisplatin-induced apoptosis in rat dorsal root ganglion neurons is associated with attempted entry into the cell cycle. *Journal of Clinical Investigation,* Vol. 101, No. 12, pp. 2842-2850, ISSN 0021-9738

Gilles-Amar, V., Garcia, M.L., Sebille, A., Maindrault-Goebel, F., Louvet, C., Beerblock, K., Krulik, M. & Gramont, A.D. (1999). 1999 ASCO Annual Meeting.

Gradishar, W.J., Stephenson, P., Glover, D.J., Neuberg, D.S., Moore, M.R., Windschitl, H.E., Piel, I. & Abeloff, M.D. (2001). A Phase II trial of cisplatin plus WR-2721 (amifostine) for metastatic breast carcinoma: an Eastern Cooperative Oncology Group Study (E8188). *Cancer,* Vol. 92, No. 10, pp. 2517-2522, ISSN 0008-543X

Gregg, R.W., Molepo, J.M., Monpetit, V.J., Mikael, N.Z., Redmond, D., Gadia, M. & Stewart, D.J. (1992). Cisplatin neurotoxicity: the relationship between dosage, time, and platinum concentration in neurologic tissues, and morphologic evidence of toxicity. *Journal of Clinical Oncology,* Vol. 10, No. 5, pp. 795-803, ISSN 0732-183X

Grothey, A. & Schmoll, H.J. (2001). New chemotherapy approaches in colorectal cancer. *Current Opinion in Oncology,* Vol. 13, No. 4, pp. 275-286, ISSN 1040-8746

Grothey, A. (2003). Oxaliplatin-safety profile: neurotoxicity. *Seminars in Oncology,* Vol. 30, No. 4 Suppl 15, pp. 5-13, ISSN 0093-7754

Grothey, A., Nikcevich, D.A., Sloan, J.A., Kugler, J.W., Silberstein, P.T., Dentchev, T., Wender, D.B., Novotny, P.J., Chitaley, U., Alberts, S.R. & Loprinzi, C.L. (2011). Intravenous calcium and magnesium for oxaliplatin-induced sensory neurotoxicity in adjuvant colon cancer: NCCTG N04C7. *Journal of Clinical Oncology,* Vol. 29, No. 4, pp. 421-427, ISSN 1527-7755

Hah, S.S., Stivers, K.M., de Vere White, R.W. & Henderson, P.T. (2006). Kinetics of carboplatin-DNA binding in genomic DNA and bladder cancer cells as determined by accelerator mass spectrometry. *Chemical Research in Toxicology,* Vol. 19, No. 5, pp. 622-626, ISSN 0893-228X

Hart, I.K., Waters, C., Vincent, A., Newland, C., Beeson, D., Pongs, O., Morris, C. & Newsom-Davis, J. (1997). Autoantibodies detected to expressed K+ channels are implicated in neuromyotonia. *Annals of Neurology,* Vol. 41, No. 2, pp. 238-246, ISSN 0364-5134

Hausheer, F.H., Kanter, P., Cao, S., Haridas, K., Seetharamulu, P., Reddy, D., Petluru, P., Zhao, M., Murali, D., Saxe, J.D., Yao, S., Martinez, N., Zukowski, A. & Rustum, Y.M. (1998). Modulation of platinum-induced toxicities and therapeutic index: mechanistic insights and first- and second-generation protecting agents. *Seminars in Oncology,* Vol. 25, No. 5, pp. 584-599, ISSN 0093-7754

Hausheer, F.H., Schilsky, R.L., Bain, S., Berghorn, E.J. & Lieberman, F. (2006). Diagnosis, management, and evaluation of chemotherapy-induced peripheral neuropathy. *Seminars in Oncology,* Vol. 33, No. 1, pp. 15-49, ISSN 0093-7754

Henningsson, A., Karlsson, M.O., Vigano, L., Gianni, L., Verweij, J. & Sparreboom, A. (2001). Mechanism-based pharmacokinetic model for paclitaxel. *Journal of Clinical Oncology,* Vol. 19, No. 20, pp. 4065-4073, ISSN 0732-183X

Hensley, M.L., Schuchter, L.M., Lindley, C., Meropol, N.J., Cohen, G.I., Broder, G., Gradishar, W.J., Green, D.M., Langdon, R.J., Jr., Mitchell, R.B., Negrin, R., Szatrowski, T.P., Thigpen, J.T., Von Hoff, D., Wasserman, T.H., Winer, E.P. & Pfister, D.G. (1999). American Society of Clinical Oncology clinical practice guidelines for the use of chemotherapy and radiotherapy protectants. *Journal of Clinical Oncology,* Vol. 17, No. 10, pp. 3333-3355, ISSN 0732-183X

Hilkens, P.H. & ven den Bent, M.J. (1997). Chemotherapy-induced peripheral neuropathy. *Journal of the Peripheral Nervous System,* Vol. 2, No. 4, pp. 350-361, ISSN 1085-9489

Hochster, H.S., Grothey, A. & Childs, B.H. (2007). Use of calcium and magnesium salts to reduce oxaliplatin-related neurotoxicity. *Journal of Clinical Oncology,* Vol. 25, No. 25, pp. 4028-4029, ISSN 1527-7755

Holmes, J., Stanko, J., Varchenko, M., Ding, H., Madden, V.J., Bagnell, C.R., Wyrick, S.D. & Chaney, S.G. (1998). Comparative neurotoxicity of oxaliplatin, cisplatin, and ormaplatin in a Wistar rat model. *Toxicological Sciences,* Vol. 46, No. 2, pp. 342-351, ISSN 1096-6080

Hovestadt, A., van der Burg, M.E., Verbiest, H.B., van Putten, W.L. & Vecht, C.J. (1992). The course of neuropathy after cessation of cisplatin treatment, combined with Org 2766 or placebo. *Journal of Neurology,* Vol. 239, No. 3, pp. 143-146, ISSN 0340-5354

Johnson, D.C., Ramos, C., Szubert, A.J., Gregory, W.M., Child, A.J., Davies, F.E., Durie, B.G.M., Van Ness, B.G. & Morgan, G.J. (2008). Genetic variation in ADME genes is associated with thalidomide-related peripheral neuropathy in multiple myeloma patients. *Blood (ASH Annual Meeting Abstracts),* Vol. 112, No. 11, pp. 1675.

Kannarkat, G., Lasher, E.E. & Schiff, D. (2007). Neurologic complications of chemotherapy agents. *Current Opinion in Neurology,* Vol. 20, No. 6, pp. 719-725, ISSN 1350-7540

Kartalou, M. & Essigmann, J.M. (2001). Recognition of cisplatin adducts by cellular proteins. *Mutation Research,* Vol. 478, No. 1-2, pp. 1-21, ISSN 0027-5107

Katsumata, N. (2003). Docetaxel: an alternative taxane in ovarian cancer. *British Journal of Cancer,* Vol. 89 Suppl 3, No., pp. S9-S15, ISSN 0007-0920

Kocer, B., Sucak, G., Kuruoglu, R., Aki, Z., Haznedar, R. & Erdogmus, N.I. (2009). Clinical and electrophysiological evaluation of patients with thalidomide-induced neuropathy. *Acta Neurologica Belgica,* Vol. 109, No. 2, pp. 120-126, ISSN 0300-9009

Kowalski, R.J., Giannakakou, P. & Hamel, E. (1997). Activities of the microtubule-stabilizing agents epothilones A and B with purified tubulin and in cells resistant to paclitaxel (Taxol(R)). *Journal of Biological Chemistry,* Vol. 272, No. 4, pp. 2534-2541, ISSN 0021-9258

Krarup, C. (1999). Pitfalls in electrodiagnosis. *Journal of Neurology,* Vol. 246, No. 12, pp. 1115-1126, ISSN 0340-5354

Krarup-Hansen, A., Rietz, B., Krarup, C., Heydorn, K., Rorth, M. & Schmalbruch, H. (1999). Histology and platinum content of sensory ganglia and sural nerves in patients treated with cisplatin and carboplatin: an autopsy study. *Neuropathology and Applied Neurobiology,* Vol. 25, No. 1, pp. 29-40, ISSN 0305-1846

Krishnan, A.V., Goldstein, D., Friedlander, M. & Kiernan, M.C. (2005). Oxaliplatin-induced neurotoxicity and the development of neuropathy. *Muscle and Nerve,* Vol. 32, No. 1, pp. 51-60, ISSN 0148-639X

Labie, C., Lafon, C., Marmouget, C., Saubusse, P., Fournier, J., Keane, P.E., Le Fur, G. & Soubrie, P. (1999). Effect of the neuroprotective compound SR57746A on nerve growth factor synthesis in cultured astrocytes from neonatal rat cortex. *British Journal of Pharmacology,* Vol. 127, No. 1, pp. 139-144, ISSN 0007-1188

Landowski, T.H., Megli, C.J., Nullmeyer, K.D., Lynch, R.M. & Dorr, R.T. (2005). Mitochondrial-mediated disregulation of Ca2+ is a critical determinant of Velcade (PS-341/bortezomib) cytotoxicity in myeloma cell lines. *Cancer Research,* Vol. 65, No. 9, pp. 3828-3836, ISSN 0008-5472

Lanzani, F., Mattavelli, L., Frigeni, B., Rossini, F., Cammarota, S., Petrò, D., Jann, S., Cavaletti, G. (2008). Role of a pre-existing neuropathy on the course of bortezomib-induced peripheral neurotoxicity. *J. Peripher. Nerv. Syst.* 13, 267–274.

Lauria, G. (2005). Small fibre neuropathies. *Curr. Opin. Neurol.* 18, 591–597.

Lemaire, L., Fournier, J., Ponthus, C., Le Fur, Y., Confort-Gouny, S., Vion-Dury, J., Keane, P. & Cozzone, P.J. (2002). Magnetic resonance imaging of the neuroprotective effect of xaliproden in rats. *Investigative Radiology,* Vol. 37, No. 6, pp. 321-327, ISSN 0020-9996

Leong, S.S., Tan, E.H., Fong, K.W., Wilder-Smith, E., Ong, Y.K., Tai, B.C., Chew, L., Lim, S.H., Wee, J., Lee, K.M., Foo, K.F., Ang, P. & Ang, P.T. (2003). Randomized double-blind trial of combined modality treatment with or without amifostine in unresectable stage III non-small-cell lung cancer. *Journal of Clinical Oncology,* Vol. 21, No. 9, pp. 1767-1774, ISSN 0732-183X

Lersch, C., Schmelz, R., Eckel, F., Erdmann, J., Mayr, M., Schulte-Frohlinde, E., Quasthoff, S., Grosskreutz, J. & Adelsberger, H. (2002). Prevention of oxaliplatin-induced peripheral sensory neuropathy by carbamazepine in patients with advanced colorectal cancer. *Clinical Colorectal Cancer,* Vol. 2, No. 1, pp. 54-58, ISSN 1533-0028

Lipton, R.B., Apfel, S.C., Dutcher, J.P., Rosenberg, R., Kaplan, J., Berger, A., Einzig, A.I., Wiernik, P. & Schaumburg, H.H. (1989). Taxol produces a predominantly sensory neuropathy. *Neurology,* Vol. 39, No. 3, pp. 368-373, ISSN 0028-3878

Lobert, S., Vulevic, B. & Correia, J.J. (1996). Interaction of vinca alkaloids with tubulin: a comparison of vinblastine, vincristine, and vinorelbine. *Biochemistry,* Vol. 35, No. 21, pp. 6806-6814, ISSN 0006-2960

Maindrault-Goebel, F., de Gramont, A., Louvet, C., Andre, T., Carola, E., Mabro, M., Artru, P., Gilles, V., Lotz, J.P., Izrael, V. & Krulik, M. (2001). High-dose intensity oxaliplatin added to the simplified bimonthly leucovorin and 5-fluorouracil regimen as second-line therapy for metastatic colorectal cancer (FOLFOX 7). *European Journal of Cancer,* Vol. 37, No. 8, pp. 1000-1005, ISSN 0959-8049

Makino, H. (2004). Treatment and care of neurotoxicity from taxane anticancer agents. *Breast Cancer,* Vol. 11, No. 1, pp. 100-104, ISSN 1340-6868

Masuda, N., Negoro, S., Hausheer, F., Nakagawa, K., Matsui, K., Kudoh, S., Takeda, K., Yamamoto, N., Yoshimura, N., Ohashi, Y. & Fukuoka, M. (2011). Phase I and pharmacologic study of BNP7787, a novel chemoprotector in patients with advanced non-small cell lung cancer. *Cancer Chemotherapy and Pharmacology,* Vol. 67, No. 3, pp. 533-542, ISSN 1432-0843

Masurovsky, E.B., Peterson, E.R., Crain, S.M. & Horwitz, S.B. (1983). Morphological alterations in dorsal root ganglion neurons and supporting cells of organotypic mouse spinal cord-ganglion cultures exposed to taxol. *Neuroscience,* Vol. 10, No. 2, pp. 491-509, ISSN 0306-4522

McDonald, E.S., Randon, K.R., Knight, A. & Windebank, A.J. (2005). Cisplatin preferentially binds to DNA in dorsal root ganglion neurons in vitro and in vivo: a potential mechanism for neurotoxicity. *Neurobiology of Disease,* Vol. 18, No. 2, pp. 305-313, ISSN 0969-9961

McKeage, M.J. (1995). Comparative adverse effect profiles of platinum drugs. *Drug Safety,* Vol. 13, No. 4, pp. 228-244, ISSN 0114-5916

McKeage, M.J., Hsu, T., Screnci, D., Haddad, G. & Baguley, B.C. (2001). Nucleolar damage correlates with neurotoxicity induced by different platinum drugs. *British Journal of Cancer,* Vol. 85, No. 8, pp. 1219-1225, ISSN 0007-0920

McWhinney, S.R., Goldberg, R.M. & McLeod, H.L. (2009). Platinum neurotoxicity pharmacogenetics. *Molecular Cancer Therapeutics,* Vol. 8, No. 1, pp. 10-16, ISSN 1535-7163

Meijer, C., de Vries, E.G., Marmiroli, P., Tredici, G., Frattola, L. & Cavaletti, G. (1999). Cisplatin-induced DNA-platination in experimental dorsal root ganglia neuronopathy. *Neurotoxicology,* Vol. 20, No. 6, pp. 883-887, ISSN 0161-813X

Meininger, V., Bensimon, G., Bradley, W.R., Brooks, B., Douillet, P., Eisen, A.A., Lacomblez, L., Leigh, P.N. & Robberecht, W. (2004). Efficacy and safety of xaliproden in amyotrophic lateral sclerosis: results of two phase III trials. *Amyotrophic Lateral Sclerosis and Other Motor Neuron Disorders,* Vol. 5, No. 2, pp. 107-117, ISSN 1466-0822

Meregalli, C., Canta, A., Carozzi, V.A., Chiorazzi, A., Oggioni, N., Gilardini, A., Ceresa, C., Avezza, F., Crippa, L., Marmiroli, P. & Cavaletti, G. (2010). Bortezomib-induced painful neuropathy in rats: a behavioral, neurophysiological and pathological study in rats. *European Journal of Pain,* Vol. 14, No. 4, pp. 343-350, ISSN 1532-2149

Mileshkin, L. & Prince, H.M. (2006). The troublesome toxicity of peripheral neuropathy with thalidomide. *Leuk Lymphoma,* Vol. 47, No. 11, pp. 2276-2279, ISSN 1042-8194

Mileshkin, L., Stark, R., Day, B., Seymour, J.F., Zeldis, J.B. & Prince, H.M. (2006). Development of neuropathy in patients with myeloma treated with thalidomide: patterns of occurrence and the role of electrophysiologic monitoring. *Journal of Clinical Oncology,* Vol. 24, No. 27, pp. 4507-4514, ISSN 1527-7755

Mitchell, P., Goldstein, D., Michael, M., Beale, P., Friedlander, M., Zalcberg, J., Clarke, S. & White, S. (2005). Addition of gabapentin (G) to a modified FOLFOX regimen does not reduce neurotoxicity in patients (pts) with advanced colorectal cancer (CRC). *Journal of Clinical Oncology,* Vol. 23, pp. 266s (Abstract 3581).

Mohty, B., El-Cheikh, J., Yakoub-Agha, I., Moreau, P., Harousseau, J.L. & Mohty, M. (2010). Peripheral neuropathy and new treatments for multiple myeloma: background and practical recommendations. *Haematologica,* Vol. 95, No. 2, pp. 311-319, ISSN 1592-8721

Montagut, C., Rovira, A. & Albanell, J. (2006). The proteasome: a novel target for anticancer therapy. *Clinical and Translational Oncology,* Vol. 8, No. 5, pp. 313-317, ISSN 1699-048X

Moore, D.H., Donnelly, J., McGuire, W.P., Almadrones, L., Cella, D.F., Herzog, T.J. & Waggoner, S.E. (2003). Limited access trial using amifostine for protection against cisplatin- and three-hour paclitaxel-induced neurotoxicity: a phase II study of the Gynecologic Oncology Group. *Journal of Clinical Oncology,* Vol. 21, No. 22, pp. 4207-4213, ISSN 0732-183X

Muthuraman, A., Singh, N. & Jaggi, A.S. (2011). Protective effect of Acorus calamus L. in rat model of vincristine induced painful neuropathy: An evidence of anti-inflammatory and anti-oxidative activity. *Food and Chemical Toxicology,* Epub ahead of print, pp., 1873-6351

New, P.Z., Jackson, C.E., Rinaldi, D., Burris, H. & Barohn, R.J. (1996). Peripheral neuropathy secondary to docetaxel (Taxotere). *Neurology,* Vol. 46, No. 1, pp. 108-111, ISSN 0028-3878

Nikcevich, D.A., Grothey, A., Sloan, J.A., Kugler, J.W., Silberstein, P.T., Dentchev, T., Wender, D.B., Novotny, P.J., Windschitl, H.E. & Loprinzi, C.L. (2008). Effect of intravenous calcium and magnesium (IV CaMg) on oxaliplatin-induced sensory neurotoxicity (sNT) in adjuvant colon cancer: Results of the phase III placebo-controlled, double-blind NCCTG trial N04C7. *Journal of Clinical Oncology,* Vol. 26, No. May 20 Supplement, pp. Abstract 4009.

Openshaw, H., Beamon, K., Synold, T.W., Longmate, J., Slatkin, N.E., Doroshow, J.H., Forman, S., Margolin, K., Morgan, R., Shibata, S. & Somlo, G. (2004). Neurophysiological study of peripheral neuropathy after high-dose Paclitaxel: lack of neuroprotective effect of amifostine. *Clinical Cancer Research,* Vol. 10, No. 2, pp. 461-467, ISSN 1078-0432

Pal, P.K. (1999). Clinical and electrophysiological studies in vincristine induced neuropathy. *Electromyography and Clinical Neurophysiology,* Vol. 39, No. 6, pp. 323-330, ISSN 0301-150X

Park, S.B., Lin, C.S., Krishnan, A.V., Goldstein, D., Friedlander, M.L. & Kiernan, M.C. (2009). Oxaliplatin-induced lhermitte's phenomenon as a manifestation of severe generalized neurotoxicity. *Oncology,* Vol. 77, No. 6, pp. 342-348, ISSN 1423-0232

Park, B.Y., Park, S.H., Kim, W.M., Yoon, M.H. & Lee, H.G. (2010). Antinociceptive Effect of Memantine and Morphine on Vincristine-induced Peripheral Neuropathy in Rats. *Korean Journal of Pain,* Vol. 23, No. 3, pp. 179-185, ISSN 2093-0569

Parker, A.R., Petluru, P.N., Wu, M., Zhao, M., Kochat, H. & Hausheer, F.H. (2010). BNP7787-mediated modulation of paclitaxel- and cisplatin-induced aberrant microtubule protein polymerization in vitro. *Molecular Cancer Therapeutics,* Vol. 9, No. 9, pp. 2558-2567, ISSN 1538-8514

Parkin, D.M., Bray, F., Ferlay, J., Pisani, P. (2005). CA Cancer J Clin., 55, 74.

Peltier, A.C. & Russell, J.W. (2002). Recent advances in drug-induced neuropathies. *Current Opinion in Neurology,* Vol. 15, No. 5, pp. 633-638, ISSN 1350-7540

Persohn, E., Canta, A., Schoepfer, S., Traebert, M., Mueller, L., Gilardini, A., Galbiati, S., Nicolini, G., Scuteri, A., Lanzani, F., Giussani, G. & Cavaletti, G. (2005).

Morphological and morphometric analysis of paclitaxel and docetaxel-induced peripheral neuropathy in rats. *European Journal of Cancer,* Vol. 41, No. 10, pp. 1460-1466, ISSN 0959-8049

Poruchynsky, M.S., Sackett, D.L., Robey, R.W., Ward, Y., Annunziata, C. & Fojo, T. (2008). Proteasome inhibitors increase tubulin polymerization and stabilization in tissue culture cells: a possible mechanism contributing to peripheral neuropathy and cellular toxicity following proteasome inhibition. *Cell Cycle,* Vol. 7, No. 7, pp. 940-949, ISSN 1551-4005

Postma, T.J., Benard, B.A., Huijgens, P.C., Ossenkoppele, G.J. & Heimans, J.J. (1993). Long-term effects of vincristine on the peripheral nervous system. *Journal of Neuro-Oncology,* Vol. 15, No. 1, pp. 23-27, ISSN 0167-594X

Postma, T.J., Heimans, J.J., Muller, M.J., Ossenkoppele, G.J., Vermorken, J.B. & Aaronson, N.K. (1998). Pitfalls in grading severity of chemotherapy-induced peripheral neuropathy. *Annals of Oncology,* Vol. 9, No. 7, pp. 739-744, ISSN 0923-7534

Potti, A., Dressman, H.K., Bild, A., Riedel, R.F., Chan, G., Sayer, R., Cragun, J., Cottrill, H., Kelley, M.J., Petersen, R., Harpole, D., Marks, J., Berchuck, A., Ginsburg, G.S., Febbo, P., Lancaster, J. & Nevins, J.R. (2006). Genomic signatures to guide the use of chemotherapeutics. *Nature Medicine,* Vol. 12, No. 11, pp. 1294-1300, ISSN 1078-8956

Quasthoff, S. & Hartung, H.P. (2002). Chemotherapy-induced peripheral neuropathy. *Journal of Neurology,* Vol. 249, No. 1, pp. 9-17, ISSN 0340-5354

Roberts, J.A., Jenison, E.L., Kim, K., Clarke-Pearson, D. & Langleben, A. (1997). A randomized, multicenter, double-blind, placebo-controlled, dose-finding study of ORG 2766 in the prevention or delay of cisplatin-induced neuropathies in women with ovarian cancer. *Gynecologic Oncology,* Vol. 67, No. 2, pp. 172-177, ISSN 0090-8258

Rowinsky, E.K., Cazenave, L.A. & Donehower, R.C. (1990). Taxol: a novel investigational antimicrotubule agent. *Journal of the National Cancer Institute,* Vol. 82, No. 15, pp. 1247-1259, ISSN 0027-8874

Saadati, H. & Saif, M.W. (2009). Oxaliplatin-induced hyperexcitability syndrome in a patient with pancreatic cancer. *JOP,* Vol. 10, No. 4, pp. 459-461, ISSN 1590-8577

Sahenk, Z., Brady, S.T. & Mendell, J.R. (1987). Studies on the pathogenesis of vincristine-induced neuropathy. *Muscle and Nerve,* Vol. 10, No. 1, pp. 80-84, ISSN 0148-639X

Sahenk, Z., Barohn, R., New, P. & Mendell, J.R. (1994). Taxol neuropathy. Electrodiagnostic and sural nerve biopsy findings. *Archives of Neurology,* Vol. 51, No. 7, pp. 726-729, ISSN 0003-9942

Saika, F., Kiguchi, N., Kobayashi, Y., Fukazawa, Y., Maeda, T., Ozaki, M. & Kishioka, S. (2009). Suppressive effect of imipramine on vincristine-induced mechanical allodynia in mice. *Biological and Pharmaceutical Bulletin,* Vol. 32, No. 7, pp. 1231-1234, ISSN 0918-6158

Schmidinger, M., Budinsky, A.C., Wenzel, C., Piribauer, M., Brix, R., Kautzky, M., Oder, W., Locker, G.J., Zielinski, C.C. & Steger, G.G. (2000). Glutathione in the prevention of cisplatin induced toxicities. A prospectively randomized pilot trial in patients with head and neck cancer and non small cell lung cancer. *Wiener Klinische Wochenschrift,* Vol. 112, No. 14, pp. 617-623, ISSN 0043-5325

Screnci, D. & McKeage, M.J. (1999). Platinum neurotoxicity: clinical profiles, experimental models and neuroprotective approaches. *Journal of Inorganic Biochemistry,* Vol. 77, No. 1-2, pp. 105-110, ISSN 0162-0134

Sghirlanzoni, A., Pareyson, D. & Lauria, G. (2005). Sensory neuron diseases. *Lancet Neurol.* 4,349–361.

Shemesh, O.A. & Spira, M.E. (2010). Paclitaxel induces axonal microtubules polar reconfiguration and impaired organelle transport: implications for the pathogenesis of paclitaxel-induced polyneuropathy. *Acta Neuropathologica,* Vol. 119, No. 2, pp. 235-248, ISSN 1432-0533

Shy, M.E., Frohman, E.M., So, Y.T., Arezzo, J.C., Cornblath, D.R., Giuliani, M.J., Kincaid, J.C., Ochoa, J.L., Parry, G.J. & Weimer, L.H. (2003). Quantitative sensory testing: report of the Therapeutics and Technology Assessment Subcommittee of the American Academy of Neurology. *Neurology,* Vol. 60, No. 6, pp. 898-904, ISSN 1526-632X

Silverman, L.C.L., Kadambi, V.J., Decoster, R., Vynckier, A., Jortner, B. & Alden, C.L. (2006). Model for proteasome inhibition associated peripheral neuropathy. *Toxicologic Pathology [Abstract],* Vol. 34(989)

Susman, E. (2006). Xaliproden lessens oxaliplatin-mediated neuropathy. *Lancet Oncology,* Vol. 7, No. 4, pp. 288, ISSN 1470-2045

Ta, L.E., Espeset, L., Podratz, J. & Windebank, A.J. (2006). Neurotoxicity of oxaliplatin and cisplatin for dorsal root ganglion neurons correlates with platinum-DNA binding. *Neurotoxicology,* Vol. 27, No. 6, pp. 992-1002, ISSN 0161-813X

Tankanow, R.M. (1998). Docetaxel: a taxoid for the treatment of metastatic breast cancer. *American Journal of Health-System Pharmacy,* Vol. 55, No. 17, pp. 1777-1791, ISSN 1079-2082

Tanner, K.D., Levine, J.D. & Topp, K.S. (1998). Microtubule disorientation and axonal swelling in unmyelinated sensory axons during vincristine-induced painful neuropathy in rat. *Journal of Comparative Neurology,* Vol. 395, No. 4, pp. 481-492, ISSN 0021-9967

Tarlaci, S. (2008). Vincristine-induced fatal neuropathy in non Hodgkin's lymphoma. *Neurotoxicology,* Vol. 29, No. 4, pp. 748-749, ISSN 0161-813X

ten Tije, A.J., Verweij, J., Loos, W.J. & Sparreboom, A. (2003). Pharmacological effects of formulation vehicles: implications for cancer chemotherapy. *Clinical Pharmacokinetics,* Vol. 42, No. 7, pp. 665-685, ISSN 0312-5963

Thompson, S.W., Davis, L.E., Kornfeld, M., Hilgers, R.D. & Standefer, J.C. (1984). Cisplatin neuropathy. Clinical, electrophysiologic, morphologic, and toxicologic studies. *Cancer,* Vol. 54, No. 7, pp. 1269-1275, ISSN 0008-543X

Topp, K.S., Tanner, K.D. & Levine, J.D. (2000). Damage to the cytoskeleton of large diameter sensory neurons and myelinated axons in vincristine-induced painful peripheral neuropathy in the rat. *Journal of Comparative Neurology,* Vol. 424, No. 4, pp. 563-576, ISSN 0021-9967

Toyooka, K. & Fujimura, H. (2009). Iatrogenic neuropathies. *Current Opinion in Neurology,* Vol. 22, No. 5, pp. 475-479, ISSN 1473-6551

Tredici, C., Braga, M., Nicolini, G., Miloso, M., Marmiroli, P., Schenone, A., Nobbio, L., Frattola, L. & Cavaletti, G. (1999). Effect of recombinant human nerve growth factor on cisplatin neurotoxicity in rats. *Experimental Neurology,* Vol. 159, No. 2, pp. 551-558, ISSN 0014-4886

Trobaugh-Lotrario, A.D., Smith, A.A. & Odom, L.F. (2003). Vincristine neurotoxicity in the presence of hereditary neuropathy. *Medical and Pediatric Oncology,* Vol. 40, No. 1, pp. 39-43, ISSN 0098-1532

Una, E. (2010). Atypical presentation of acute neurotoxicity secondary to oxaliplatin. *Journal of Oncology Pharmacy Practice,* Vol. 16, No. 4, pp. 280-282, ISSN 1477-092X

U.S. Food and Drug Administration. (n.d.) FDA Oncology Tools Product Label Details in Conventional Order for Oxaliplatin. Available from http://www.accessdata.fda.gov/scripts/cder/onctools/labels.cfm?GN=oxaliplatin

U.S. Food and Drug Administration. (2009). Guidance for industry. Patient-reported outcome measures: use in medical product development to support labeling claims. Available from http://www.fda.gov/downloads/Drugs/GuidanceCompliance%20RegulatoryInformation/Guidances/UCM193282.pdf%20(2009)

Vahdat, L., Papadopoulos, K., Lange, D., Leuin, S., Kaufman, E., Donovan, D., Frederick, D., Bagiella, E., Tiersten, A., Nichols, G., Garrett, T., Savage, D., Antman, K., Hesdorffer, C.S. & Balmaceda, C. (2001). Reduction of paclitaxel-induced peripheral neuropathy with glutamine. *Clinical Cancer Research,* Vol. 7, No. 5, pp. 1192-1197, ISSN 1078-0432

van der Hoop, R.G., Vecht, C.J., van der Burg, M.E., Elderson, A., Boogerd, W., Heimans, J.J., Vries, E.P., van Houwelingen, J.C., Jennekens, F.G., Gispen, W.H. & et al. (1990). Prevention of cisplatin neurotoxicity with an ACTH(4-9) analogue in patients with ovarian cancer. *New England Journal of Medicine,* Vol. 322, No. 2, pp. 89-94, ISSN 0028-4793

Verdu, E., Vilches, J.J., Rodriguez, F.J., Ceballos, D., Valero, A. & Navarro, X. (1999). Physiological and immunohistochemical characterization of cisplatin-induced neuropathy in mice. *Muscle and Nerve,* Vol. 22, No. 3, pp. 329-340, ISSN 0148-639X

Verstappen, C.C., Koeppen, S., Heimans, J.J., Huijgens, P.C., Scheulen, M.E., Strumberg, D., Kiburg, B. & Postma, T.J. (2005). Dose-related vincristine-induced peripheral neuropathy with unexpected off-therapy worsening. *Neurology,* Vol. 64, No. 6, pp. 1076-1077, ISSN 1526-632X

Wang, D. & Lippard, S.J. (2005). Cellular processing of platinum anticancer drugs. *Nature Reviews. Drug Discovery,* Vol. 4, No. 4, pp. 307-320, ISSN 1474-1776

Wilson, R.H., Lehky, T., Thomas, R.R., Quinn, M.G., Floeter, M.K. & Grem, J.L. (2002). Acute oxaliplatin-induced peripheral nerve hyperexcitability. *Journal of Clinical Oncology,* Vol. 20, No. 7, pp. 1767-1774, ISSN 0732-183X

Windebank, A.J. & Grisold, W. (2008). Chemotherapy-induced neuropathy. *Journal of the Peripheral Nervous System,* Vol. 13, No. 1, pp. 27-46, ISSN 1529-8027

Wolf, S., Barton, D., Kottschade, L., Grothey, A. & Loprinzi, C. (2008). Chemotherapy-induced peripheral neuropathy: prevention and treatment strategies. *European Journal of Cancer,* Vol. 44, No. 11, pp. 1507-1515, ISSN 0959-8049

Wong, G.Y., Michalak, J.C., Sloan, J.A., Mailliard, J.A., Nikcevich, D.A., Novotny, P.J., Warner, D.O., Kutteh, L., Dakhil, S.R. & Loprinzi, C.L. (2005). A phase III double blinded, placebo controlled, randomized trial of gabapentin in patients with chemotherapy-induced peripheral neuropathy: A North Central Cancer Treatment Group Study. *Journal of Clinical Oncology,* Vol. 23, pp. 729s (Abstract 8001).

Zhu, C., Raber, J. & Eriksson, L.A. (2005). Hydrolysis process of the second generation platinum-based anticancer drug cis-amminedichlorocyclohexylamineplatinum(II). *Journal of Physical Chemistry. B,* Vol. 109, No. 24, pp. 12195-12205, ISSN 1520-6106

Zielasek, J., Martini, R., Suter, U. & Toyka, K.V. (2000). Neuromyotonia in mice with hereditary myelinopathies. *Muscle and Nerve,* Vol. 23, No. 5, pp. 696-701, 0148-639X

14

Basics of Peripheral Nerve Injury Rehabilitation

Reza Salman Roghani[1] and Seyed Mansoor Rayegani[2]
[1]*University of Social Welfare and Rehabilitation, Tehran,*
[2]*Shahid Beheshti University of Medical Science, Tehran,*
Iran

1. Introduction

The study of *peripheral nerve injury, repair & rehabilitation* began during the American Civil War and has since expanded to not only include to extensive characterization of the processes and factors that contribute to nerve regeneration and reinnervation, but also to determining therapies that enhance nerve regeneration such as physical modalities, rehabilitation consideration and recently biological conduits and administration of growth promoting molecules.[1] Rehabilitation medicine is a branch of medicine that aims to enhance and restore functional ability and quality of life to those with physical impairments or disabilities. Functional disability due to nerve lesions is completely related to the severity, type and location of nerve lesions. So, before starting any rehabilitation program for patients with nerve injury, deep knowledge of lesion's type and denervation consequences is necessary.

2. Peripheral nerve injury classification

Classification of peripheral nerve injury has an important role in prognosis prediction and treatment strategy determination. Classification of nerve injury was described by Seddon in 1943 and by Sunderland in 1951. In brief it classified to mild, moderate and severe injuries resembling pathologic terms of neurapraxia, axonotmesis and neurotmesis consequently. In the first one the nerve remains intact but signaling ability is damaged, in the second degree the axon is damaged but the surrounding connective tissue remains intact and in the last one both the axon and connective tissue are damaged. [2, 3] the most common etiology for these three types of injury is entrapment neuropathies, blunt and sharp trauma consequently.

3. Peripheral nerve injury consequences

The effects of peripheral nerve injuries are vary depending on the cause and severity of the injury. These are Pain (ranging from a tingling to intense burning pain), numbness or altered sensations, muscle weakness in the affected body part, loss of function (eg. a hand or leg being difficult to use whilst performing tasks), Loss of active movement (eg. wrist drop and foot drop) joint stiffness and skin sores and finally emotional stress.

4. Rehabilitation medicine in brief

Rehabilitation medicine in nerve injuries is a non surgical, comprehensive management of injury consequences, controlling positive disturbing symptoms such as pain, preventing long term deformities such as contractures and utilizing proper techniques and modalities to enhance nerve repair and recovery. Following we will discuss the program in detail.

5. Pain management

Pain is one of the most common and annoying consequences of nerve damage. For the first time massive spontaneous discharges was reported in L4 and 5 dorsal rootlets after producing an experimental sciatic nerve lesion of a rabbit. Since then many mechanisms proposed as the etiology of neuropathic pain but the most recent and acceptable one is dramatic and robust chemical changes occurring in dorsal root ganglions after peripheral nerve damage, which is a new generator and presumably contribute in the process of neuropathic pain. There are also other mechanisms in dorsal column of cord and brain which are proposed as contributors to neuropathic pain. This pain management is an interdisciplinary approach centered by pharmacological treatments.[4] New treatment strategies for neuropathic pain are mainly invented considering the changes in central nervous system. [5] Anticonvulsants and tri-cyclic anti depressants are the most popular drugs for neuropathic pain.[6] Complete relief is very difficult and only 40-60% of patients achieves partial relief. [7] Other modalities which have some role in neuropathic pain management are yoga, massage, meditation, cognitive exercise, acupuncture and Trans-cutaneous electrical nerve stimulation (TENS). [8]

6. Sensation deficit and relearning

Body image, objects' shape and texture recognition and avoiding hazardous objects are the principles roles of an intact sensation. Sensory stimuli are also send a feedback to motor system for proper adjustment in function. Contra lateral somatosensory cortex play as a central processing unit for almost all of these functions. Following a peripheral nerve injury one or all of above mentioned functions may be impaired based on the severity of insult. Complete injury of a major nerve or its sensory part turns off related contra lateral somatosensory cortex until reinnervation or repair is occurred. In this scene all of five principles sensory functions being impaired. If reinnervation occurs in a disorganized pattern the sensory cortex faced a new pattern of input which is usually unknown. This is the basis of sensory rehabilitation or re-familiarization even with a successful surgical nerve repair. Shape and texture relearning with open eye and stimulating deep receptor by rough objects are helpful methods of proper reorganization [fig1]. (Rosén et al., 2003; Lundborg, 2004) large nerves injury such as sciatic in lower extremities' nerve and also more widespread nerve lesions such as neuropathies have a profound effect on all sensation and motor related functions but proprioception is one of the most important one. Proprioception is defined as sensing the body movements and awareness of posture, enabling the person to orient itself in space without visual clues.[9] Proprioception is what allows someone to walk in complete darkness or driving with only looking the road without losing balance or control. During the learning of any new skills or relearning old one such as a sport activity, or an art, it is usually necessary to become familiar with some proprioceptive tasks specific to that activity.

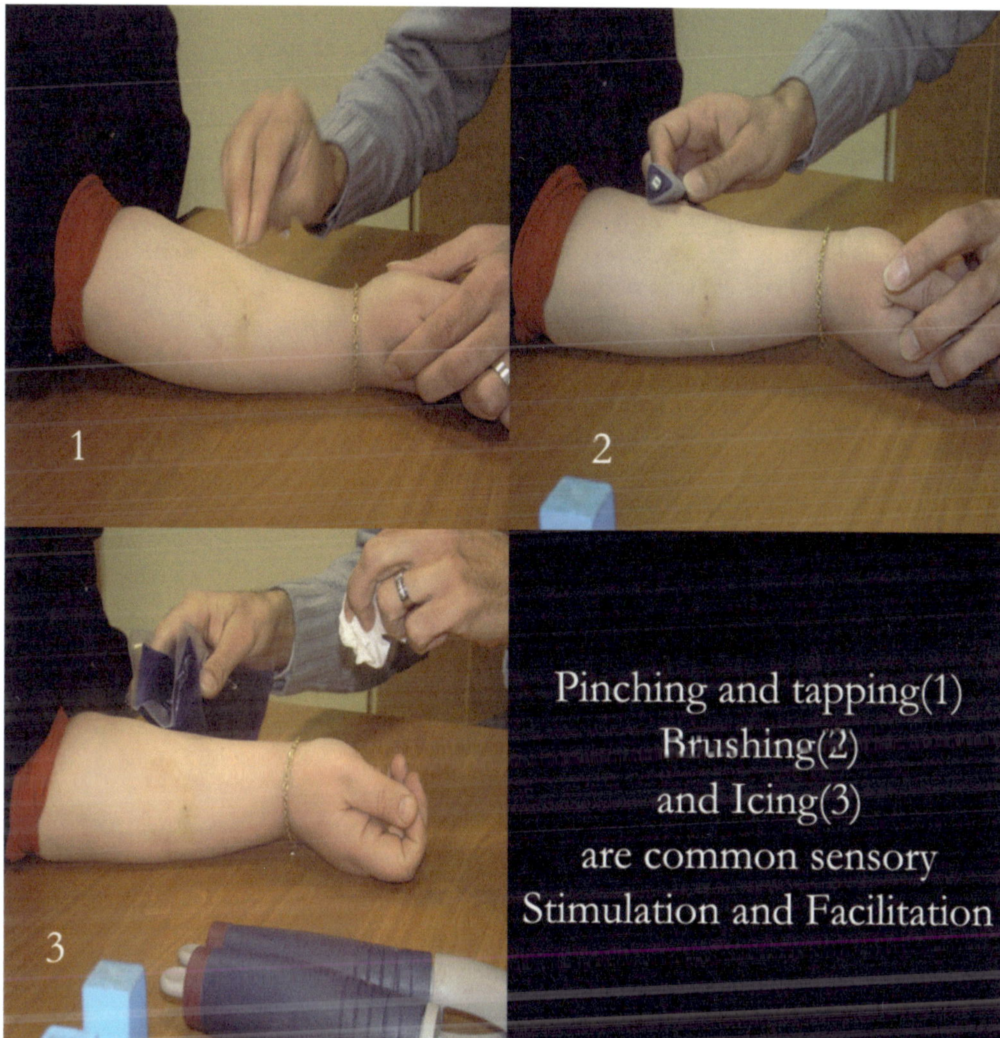

Fig. 1. Sensory stimulation and facilitation by Reza S Roghani, Rehabilitation University, Tehran, Iran

The proprioceptive sense can be sharpened through Juggling trains reaction time, spatial location, and efficient movement. Standing on a balance board is often used to retrain or increase proprioception abilities, particularly as physical therapy for ankle, knee and its nerve injuries. Advanced balance abilities which are used usually for athletes following nerve repair could be achieved by Yoga, Wing Chun and Tai-chi . There are even specific devices designed for proprioception training, such as the exercise ball, which works on balancing the abdominal and back muscles which may be impaired in nerve's root injuries. [10, 11]

7. Muscle weakness

Major peripheral nerve injuries are usually leading to severe muscle atrophy and significant functional deficits. The neuromuscular junction undergoes significant changes after nerve injury and is the most critical point for functional recovery even after proper nerve regeneration .[12] Several methods are proposed for functional recovery and prevent muscle wasting. One of them is electrical stimulation which has a great controversy regarding beneficial effects in nerve regrowth [13] or diminish the speed and accuracy of reinnervation. [14] Another modality, is low level laser therapy or phototherapy which has promising effects in nerve re growth.[15] Muscle care following nerve injury is essential and includes protection against cold and heat exposures, minor trauma and overstretching by gravity. The key point is keeping muscles in a normal physiological length to prevent vascular and lymphatic stasis, contractures, and joint stiffness. Modalities which have significant role to achieve above goals are warmth, massage and passive movements, bandaging, ultrasound therapy, hydrotherapy and splints.

Static and detachable splints [fig2] is useful mechanical devices to give rest to the paralyzed muscles and joints, preventing overstretching and shortening and to allow exercises and other therapeutic methods to be given regularly for preventing complications of continued immobilization.[16]

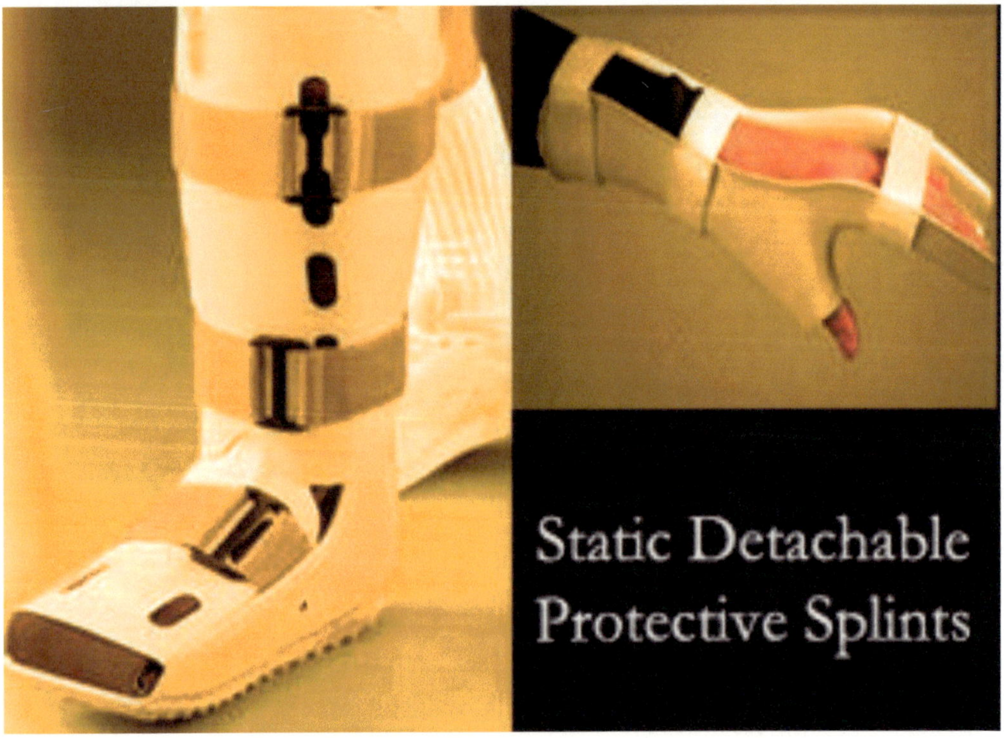

Fig. 2. Static and detachable splints by Reza S Roghani, Rehabilitation University, Tehran, Iran

8. Loss of function

Functional loss is a direct effect of sensory and motor deficit following nerve injury. cortical sensory synaptic changes due to miss stimulation of peripherals, starting immediately after nerve injury leads to remapping of central sensory system makes re learning and proper functional recovery difficult. New trends in nerve injury rehabilitation focus on manipulation of central nervous processes rather than peripheral factors. Using the brain capacity for Visio-tactile and audio-tactile interaction and fine motor relearning [fig3] is the main concept for maintaining sensory cortex and periphery relationship in the initial phase following nerve injury and repair. After initiation of nerve re-growth, anesthesia of intact peripheral skin with topical agents especially during sensory relearning sessions is a new method to prevent early changes until sensory recovery completes and relearning process made possible. [17, 18] another issue in proper functional recovery is neuromuscular junction instability immediately after denervation which is hard to stabilized properly even after repair and complete regeneration. It is more present in more complex and fine tasks. Rehabilitation protocols that focus on relearning programs of fine tasks address this issue and increase the chance of functional outcome improvement after nerve repair. [18]

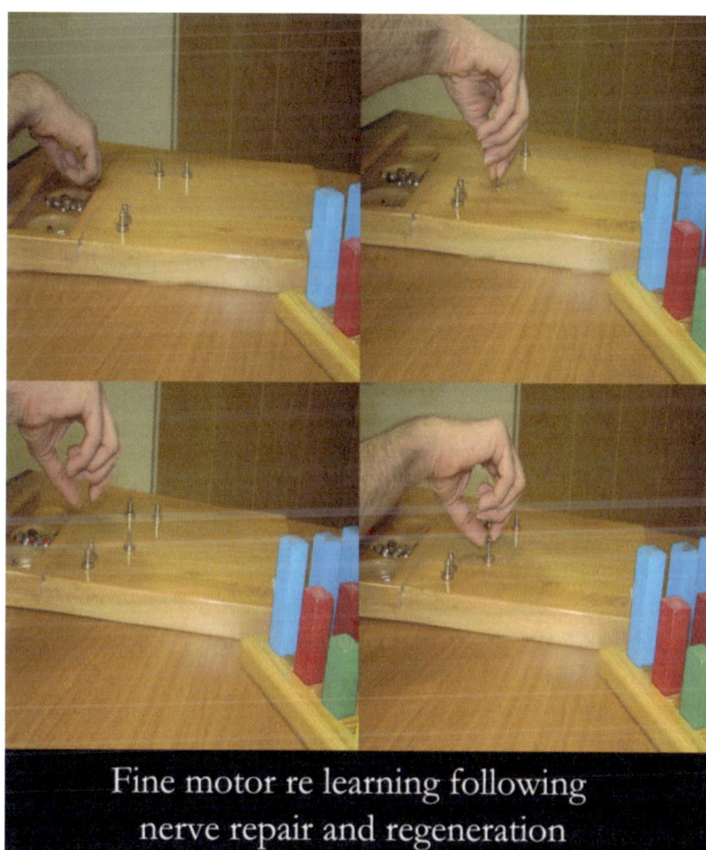

Fig. 3. Fine motor re learning following nerve repair and regeneration by Reza S Roghani, Rehabilitation University, Tehran, Iran

9. Joint stiffness

The insensitive joints and ligaments and other surrounding tissues which are affected by the injury to all or some supplying nerves are at the risk of stiffness, shortening and finally contracture. Regular daily massage, passive motion in full range at least one time per day and protective detachable static splints could prevent these complications. In case of joint stiffness dynamic splints and physical modalities such as ultrasound and laser [Fig4] will help to regain the softening and range of motion. [19]

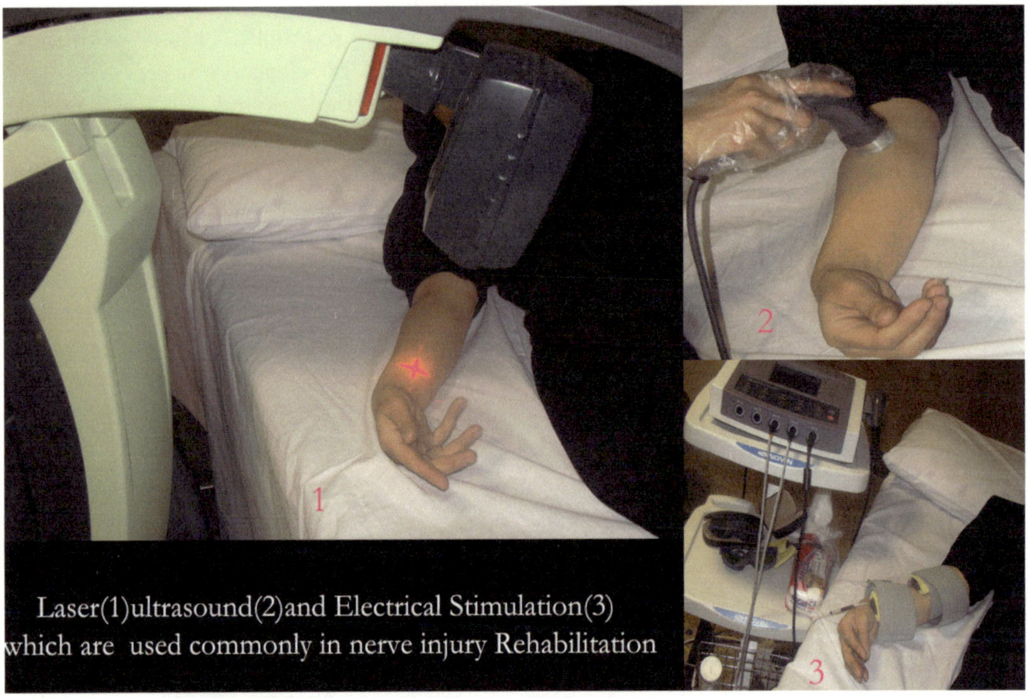

Fig. 4. Common modalities in nerve injury rehabilitation by Reza S Roghani, Rehabilitation University, Tehran, Iran

10. Care of denervated skin

Proper hot and sharp objects handling, take care of nails, avoiding long term cold weather exposure, and well padded splints use are the corner stone of denervated skin care. Skin also should be cleaned with mild soap and warm water and gently patted dry. Locations is vulnerable to excess moisture can be protected with talcum powder and too dry area should have lotion applied. Direct or using a mirror for daily skin inspection is important to identify vulnerable areas for sores such as high pressure points under splints.[20]

11. Emotional stress

Severe pain and paralysis accompanying nerve injury usually lead to cognitive problem; sleep disorder and anxiety reduce quality of life and hamper efficient medical treatment. [21] Alteration of extracellular glycine concentration in related spinal cord and brain cortex develop mechanical hypersensitivity after peripheral nerve injury may exhibit impaired recognition ability and may be the main mechanism of long lasting pain and a source of emotional stress. If it is not addressed properly and as soon as possible it may lead to chronic hippocampal plasticity and develop chronic pain.[22] Cognitive rehabilitation programs would address mood disturbance, enhance functional outcome and also prevent or decline chronic pain following nerve injury and repair. [23]

12. References

[1] Campbell, W.W., *Evaluation and management of peripheral nerve injury.* Clinical Neurophysiology, 2008. 119: p. 1951-1965.

[2] Sunderland, S., *A classification of peripheral nerve injuries producing loss of function.* Brain, 1951. 74: p. 491-516.

[3] Seddon, H., *Three types of nerve injuries.* Brain, 1943. 66: p. 237.

[4] Hökfelt, T., et al., eds. *Central consequences of peripheral nerve.* Neuropathic pain. 2005.

[5] Baron, R., A. Binder, and G. Wasner, *Neuropathic pain: diagnosis, pathophysiological mechanisms, and treatment.* Lancet Neurol, 2010. 9(8): p. 807-19.

[6] Selph, S., et al., *Drug Class Review: Neuropathic Pain.* 2011.

[7] O'Connor, A.B. and R.H. Dworkin, *Treatment of neuropathic pain: an overview of recent guidelines.* Am J Med, 2009. 122(10 Suppl): p. S22-32.

[8] Yameen, F., et al., *Efficacy of transcutaneous electrical nerve stimulation and its different modes in patients with trigeminal neuralgia.* J Pak Med Assoc, 2011. 61(5): p. 437-9.

[9] Mosby, *properioception* 8th edition ed. Medica Dictionary. 2009: elsevier.

[10] Salsabili, H., et al., *Dynamic stability training improves standing balance control in neuropathic patients with type 2 diabetes.* J Rehabil Res Dev, 2011. 48(7): p. 775-86.

[11] Bullinger, K.L., et al., *Permanent central synaptic disconnection of proprioceptors after nerve injury and regeneration. II. Loss of functional connectivity with motoneurons.* J Neurophysiol, 2011. 106(5): p. 2471-85.

[12] Kang, J.R., D.P. Zamorano, and R. Gupta, *Limb salvage with major nerve injury: current management and future directions.* J Am Acad Orthop Surg, 2011. 19 Suppl 1: p. S28-34.

[13] Gordon, T., O.A. Sulaiman, and A. Ladak, *Chapter 24: Electrical stimulation for improving nerve regeneration: where do we stand?* Int Rev Neurobiol, 2009. 87: p. 433-44.

[14] Gigo-Benato, D., et al., *Electrical stimulation impairs early functional recovery and accentuates skeletal muscle atrophy after sciatic nerve crush injury in rats.* Muscle Nerve, 2011. 41(5): p. 685-93.

[15] Rochkind, S., S. Geuna, and A. Shainberg, *Chapter 25: Phototherapy in peripheral nerve injury: effects on muscle preservation and nerve regeneration.* Int Rev Neurobiol, 2009. 87: p. 445-64.

[16] Campbell, W.W., *Evaluation and management of peripheral nerve injury.* Clin Neurophysiol, 2008. 119(9): p. 1951-65.

[17] Rosen, B. and G. Lundborg, *Sensory re-education after nerve repair: aspects of timing.* Handchir Mikrochir Plast Chir, 2004. 36(1): p. 8-12.

[18] Lundborg, G. and B. Rosen, *Hand function after nerve repair.* Acta Physiol (Oxf), 2007. 189(2): p. 207-17.

[19] Krosl, W., *[To treat or prevent joint stiffness. (Problem of organization)].* Riv Infort Mal Prof, 1961. 48: p. 83-9.

[20] Dealey, C., *Skin care and pressure ulcers.* Advances in Skin & Wound Care, 2009. 22.

[21] Novak, C.B., et al., *Biomedical and psychosocial factors associated with disability after peripheral nerve injury.* J Bone Joint Surg Am, 2011. 93(10): p. 929-36.

[22] Kodama, D., H. Ono, and M. Tanabe, *Increased hippocampal glycine uptake and cognitive dysfunction after peripheral nerve injury.* Pain, 2011. 152(4): p. 809-17.

[23] Mahmoudaliloo, M., et al., *The correlation of cognitive capacity with recovery of hand sensibility after peripheral nerve injury of upper extremity.* NeuroRehabilitation, 2011. 29(4): p. 373-9.

15

Median and Ulnar Nerves Traumatic Injuries Rehabilitation

Rafael Inácio Barbosa, Marisa de Cássia Registro Fonseca, Valéria Meirelles Carril Elui, Nilton Mazzer and Cláudio Henrique Barbieri
University of São Paulo
Brazil

1. Introduction

Peripheral nerves are structures that suffer injuries similar to those seen in other tissues, resulting in important motor and sensory disabilities. It is estimated that the incidence of traumatic lesions is as high as 500.000 cases per year in some countries, where 2,8% of the patients become permanently disabled due to prolonged nerve regeneration time (Noble et al., 1998; Rodrígues et al., 2004)

Injuries to the peripheral nerve system can cause significant motor and sensory changes, which are classified, by Seddon, as neuropraxis, axonotmesis, and neurotmesis (Fonseca et al., 2006; Lundborg, 2000; Novak & Mackinnon, 2005).

The causes of peripheral nerve system injuries include cutting wounds, firearm lesions, injuries due to temperature changes, prolonged or acute compressions, mechanical traction, infectious and toxic causes. There are also different injuries mechanisms such as laceration, avulsion, section, stretching, compression and crushing. These injuries can damage the tissue integrity, causing important dysfunctions in the innervated structures of the damaged nerve, with consequent changes in the nerve pathway and axonal transport (Dahlin, 2004; Marcolino et al., 2008; Sulaiman & Gordon, 2000).

2. Median and ulnar nerve injuries

The traumatic transaction of median or ulnar nerve in the hand usually results in impairment of function and represents a major problem for the patient. Traffic accidents and glass injury are common causes of fracture or tendon and nerves lacerations in young people (Fonseca et al., 2006).

Median nerve injury can cause palsy disfunction in thenar muscles and sensitive alteration of thumb, 2nd and 3rd fingers and radial portion of anular finger.

At wrist level can be affected the following muscles: abductor pollicis brevis, superficial portion of brevis flexor of the thumb, opponents and 1st and 2nd lumbricals, and can cause the fingers claw. When more proximal lesions occurs (arm, elbow or cervical area) extrinsic muscles are also involved as: flexor pollicis longus, radial portion of profundus fingers flexors, superficiallis fingers flexors, pronators, flexor radiallis carpi and palmar longus. Such alterations can lead to a manipulative dysfunction of small and greater objects. (Colli et al., 2003).

Ulnar nerve injuries cause palsy and hypotrophy in intrinsic hand muscles, palmar and dorsal interosseous, ulnar fingers lumbricals, hypothenar eminency, thumb adutor and thumb flexor brevis profundus, which results in a deformity characterized as ulnar claw hand (Figure 1). A typical deformity at 5th finger in hyperabduction can also be present what usually happens because of the imbalance between intrinsic and extrinsic muscles. Hypoesthesia or anesthesia can be present at the 4th and 5th fingers. In proximal lesions, the muscles ulnar carpi flexor and profundus flexor of 4th and 5th fingers are affected. The most incapacity in that case is the reduction in grip strength. This is mainly attributed to failure in fingers abduction, damaging circumduction of a object in the act of prehension. The inefficiency action of the adductor muscles of the thumb also hinders the pinch execution (Pereira et al., 2003).

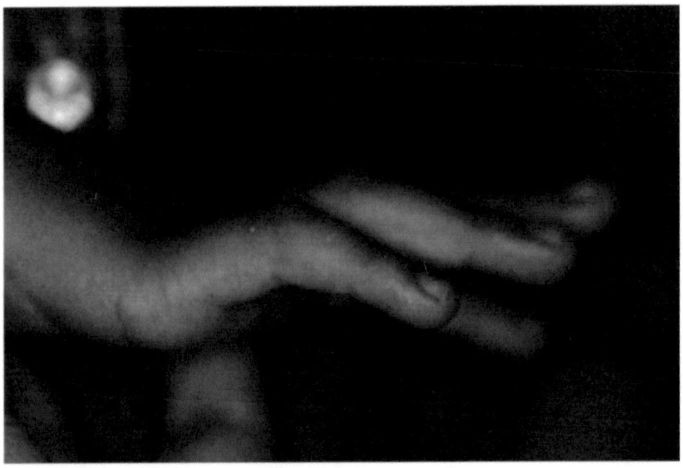

Fig. 1. Ulnar claw hand in patient with ulnar nerve injury.

3. Physical and functional assessment

Through standardized assessment and analysis of physical disability, therapists and surgeons seek to determine the quality of results after surgery or to schedule and monitor the rehabilitation process in any disease, such as a traumatic nerve injury or compression syndrome, for example, thereby allowing, comparisons between different groups of patients (Amadio, 2001; Gianini, 2007; Macdermid, 2011). New protocols have been developed and validated regarding evaluation items related to symptoms, dysfunction, disability and quality of life related to a disease, based on the World Health Organization concept. (Padua et al., 2007).

An early accurate diagnosis in all peripheral nerve injury is essential to determine the prognosis and treatment plan, which could be surgical or conservative.

In some cases are necessary complementary exams like images searching for nerve structures pathological alterations. To evaluate only the anatomy of the nervous structures, sometimes resulting in false-negative or false-positive diagnosis. In order to have a more accurate diagnosis and obtain more reliable information about the location, severity and prognosis of peripheral nerve injury, is fundamental to perform an electroneuromyography exam. This exam is a type of electrodiagnostic that investigate the existence of any alterations in the motor unit or in its components.

Sensory and motor hand assessment after a complex hand injury are made by several methods and tools (Aulicino, 2002; Bell-krotoski & Buford, 1997; Byl et al., 2002; Dannenbaum et al., 2002; Davis et al., 1999; Fess, 1995, 2011; Hagander et al., 2000; Jerosch-Herold, 2005; Lundborg & Rosén, 2007; Macey et al., 1995; Novak, 2001; Patel & Bassin, 1999; Polatkan et al., 1998; Rosén, 1996; Rosén & Lundborg, 2000; Rosén & Lundborg, 2001; Roséntal et al., 2000).

The Semmes-Weinstein monofilaments (Figure 2) are objective and semi-quantitative measurement instruments for assessment the skin peripheral innervations. It is considered a test of sensory threshold that evaluate the group of slowly adapting fibers. It is easy to apply, providing the mapping of sensory dermatomes, and can be used with reliability and repeatability. (Bell-Krotoski, 2002; Bell-Krotoski, 2011).

The two points discrimination test (2PD) (Figure 2) evaluates the density of reinnervation of large myelinated fibers of the skin receptors, through a pressure-specific sensory device (Aszmann & Dellon, 1998). This test correlates with nerve conduction velocity, although this depends on several factors such as age (Kaneko et al., 2005) and should be accompanied by a description of how the test was performed to quantify the tactile discrimination, in association of others tests (Jerosch-Herold, 2000; Jerosch-Herold, 2003; Lundborg & Rosén, 2004).

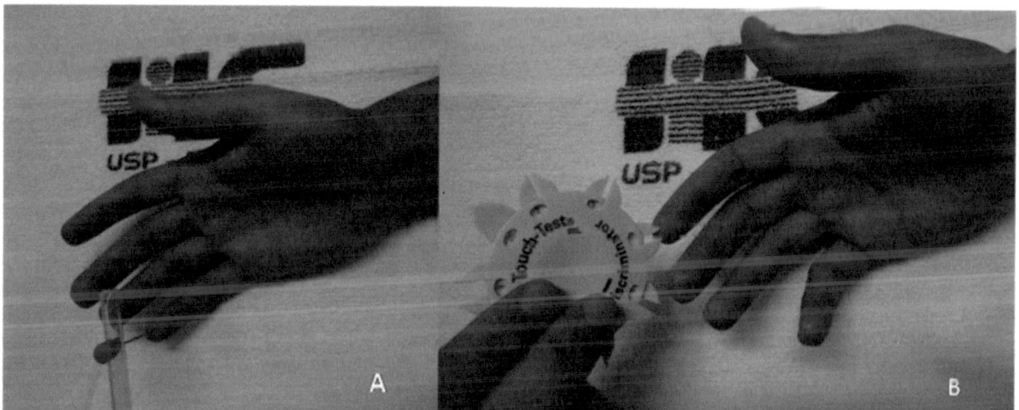

Fig. 2. Sensation assessment: Semmes-Weinstein monofilaments (A) and two points discrimination test (B)

The prehension and pinch muscle strength are evaluated using the Jamar™ and Pinch Gauge™ dynamometer. The nominal value of isometric force is measured in kilograms, and the examined limb position follows the norms established by the American Association of Hand Surgery and the American Association of Hand Therapists (Abdalla & Brandão, 2005). Manual muscle testing is also useful in motor nerve recovery evaluation (Macdermid, 2005).

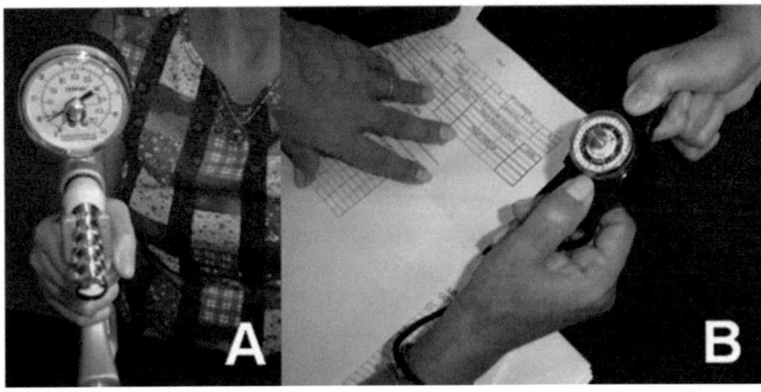

Fig. 3. The Jamar™ (A) and Pinch Gauge™ (B) dynamometers.

Nerve repair is a specific situation that needs a specific available scale relating activity and participation allied with motor, sensation and discomfort dysfunction (Macdermid, 2005).

Rosén et al. (1996) in their study highlighted four aspects in the recovery of hand function after a nerve injury, the more effective tests and its correlation with function. Through the calculating of data collection from various evaluation items in median or ulnar nerve injury in adults, an index called Rosén Score was validated (Rosén, 2000, 2003). It comprises several items divided into three areas: sensory, motor and pain/discomfort. These are related to pain sensitivity, motor function, muscle strength, function and identification of shapes and textures.

These include mapping of sensory threshold that is accomplished through the use of the technique of esthesiometry on key points of sensory dermatomes related to nerves evaluated. The assessment of tactile gnosis is made by the Weber Disk Discriminator™ (D2P), the shape and texture identification through the STI-test™ (Figure 4) (Rosén et al., 1998, 2000, 2003).

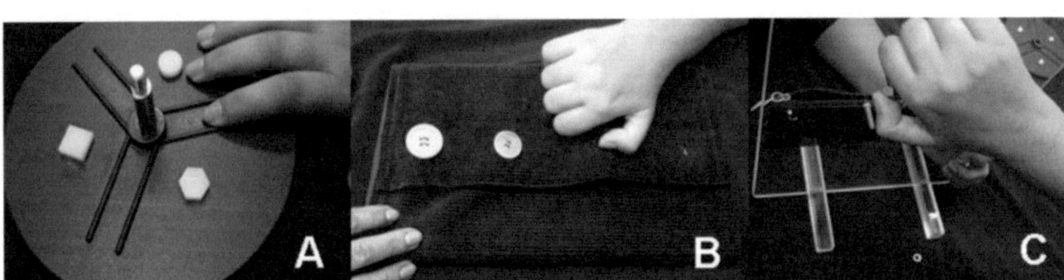

Fig. 4. The STI-test™, developed and validated for the identification of shapes and textures (A), Some itens off Sollerman test to evaluate the sensory integration motor function (B and C).

For the motor area, maximal isometric grip and pinch of the fingers are evaluated with the use of isometric grip strength using the Jamar™ and Pinch Gauge™ and functional manual muscle test is applied for palmar abduction, radial abduction of the second digit and adduction and abduction fifth digit (Brandsma et al., 1995).

The pain and cold discomfort are analyzed using a specific scale. To evaluate the sensory integration and motor function are applied four issues from Sollerman test (Figure 4)

(Sollerman & Ejeskär, 1995). Thus, through this index is possible to monitor the progress of each patient after a specific rehabilitation process.

The esthesiometry test and identification of texture and shape test (STI-test™) have psychometric properties evaluated and quantified and are considered tests with standardized criteria (Rosén & Lundborg, 1998; Rosén, 2003; Jerosch-Herold, 2005).

The assessment of disability, progression, symptom relief and functional improvement due to disease or trauma remains a challenge. Several tools have been developed, either for dysfunction or for specific body segment analysis (Amadio, 2001, Heras-Palou et al., 2003; Macdermid, 2002, 2011a, 2011b).

The DASH questionnaire (Disabilities of the Arm, Shoulder and Hand) was developed in a multidisciplinary effort, based on questionnaires previously tested and is clinically useful for the entire upper limb in relation to their function. It is used for evaluation of single or multiple disorders. It is a disability questionnaire with 30 items related to activities of daily living, social integration, work and leisure. This questionnaire evaluates symptoms and physical function, with five response options for each item, totalizing 100 points. The higher the value, the greater the dysfunction (Beaton et al., 2001). This questionnaire is validated for several countries (Padua et al. 2003; Macdermid et al., 2004; Orfale et al., 2005; Themistocleous et al.,2006).

The evaluation process starts in the first visit but need to be repeated by times. It is crucial because can give the therapist the actual status of the regeneration process and prognosis but more than that, helps the therapist to educate the patient in a way he/she can understand what is happening and can occurs, give them a feedback, motivation and also a evidence bases for the therapist to change the treatment plan. It is a long rehabilitation period and the patient education is one of the keys for success and the focus must be in nerve regeneration process and brain interaction bringing the patient into his treatment and responsible for his rehabilitation.

4. Rehabilitation after peripheral nerve repair in the hand

The traumatic transection of median or ulnar nerve in the hand usually results in function impairment and represents a major problem for the patient. It can cause different levels of motor and sensitive dysfunction, as protective sensation, tactil discrimination, pain, disestesia, cold intolerance and uncoordinated grip strength. (Novak, 2001; Lundborg, 2000, Lundborg & Rosén, 2007). This kind of injury is common in the upper extremity of young male (Noble et al. , 1998).

The use of exercises post-immobilization period aim recover the motion and muscle function lost during the phase of immobilization. For example, with a low median and/or ulnar nerve repair, usually the wrist is positioned in flexion during the immobilization period and the patient may have restricted wrist flexion when permitted to begin exercises. Exercises are directed at gradually recovering of wrist extension and all fingers movement, generally starting with active range of motion (ROM). Passive and active-assisted ROM exercises are introduced depending on the patient´s progress as well as on specific precautions relevant to the individual cases.

In recovery phase, before an evidence of muscle reinnervation, passive exercises are important to maintain joint ROM and muscle-tendon length.

The motor retraining begins at the earliest evidence of muscle reinervation and progressive resistive exercise is also used to increase strength and endurance in muscle. Key exercises for median nerve injury involve the tenar intrinsic muscles and finger abduction an adduction exercises are key with ulnar nerve injury and also the intrinsic plus exercise.

The use of splints in peripheral-nerve injury to the hand, follow some principles like: to keep the denervated muscles from remaining in an overstreched position; to prevent a joint stiffness; the development of strong movement substitution patterns and to maximize functional use of the hand (Colditz, 2002).

The goal in splinting a low lesion of ulnar nerve is to prevent a overstretching of the denervated intrinsic muscles of ring and little fingers. Any splint that blocks the MP joints in slight flexion prevent de claw deformity by forcing the extrinsic extensor to transmit force into the dorsal hood mechanism of the finger (Figure 5). High ulnar palsy lesions are commonly a result of trauma at or above de elbow and cause the palsy in flexor digitorum profundi associated with a absence of the all intrinsic muscles of the ring and little fingers. For this reason, clawing in the high ulnar nerve lesion is rarely present (Colditz, 2002).

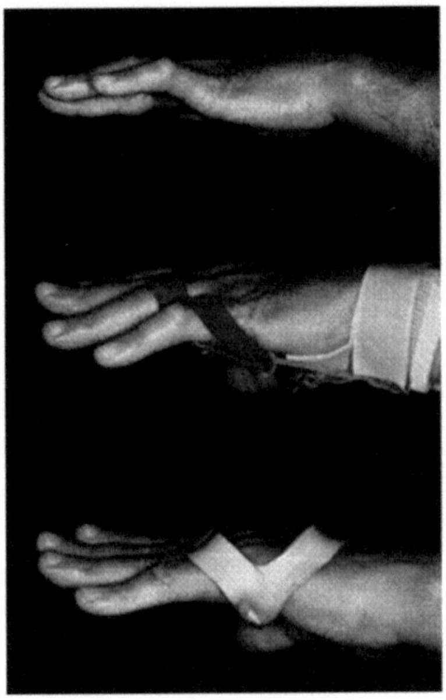

Fig. 5. Examples of splints for ulnar claw hand, whit blocks hyperextension of the metacarpophalangeal joints and allows full flexion off all fingers joints.

The deformity of the median nerve injury occurs with the flattening of the thenar eminence, with the thumb next to the palm of the hand, resulting in loss of opposition and palmar abduction. The goal of splinting is the maintenance of the first space, placing the thumb in palmar abduction and the indicator in opposition that could be indicated for night time (A) and promote function use of the hand during the day time (B) (Figure 6).

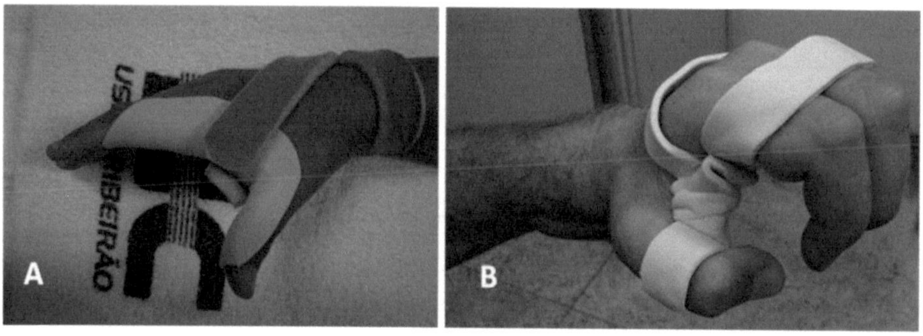

Fig. 6. Example of splint for median nerve injury (A) and median/ulnar nerve injury (B).

The number and type of regenerate nervous fibers as well the new connections after reparation or nerve reconstruction are quite different as original. The same stimuli will generate confusing sensorial impulses, sometimes painful or hard to interpret (Dellon, 1982, 1997). In consequence of axonal growth to other directions than original and due to remapping of cortical representation, the hand "talks another language to the brain", being necessary a time for sensory re-education in order to regain functional sensation as described, Dellon (1982) and Callahan (1990).

According to these programs the stimulation are started only when some return of sensitivity of the hand happens, usually several months after suture (Dellon, 1997). However, when evaluating recovery of tactile gnosis, which is the ability to discriminate objects, the result is disappointing (Fonseca et al. 2003; Rosén & Lundborg, 2001). One reason for these bad results is the long absence of sensitivity that allows a disfunctional reorganization and change in the cortical map of the hand in the brain.

Sensory re education is a process of reprogramming the brain trough a new learning process with progressive challenges, exploring the aid of vision trough exercises with opened and closed eyes. (Lundborg, 2000; Lundborg & Rosén, 2007). The proposed alternative sensory stimuli feed the somatosensory cortex and is essential to preserve the cortical map of the hand and to facilitate sensory recovery. (Rosén & Lundborg, 2003).

Changes in cerebral cortex starts early after the lesion resulting in overlapping of adjacent cortical areas in response to absence of stimuli in injury nerve representation area. (Lundborg, 2000). In the early post-operative phase, mechanoreceptors in the hand, as well the cerebral cortex are intact, but functional properties of the communication system and peripheral nerve are lost (Lundborg, 1988). So, in case of absence of peripheral stimuli, a week is sufficient to alter neighboring cortical areas (Lundborg, 2000).

Several studies describe physiologic changes after peripheral nerve injury and its consequences in short and long term showed that relearning process is facilitated by sensory re-education programs (Lundborg, 2000; Dellon, 1982, 1997; Rosén & Lundborg, 2000).

Monkey experiments demonstrated that tasks executed by hands or even by the observation of other actions performed can activate pre-motor cortex neurons (Di Pellegrino et al, 1992; Di Pellegrino, Wise, 1993; Rizzolatti et al., 2001). Another study in humans through cortical image reveled that tactile hand stimulation activates areas of somatosensorial cortex (Hansson et al., 2004).

The observation of a tactile stimuli in the hand through mirror can hypothetically active neurons in somatosensorial cortex, so early re-education helps to preserve cortical representation and reduce or inhibit cortical "bad" reorganization that could occur without interventions (Lundborg & Richard, 2003; Merzenich & Jenkins, 1993; Rosén et al., 2003; Pons et al., 1991; Buccino et al., 2004; Rizzolatti & Craighero, 2004; Rizzolatti et al., 1998).

Rosén and Lundborg (1999), reports a case using the concept of artificial sensation based in substitution touch from hearing. They used a tactile glove with microphones over the fingertips which were introduced as the patient could move his hand, with five weeks postoperatively. The microphone captured the sound produced by the manipulation of objects and then was amplified for the patient to "hear" what the injury hand feels (Rosen & Lundborg, 2003). With the same goal of preserving the cortical map, case studies were performed with the use of mirror, which was established in the fourth week after surgery, replacing the visual stimulus by touch. A mirror was placed vertically in front of the patient to reflect the full innervated hand, thus the patient would receive the stimuli with the perception that the sensitivity of the damaged hand remains intact (Rosen & Lundborg, 2005).

Besides wide literature involving new rehabilitation and surgical concepts, there is still not a single technique that ensures the full recovery of tactile discrimination of the hand of an adult after a peripheral nerve injury (Lundborg & Rosén, 2007). Therefore, new strategies for sensory re-education could be adapted to the sensory and functional recovery after repair (Lundborg & Richard, 2003).

Methods such as the mirror and the sensory glove allow sensory reeducation is started early, before some innervation is noticed. Both studies showed favorable results for early realization of stimuli to keep the cortical areas and accelerate the return of sensitivity, although further investigations are needed with larger groups of individuals (Rosen & Lundborg, 2003, 2005).

4.1 Therapeutic modalities

The use of therapeutic modalities for peripheral nerve system regeneration is currently investigated. Low-power laser (Barbosa et al., 2010a, 2010b; Marcolino et al., 2010), ultrasound (Monte Raso et al., 2005) and electric stimulation (Mendonça et al., 2003) have been used for accelerating regenerative processes in order to achieve early functional recovery.

Low-power laser has been used in several clinical and experimental research studies on peripheral nerve system injuries because it promotes microcirculation stimulus through paralysis of pre-capillary sphincters, induction of arteriolar and capillary vasodilatation, and vascular neoformation, thus leading to an increase in blood flow in the irradiated area. This procedure promotes changes in enzymatic reactions by inhibiting both synthesis of prostaglandins and release of autacoids. Low-power laser has also been employed for healing different types of tissues, because it stimulates the production of adenosine triphosphate (ATP), which enhances the cells' mitotic activity (Karu et al., 1995, 2004; Khullar et al., 1995; Kitchen & Partridge, 1991; Manteifel et al., 1997; Schindl et al., 1999). Several studies using different methodologies to assess the use of low-power laser for treating peripheral nerve system injuries are currently being carried out. The use of different laser models depends on variables such as wavelength (632–904 nm), energy, density, duration, mechanism, type of injury and its treatment. Several parameters, such as wavelength, energy density, laser pulse and potency, have been used to stimulate regeneration and accelerate functional recovery of peripheral nerves (Belchior et al., 2009; Mohammed et al., 2007; Rochkind et al., 1987; Reis et al., 2009; Walsh et al., 2000).

In general, studies on laser therapy using continuous emissions had positive outcomes for peripheral nerve regeneration. However, Bagis et al. (2003) observed no benefit from using low-power laser for nerve injuries.

The interaction between laser and molecules depends on several physical parameters and is evident in the relationship between wavelength and biological response. The activation pathways proposed for low-level laser therapy (LLLT) take into account its action on the chromophores located in the mitochondria and the cell membrane. Red light has a preferred share in the mitochondria and infrared chromophores in the cell membrane (Amat et al., 2006). Therefore, the therapeutic effects are specific, which suggests that there is the possibility of using wavelengths defined with the aim of increasing a particular biological response.

The biological action of laser radiation in the visible region of light, and its clinical application, is based on three reactions: (1) photodynamic action on membranes, accompanied by intracellular calcium increase and cell stimulation; (2) photoreactivation of Cu-Zn superoxide dismutase (SOD); and (3) photolysis of the metal complexes of nitric oxide with release of this vasodilator. It was postulated that these three effects underlie the indirect bactericidal, regenerative, and vasodilatory actions of laser radiation (Vladimirov et al., 2004). It can be considered that the improvement in motor response obtained with a wavelength of 660 nm can be related to the phenomenon of photoreactivation of cellular superoxide dismutase (Cu-Zn-SOD), observed with the helium–neon (He–Ne) laser in wound healing. Radiation of exudates with an He–Ne laser also suppressed luminescence, the laser light thus acting as catalase or superoxide dismutase. It would be natural to suggest that the activity of catalase or superoxide dismutase in exudates was initially reduced under some conditions and that laser radiation reactivated one of those enzymes (Romm et al., 1986). It should be noted that both enzymes absorb at the He–Ne laser wavelength of 633 nm.

Another well studied activity, which might be related to the results, is associated with the production of ATP. In animal cells the sodium–potassium (Na+ K+ gradient controls cell volume, drives the active transport of sugars and amino acids, and renders nerve and muscle cells electrically excitable. The fact that more than one-third of the ATP consumed by an animal at rest is used to operate this pump underscores the importance of this mechanism (Pedersen & Carafoli, 1987). It must be considered that cytochrome-c oxidase is the photoreceptor in the red region of the spectrum and is responsible for activating the synthesis of ATP and, consequently, cell metabolism (Manteifel & Karu, 2005). The ability of the cell to have a greater energy intake during the repair process might be related to the better response observed in the group treated with laser 660 nm, since the mitochondria selectively absorb that wavelength. Visible wavelengths (632.8 nm) are reported to increase the activity of Na+-K+ ATPase in erythrocytes (Kilanczyk et al., 2002). In cells that do have mitochondria, the operation of the Na+-K+ ATPase without ATP due to irradiation in concrete cellular metabolic states will lead to an increase in cellular ATP concentration, and, therefore, ATP synthesis will stop. This hypothesis is supported by the experimental observation that the substance that blocks the Na+-K+ ATPase stops mitochondrial respiration by increasing cellular ATP concentration (Karu et al., 2004). The authors also mention that nitric oxide is associated with stimulation of mitochondria biogenesis, increased microcirculation and apoptosis. Bolognani et al. (1992) found that myosin ATPase previously inactivated by carbon dioxide (CO2) gas could be partially reactivated after irradiation with He-Ne (632.8 nm). In this context, it is suggested that increased mitochondrial ATP might have promoted a more restorative response in the peripheral nerve, thus enabling better functional recovery.

Morphological changes in the mitochondria of lymphocytes were also observed after radiation with red laser, as well as the proliferation of mononuclear cells, responses that might be beneficial in the process of tissue repair (Gulsoy et al., 2006; Karu, 1992).

For all effects presented, the use of low-power laser should be considered in case of injuries of the peripheral nervous system.

Is well known nowadays that physical agents like electricity, magnetic field and ultrasound may positively influence the outcome of the healing process of different tissues like skin, bone, muscles and tendons and peripheral nerves (Brighton, 1981; Mendonça et al., 2003; Pomeranz et al., 1984).

Ultrasound have been studied in the area of enhancing recovery after peripheral nerve injury: 1) reducing pain and improving function with entrapment neuropathies, and 2) facilitating regeneration. Regarding the therapeutic ultrasound, the first investigations were addressed only at the alterations induced in the conduction velocity of the ulnar and radial superficial sensory nerves, with the demonstration that conduction velocity increases or decreases depending on the intensity and period of ultrasound application, a fact attributed to the thermal or mechanical effects of the ultrasound (Farmer, 1986; Halle et al., 1981; Moore et al., 2000). Despite the wide use of therapeutic ultrasound to treat a wide variety of pathologic conditions of the musculoskeletal system, very little is known about its effects upon damaged peripheral nerves. However, some evidence has been produced that peripheral nerves somehow respond to ultrasound irradiation, although the results of previous investigations were somewhat inconclusive, particularly in what refers to the application in humans.

Lowdon et al.. (1988) investigated the role of therapeutic ultrasound irradiation in the regeneration of the tibial nerve of rats following a compression lesion, using continuous irradiation (1 MHz, 0.5 and 1 W/cm^2, 1 min application, three times a week, 2–3 weeks) over the lesion site, and demonstrated that the conduction velocity recovered significantly earlier with the intensity of 0.5 W/cm^2 and significantly later with the intensity of 1 W/cm^2, as compared to non-irradiated nerves. They concluded that irradiation with low intensity therapeutic ultrasound can improve regeneration of a peripheral nerve with a compressive lesion, but a delayed regeneration can result from high intensity irradiation. A similar effect was demonstrated in rats whose sciatic nerve was submitted to a crush injury at its midportion followed by irradiation with therapeutic ultrasound of different intensity, frequency and duration, applied three times a week for 1 month. Regeneration of the nerve was enhanced with 0.25 W/cm^2 intensity and 2.25MHz frequency (Mourad et al., 2001).

Authors showed that ultrasound intensities as low as 0.5 W/cm^2 would be enough to accelerate regeneration of the tibial nerve after a limited lesion (moderate compression) in rats but such a low intensity would probably be useless in humans. They also suggested that nerve reaction to ultrasound would be different in damaged and intact nerves, the former being more sensitive and susceptible to the induced thermal conduction, probably the actual agent of regeneration. They were unable to suggest any other mechanism of action of the ultrasound.

There are some evidences that regeneration of the peripheral nerves can be accelerated by electric stimulation and a number of experimental studies have shown that the first signs of regeneration begin to appear by the third postoperative week and continue to happen for up to 90 days. Authors are unanimous to state that such low intensity has beneficial effect upon peripheral nerves regeneration. Although neither the intensity suggested nor the material used to make the electrodes vary from one to another. There is a controversy regarding to current intensity. Some authors used a very low current of up to 1.5 mA (Beveridge and Politis, 1988; Kerns et al., 1987, 1991; Politis et al., 1988a, 1988b; Pomeranz et al., 1984; Shen and Zhu, 1995), while others used 10 mA (McDevitt et al., 1987; Roman et al., 1987; Pomeranz & Campbell, 1993) or higher (Kerns et al., 1986, with 10 mA/cm^2). One study used rat femoral nerve model supported a continuous electrical stimulation proximal to the site of repair for accelerating axonal growth (Al-Majed et al., 2000).

5. Conclusion

Despite advances in surgical techniques over time, several cellular events and favorable clinical status should be linked and coordinated so that nerve regeneration occurs with success. In clinical practice, it's observed that the recovery of motor and sensory function still represents a challenge to reconstructive surgery and rehabilitation.

Regarding the hand sensation recovery, various sensorial re-education strategies have been introduced in the rehabilitation process with the aim of enhance patient capacity to reinterpret altered sensory stimuli due to injury sustained in the hand.

Rehabilitation is based on exercise therapy, splints and neuroplasticity principles.

This concept aim to facilitate sensory integration with the cortex area and promotes an interaction between tactile, visual and auditive stimuli, therefore represents an important tool in order to optimize sensory re-education strategies and maximize preservation of the hand's cortical map representation in the early phase following injury.

Furthermore, the use of therapeutic modalities for peripheral nerve system regeneration is currently investigated. Low-power laser, ultra-sound, and electric stimulation have been used for accelerating regenerative processes in order to achieve early functional recovery.

6. Acknowledgment

This project had financial support from the FAEPA – Hospital das Clínicas da Faculdade de Medicina de Ribeirão Preto, Brazil.

7. References

Abdalla, L. M.; Brandão, M. C. F. Forças de preensão palmar e da pinça digital. In: Recomendações para avaliação do membro superior. 2. ed. Joinville: Sociedade Brasileira de Terapia da Mão, 2005. cap. 6, p. 38-41.

Al-Majed AA, Meumann CM, Brushart TM, Gordon T. Brief electrical stimulation promotes the speed and accuracy of motor axonal regeneration. J Neurosci. 2000;20:2602–8.

Amat A, Rigau J, Waynant RW, Ilev IK, Anders JJ (2006) The electric field induced by light can explain cellular responses to electromagnetic energy: a hypothesis of mechanism. J Photochem Photobiol B 82:152–60

Amadio, P.C. Outcome assessment in Hand Surgery and Hand Therapy: An update. J. Hand Ther, v.14, p. 63-7, 2001.

Aszmann, O. C.; Dellon, L. Relationship between cutaneous pressure threshold and two-point discrimination. J. Reconst. Microsurg.; v.14, p. 417-421, 1998.

Aulicino, P.L. Clinical examination of the hand. In: HUNTER, J; MACKIN, E.J.; CALLAHAN, A.D. Rehabilitation of the hand and upper extremity. 5a. edição. St. Louis: Mosby, 2002. Cap. 8, 120-142.

Bagis, S.; Comelekoglu, U.; Coskun, B.; Milcan, A.; Buyukakilli, B.; Sahin, G. No effect of GA-AS (904 nm) laser irradiation on the intact skin of the injured rat sciatic nerve, Lasers in Medical Science, London, v. 18, p. 83–88, 2003.

Barbosa RI, Marcolino AM, Guirro RRJ, Mazzer N, Barbieri CH, Fonseca MCR (2010) Comparative effects of wavelengths of low-power laser in regeneration of sciatic nerve in rats following crushing lesion. Lasers Med Sci (2010) 25:423–430.

Barbosa RI, Marcolino AM, Guirro RRJ, Mazzer N, Barbieri CH, Fonseca MCR (2010) Efeito do laser de baixa intensidade (660 nm) na regeneração do nervo isquiático lesado em ratos. Fisioter Pesq. 2010, vol.17, n.4, pp. 294-299. ISSN 1809-2950.

Beaton, D.E.; Katz, J.N.; Fossel, A .H.; Wright, J.G.;Tarasuk, V.;Bombardier, C. Measuring the whole or the parts? Validity, reability, and responsiveness of the disabilities of the arm, shoulder and hand (DASH) outcome measure in different regions of the upper extremity. J.Hand Ther, v.14(2), p.128-146, 2001.

Belchior ACG, Reis FA, Nicolau RA, Silva IS, Pereira DM, Carvalho PTC (2009) Influence of laser (660 nm) on functional recovery of the sciatic nerve in rats following crushing lesion. Lasers Med Sci 24:893–899.

Bell-Krotoski, J.; Buford, W.L. The force-time relationship of clinically used sensory testing instruments. J.Hand Ther. , v. 10(4), p. 297-309, 1997.

Bell-Krotoski, J. Sensibility testing with the Semmes-Weinstein monofilaments. In: HUNTER, J; MACKIN, E.J.; CALLAHAN, A.D. Rehabilitation of the hand and upper extremity. 5a. edição. St. Louis: Mosby, 2002. Chap. 13, 194-213.

Beveridge JA, Politis MJ. Use of exogenous electrical current in the treatment of delayed lesions in peripheral nerves. Plast Reconstr Surg 1988;82(4):573 /7.

Bell-Krotoski, J. Sensibility Testing: History, Instrumentation, and Clinical Procedures. In: SKIRVEN, TM; LEE OSTERMAN, A.; FEDORCZYK, JM. ; AMADIO, PC. Rehabilitation of the hand and upper extremity. 6a. edição. St. Louis: Mosby, 2011. Chap. 11, 132-151.

Bolognani L, Cavalca M, Magnani C, Volpi N (1992) ATP synthesis catalysed by myosin ATPase: effect of laser and e.m. field. Laser Technol 2:115–120

Brandsma, J.W.; Schreuders, T.A.R.; Birke, J.A.; Piefer, A. Oostendorp, R. Manual muscle strength testing: Intraobserver and interobserver reliabilities for the intrinsic muscles of the hand. J. Hand Ther. , v. 8. p 185-190, 1995.

Brighton CT. Current concepts review of the treatment of non-unions with electricity. J Bone Joint Surg 1981;63A:847–51.

Buccino G, Vogt S, Ritzl A, et al. Neural circuits underlying imitation learning of hand actions: an event-related FMRI study. Neuron. 2004;42:323–334.

Bucher, C. A Survey of Current Hand Assessment Practice in the UK. Brit. J. Hand Ther. v.8 (3). p 102-109, 2003.

Byl, N.; Leano, J.; Cheney, L.K. The Byl- Cheney-Boczai Sensory Discriminator: rehability, validity and responsiveness for testing sterognosis. J. Hand Ther. , v. 15(4), p. 315-30, 2002.

Callahan, A.D. "Sensibility testing: clinical methods." Rehabilitation of the Hand:Hunter, J. et al, 35 edition. St. Louis-Toronto. C.V. Mosby Company, Chap 44, 1990.

Colli, B.O; Carlotti Júnior, C.G. (2003). Aspectos Gerais das Lesões Traumáticas Agudas dos Nervos Periféricos, In: *Nervos Periféricos, Diagnóstico e Tratamento Clínico e Cirúrgico,* Marcos Tatagiba, Nilton Mazzer, pp. 39-54, Revinter, ISBN - 85-7309-652-7, Rio de Janeiro.

Colditz, JC. Splinting the hand with a peripheral-nerve injury. In: Hunter, J; Mackin, E.J.; Callahan, A.D. Rehabilitation of the hand and upper extremity. 5a. edição. St. Louis: Mosby, 2002. Cap. 34, p. 622-34.

Dannenbaum, R.M.; Michaelsen, S.M.; Desrosiers, J.; Levin, M.F., Development and validation of two new sensory tests hand for patients with stroke. Clin. Rehabil. v. 16(6), p. 630-9, 2002.

Davis et al. Measuring disability of the upper extremity: a rationale supporting the use of a regional outcome measure. J.Hand Ther., v. 12(4), p. 269-74, 1999.

Dahlin LB (2004) The biology of nerve injury and repair. J Am Soc Surg Hand 4:143–155 Lasers Med Sci.

di Pellegrino, G., Fadiga, L., Fogassi, L., Gallese, V., Rizzolatti, G., 1992. Understanding motor events: a neurophysiological study. Exp. Brain Res. 91, 176– 180.

di Pellegrino G, Wise SP. 1993. Visuospatial vs. visuomotor activity in the premotor and prefrontal cortex of a primate. J. Neurosci. 13:1227–43.

Dellon AL, Jabaley ME. Reeducation of sensation in the hand following nerve suture. Clin Orthop. 1982;163:75-9.

Dellon AL, Sensory reeducation. In: Dellon AL, editor. Somatosensory testing and rehabilitation. Bethesda [MD, USA]: The American Occupational Therapy Association; 1997. p.246-93.

Farmer WC. Effect of intensity of ultrasound on conduction of motor axons. Phys Ther 1986;48.1233–7.

Fess, EE. Guidelines for evaluation assessment instruments. J Hand Ther. P. 144-148, 1995.

Fess, E.E. Documentation: essential elements of an upper extremity assessment battery. In: Hunter, J; Mackin, E.J., Callahan, A.D. Rehabilitation of the hand and upper extremity. 5a. edição. St. Louis: Mosby, 2002. Cap. 16, p. 263-284.

Fess, E.E. Functional tests. In: Skirven, Tm; Lee Osterman, A.; Fedorczyk, Jm. ; Amadio, Pc. Rehabilitation of the hand and upper extremity. 6a. edição. St. Louis: Mosby, 2011. Chap. 12, 152-162.

Fonseca MCR, Mazzer N, Barbieri CH, Elui VMC (2006) Hand trauma: retrospective study. Rev Bras Ortop 41:181–186

Fonseca MCR, Mazzer N, Barbieri CH, Elui VMC. (2003). Reeducação da Sensibilidade na Reabilitação da Mão, In: *Nervos Periféricos, Diagnóstico e Tratamento Clínico e*

Cirúrgico, Marcos Tatagiba, Nilton Mazzer, pp. 198-203, Revinter, ISBN - 85-7309-652-7, Rio de Janeiro.

Gianini, F. Quantitative Assessment of Historical and Objective Findings: A New Clinical Severity Scale of CTS. In: Luchetti, R, Amadio, P. Carpal Tunnel Syndrome. Springer, 2007. Cap 11, p. 82-88.

Gulsoy M, Ozer GH, Bozkulak O, Tabakoglu HO, Aktas E, Deniz G, Ertan C (2006) The biological effects of 632.8-nm low energy He-Ne laser on peripheral blood mononuclear cells in vitro. J Photochem Photobiol B 82:199–202

Hagander, L.G.; Midani, H. A .; Kuskowski, M.A .: Parry, G.J. Quantitative sensory testing: effect of site and skin temperature on thermal thresholds. Clin. Neurophysiol., v. 111(1), p. 17-22, 2000.

Halle JS, Scoville CR, Greathouse DG. Ultrasound's effect on conduction latency of superficial radial nerve in man. Phys Ther 1981;61:345–50.

Heras-Palou, C. Burke, F.D.; Dias, J.J.; Bindra, R. Outcome measurement in Hand Surgery: reporto f a consensus conference. Brit J hand Ther. V8 (2), p. 70-80, 2003.

Jerosch-Herold, C. Should sensory function after median nerve injury and repair be quantified using Two-point discrimination as the critical measure? Scand. J. Plast. Reconstr. Hand Surg. v.34, p.339-343, 2000.

Jerosch-Herold, C. A study of the relative responsiveness of five sensibility tests for assessment of recovery after median nerve injury and repair . J. Hand Surg [B]. v.28, p.255-260, 2003.

Jerosch-Herold, C. Assessment of sensibility after nerve injury and repair: a systematic review of evidence for validity, reliability and responsiveness of tests. J. Hand Surg [B]. v.3, p.252-264, 2005.

Kaneko, A; Asai, N; Kanda, T. The influence of age on pressure perception os Static an Moving two-point discrimination in normal subjects. J. Hand Ther. v. 18, p.421-425,2005.

Karu T (1992) Derepression of the genome after irradiation of human lymphocytes with HeNe laser. Laser Therapy 4:5– 24

Karu TI, Pyatibrat LV, Afanasyeva NI (2004) A novel mitochondrial signaling pathway activated by visible-to-near infrared radiation. Photochem Photobiol 80:366–372

Karu TI, Pyatibrat L, Kalendo G (1995) Irradiation with He-Ne laser increases ATP level in cells cultivated in vitro. J Photochem Photobiol B 27:219–33

Kerns JM, Fakhouri AJ, Weinrib HP, Freeman JA. Electrical stimulation of nerve regeneration in the rat: the early effects evaluated by a vibrating probe and electron microscopy. Neuroscience 1991;40(1):93 /107.

Kerns JM, Fakhouri AJ, Weinrib HP, Freeman JA. Effects of D.C. electrical stimulation on nerve regeneration in the rat sciatic nerve. Anat Rec 1986;214:64A.

Kerns JM, Pavkovic IM, Fakhouri AJ, Wickersham KL, Freeman JA´ . An experimental implant for applying a DC electrical field to peripheral nerve. J Neurosci Methods 1987;19:217 /23.

Kitchen SS, Partridge CJ (1991) A review of low level laser therapy, part I: background, physiological effects and hazards. Physiotherapy 77:161–163

Khullar SM, Brodin P, Fristad I, Kvinnsland IH (1999) Enhanced sensory reinnervation of dental target tissues in rats following low level laser (LLL) irradiation. Lasers Med Sci 14:177–184

Lowdon IMR, Seaber AV, Urbaniak JR. An improved method of recording rat tracks for measurement of the sciatic functional index of De Medinaceli. J Neurosci Meth 1988;24:279–81.

Lundborg G (2000) A 25-year perspective of peripheral nerve surgery: evolving neuroscientific concepts and clinical significance. J Hand Surg [Am] 25:391–414

Lundborg, G.; Rosén, B. The two point discrimination test- time for a re-appraisal? J. Hand Surg [B and E]. v.29B:5 , p.418-422, 2004.

Lundborg, G.; Rosén, B. Review: Hand function after nerve repair. Acta Physiol. , v. 189, p. 207-217, 2007.

Macdermid, Jc.; Fess, Ee.; Bell-Krotoski,J.; Cannon, Nm.; Evans, Rb.; Walsh, W.; Szabo, Rm.; Laseter, G.; Mackin, E.; Gettle,K.; Santore, G. A Research agenda for Hand Therapy. J. Hand Ther. v. 15, p.3-15,2002.

Macdermid, JC; Tottenham, V. Responsiveness of the Disability of the Arm, Shoulder, and Hand (DASH) and Patient-Rated Wrist/Hand Evaluation (PRWHE) in evaluating change in Hand Therapy. J. Hand Ther. v. 17, p.18-23,2004.

Macdermid, JC. The quality of clinical practice guidelines in Hand Therapy. J. Hand Ther. v. 17, p.200-209,2004.

Macdermid, JC. Measurements of health outcomes following tendon and nerve repair. J. Hand Ther. v. 18, p.297-312,2005.

Macdermid, JC. Outcomes measurement in upper extremity practice. In: Skirven, Tm; Lee Osterman, A.; Fedorczyk, Jm. ; Amadio, Pc. Rehabilitation of the hand and upper extremity. 6a. edição. St. Louis: Mosby, 2011. Chap. 16, 194-205.

Macdermid, JC. Evidence-based practice in Hand Rehabilitation. In: Skirven, Tm; Lee Osterman, A.; Fedorczyk, Jm. ; Amadio, Pc. Rehabilitation of the hand and upper extremity. 6a. edição. St. Louis: Mosby, 2011. Chap. 143, 1881-89.

Macey et al. Outcomes of hand surgery British Society for Surgery of the hand. J. Hand Surg. v. 20(6), p. 841-55, 1995.

Manteifel V, Bakeeva L, Karu T (1997) Ultrastructural changes in chondriome of human lymphocytes after irradiation with He-Ne laser: appearance of giant mitochondria. J Photochem Photobiol B 38:25–30

Manteifel VM, Karu TI (2005) Structure of mitochondria and activity of their respiratory chain in successive generations of yeast cells exposed to He-Ne laser light. Izv Akad Nauk Ser Biol 32:556–566

Marcolino AM; Barbosa RI; Fonseca MCR; Mazzer N; Elui VMC (2008) Physical therapy in brachial plexus injury: case report. Rev Fisioter Mov 21:53–61

Marcolino AM; Barbosa RI; Neves LS; Fonseca MCR. Laser de baixa intensidade (830 nm) na recuperação funcional do nervo isquiático de ratos. Acta ortop. bras., 2010, vol.18, no.4, p.207-211. ISSN 1413-7852

McDevitt L, Fortner P, Pomeranz B. Application of weak electric field to the hindpaw enhances sciatic motor nerve regeneration in the adult rat. Brain Res 1987;416:308/14.

Mendonça AC, Barbieri CH, Mazzer N (2003) Directly applied low intensity direct electric current enhances peripheral nerve regeneration in rats. J Neurosci Methods 129:183–190

Mohammed IFR, AL-Mustawfi NBV, Kaka LN (2007) Promotion of regenerative processes in injured peripheral nerve induced by low-level laser therapy. Photomed Laser Surg 25:107–111

Monte-raso VV, Barbieri CH, Mazzer N, Fazan VS (2005) Can therapeutic ultrasound influence the regeneration of peripheral nerves? J Neurosci Methods 142:185–192

Moore JH, Gieck JH, Saliba EN, Perrin DH, Ball DW, Mccue FC. The biophysical effects of ultrasound on median nerve distal latencies. Electromyogr Clin Neurophysiol 2000;40(3):169–80

Mourad PD, Lazar DA, Curra FP, Mohr BC, Andrus KC, Avelino AM, ET al. Ultrasound accelerates functional recovery after peripheral nerve damage. Neurosurgery 2001;48(5):1136–40.

Noble, J.; Munro, C.A.; Prasad, V.S.; Midha, R. Analysis of upper and lower extremity peripheral nerve injuries in a population of patients with multiple injuries. J Trauma, Oregon, v.45(1), p. 116-22, 1998.

Novak, C.B. Evaluation of hand sensibility: a review. J.Hand Ther. ,v.14(4), p.266-72, 2001.

Novak CB, Mackinnon SE (2005) Evaluation of nerve injury and nerve compression in the upper quadrant. J Hand Ther 18:230–240

Orfale, A. G.; Araújo, P. M. P.; Ferraz, M. B.; Natour, J. Translation into Brazilian Portuguese, cultural adaptation and evaluation of the reliability of the Disabilities of the Arm, Shoulder and Hand Questionnaire. Braz J Med Biol Res. , v.38, p. 293-302, 2005.

Padua, R; Padua, L; Ceccarelli, B; Romanini, E.; Zanoli, G.; Amadio, P.; Campi, A. Italian Version of the Disability of the Arm, Shoulder and Hand (dash) Questionnaire. Cross-Cultural Adaptation and Validation. J Hand Surg Eur Vol April 2003 v. 28 n2 p.179-186

Padua, R; Romanni, E; Bondi, R. Outcomes Assessment Protocols. In: Luchetti, R, Amadio, P. Carpal Tunnel Syndrome. Roma: Springer, 2007, Cap 50, p.383-391.

Patel,M.R. & Bassini, L. A comparison of five tests for determining hand sensibility. J. Reconstr. Microsurg., v. 15(7), p. 523-6, 1999.

Pedersen PL, Carafoli E (1987) Ion motive ATPase. I. Ubiquity, properties and significance to cell function. Trends Biochem Sci 12:146–150, 186–189

Polatkan,S: Orhun, E.; Polatkan, O; Nuzumlali, E.; Bayri, O. Evaluation of the improvement of sensibility after primary median repair at the wrist. Microsurg.; v.18(3), p. 192-6, 1998.

Pereira, CU; Carvalho, AF; Carvalho, MF. (2003). Exame Neurológico de Lesões do Nervo Periférico, In: *Nervos Periféricos, Diagnóstico e Tratamento Clínico e Cirúrgico,* Marcos Tatagiba, Nilton Mazzer, pp. 1-12, Revinter, ISBN – 85-7309-652-7, Rio de Janeiro

Politis MJ, Zanakis MF, Albala BJ. Mammalian optic nerve regeneration following the application of electric fields. J Trauma 1988a;28(11):1548/52.

Politis MJ, Zanakis MF, Albala BJ. Facilitated regeneration in the rat peripheral nervous system using applied electric field. J Trauma 1988b;28(9):1375/81.

Pomeranz B, Campbell J. Weak electric current accelerates motoneuron regeneration in the sciatic nerve of 10-month-old rats. Brain Res 1993;603:271 /8.

Pomeranz B, Mullen M, Markus H. Effect of applied electrical fields on sprouting of intact saphenous nerve in adult rat. Brain Res 1984;303:331–6.

Pons TP, Garraghty PE, Ommaya AK, Kaas JH, Taub E, Mishkin M. 1991. Massive cortical reorganization after sensory deafferentation in adult macaques. Science 252:1857–60.

Reis FA, Belchior ACG, Carvalho PTC, Silva BAK, Pereira DM, Silva IS, Nicolau RA (2009) Effects of laser therapy (660 nm) on recovery of the sciatic nerve in rats after injury through neurotmesis followed by epineural anastomosis. Lasers Med Sci 24:741–747.

Rizzolatti, G., Fogassi, L., Gallese, V., 2001. Neurophysiological mechanisms underlying the understanding and imitation of action. Nat. Rev. Neurosci. 2, 661–670.

Rizzolatti G, Luppino G, Matelli M. The organization of the cortical motor system: new concepts. Electroencephalogr Clin Neurophysiol. 1998;106:283–296.

Rizzolatti G, Craighero L (2004) The Mirror Neuron System. Annual Rev Neurosci 27:169–192.

Rochkind S, Barrnea L, Razon N, Bartal A, Schwartz M (1987) Stimulatory effect of He-Ne low dose laser on injured sciatic nerves of rats. Neurosurgery 20:843–847

Rodrígues, F.J.; Valero-Cabré, A.; Navarro, X. Regeneration and functional recovery following peripheral nerve injury. Drug Discov Today Dis Models, Amsterdam, v. 1, p. 177–185, 2004.

Roman GC, Strahlendorf HK, Coates PW, Rowley BA. Stimulation of sciatic nerve regeneration in the adult rat by low-intensity electric current. Exp Neurol 1987;98:222 /32.

Rosén, B. Recovery of sensory and motor function after nerve repair rationale for evaluation. J. Hand Ther. v.9(4), p. 315-27, 1996.

Rosén, B; Lundborg, G.; Abrahamsson, I.; Agberg, H.; Rosén, I. Sensory function after median nerve decompression in carpal tunnel syndrome. J Hand Surg. ,v.22B, p.602-606, 1997.

Rosén, B & Lundborg,G. A new tactile gnosis instrument in sensibility testing. J.Hand Ther. v.11, p. 251-257, 1998.

Rosén, B. The sensational hand (2000). Clinical assessment after nerve repair. Thesis, Lund University, pp. ISBN 91-628-4368-4360.

Rosén, B & Lundborg,G. A model instrument for the documentation of outcomes nerve repair. J.Hand Surg[Am]. v.25(3), p. 535-43, 2000.

Rosén, B & Lundborg, G. The long-term recovery curve in adults after median or ulnar nerve repair: a reference interval. J Hand Surg. ,v.26B, p.196-200, 2001.

Rosén, B & Lundborg,G. A new model instrument for outcome after nerve repair. Hand Clinics. v.19 p. 463-470, 2003.

Rosén, B. Inter-tester reliability of a Tactile Gnosis Test: The STI Test®. Brit. J. Hand Ther. v.8 p (3). 98-101, 2003.

Rosén, B; Balkenius, C; Lundborg,G. Sensory re-education today and tomorrow: a review of evolving concepts. Brit. J. Hand Ther. v.8 p (2). 48-56, 2003.

Rosental, T.L.; Beredjiklian, P.K.; Guyette, T.M.; Weiland, A .J. Intra and interobserver reliability of sensibility testing asymptomatic individuals. Ann. Plast. Surg., v. 44(6), p. 605-9, 2000.

Sollerman C, Ejeskär A. Sollerman hand functional test: a standardized method and its use in tetraplegic patients. Scand J Plast Reconstr Surg. 1995;29:167-176.

Schindl A, Schindl M, Schindl L, Jurecka W, Hönigsmann H, Breier F (1999) Increased dermal angiogenesis after low-intensity laser therapy for a chronic radiation ulcer determined by a video measuring system. J Am Acad Dermatol 40:481–484

Shen N, Zhu J. Experimental study using a direct current electrical field to promote peripheral nerve regeneration. J Reconstr Microsurg 1995;11(3):189/93.

Sulaiman OA, Gordon T (2000) Effects of short- and long-term Schwann cell denervation on peripheral nerve regeneration, myelination, and size. Glia 32:234–46

Themistocleous, G.S.; Goudelis, G; Kyrou, I.;Chloros, G.D.; Krokos, A; Galanos, A.; Gerostathopoulos, N.E.; Soucacos, P.N. Translation into Greek, Cross-cultural Adaptation and Validation of the Disabilities of the Arm, Shoulder, and Hand Questionnaire (DASH). J. Hand Therapy. v.2006 v.19 n.3 p.350-57

Vladimirov Yu A, Osipov AN, Klebanov GI (2004) Photobiological principles of therapeutic applications of laser radiation. Biochemistry 69:81–90

Walsh DM, Baxter GD, Allen JM (2000) Lack of effect of pulsed low-intensity infrared (820 nm) laser irradiation on nerve conduction in the human superficial radial nerve. Lasers Surg Med 26:485–490.